Psychiatric Aspects of Organ Transplantation

Psychiatric Aspects of Organ Transplantation

Edited by
John Craven
and
Gary M. Rodin

The Toronto Hospital,
University of Toronto

OXFORD · NEW YORK · TOKYO
OXFORD UNIVERSITY PRESS
1992

Oxford University Press, Walton Street, Oxford OX2 6DP

Oxford New York Toronto
Delhi Bombay Calcutta Madras Karachi
Petaling Jaya Singapore Hong Kong Tokyo
Nairobi Dar es Salaam Cape Town
Melbourne Auckland

and associated companies in
Berlin Ibadan

Oxford is a trade mark of Oxford University Press

Published in the United States
by Oxford University Press, New York

A catalogue record for this book is
available from the British Library

Library of Congress Cataloging in Publication Data
Psychiatric aspects of organ transplantation/edited by John Craven
and Gary M. Rodin.
p.   cm.
1. Transplantation of organs, tissues, etc.—Psychological
aspects. I. Craven, John, 1957– . II. Rodin, Gary.
[DNLM: 1. Organ Transplantation—psychology. WO 660 P974]
RD126.P78   1992   617.9′5′0019-dc20   91-32001
0-19-262073-8

Typeset by Joshua Associates Ltd, Oxford
Printed in Great Britain by
St Edmundsbury Press, Bury St Edmunds

Preface

The past decade has seen an exponential increase in the number and types of transplantation procedures undertaken. As a large number of patients are surviving for longer periods of time, interest has grown in the personal and psychiatric aspects of transplantation. From observations on individual patients to systematic surveys of attitudes and experiences, research suggests that the interaction of a patient, physical illness, and transplantation procedure is highly complex and intriguing. We conceived the idea of this text, believing that the time was right to review selectively the preliminary findings in this rapidly expanding field.

Our goal for compiling *Psychiatric aspects of organ transplantation* was to discusss transplantation from a variety of perspectives. Each chapter emphasizes the influence of the person on the process, and conversely, the impact of transplant on the person. We believed it useful to discuss transplantation from the vantage point of conceptual issues that apply to many types of transplant and also from the perspective of particular types of transplant. The reader who is interested in a specific type of transplant can thus easily select the relevant sections to peruse. Rather than reviewing only those topics for which there is an established literature, we have included the discussions that we view as important for the field. For example, little research on social support has been undertaken specifically in transplant patients. However, a discussion of social support and transplant is included and conceptual directions for research in this area are provided. With this approach, we hoped to synthesize the available data on the psychiatric aspects of transplant and also to encourage future work in areas where data is lacking. No effort has been made to reference every publication of relevance. Instead, chapter authors were asked to be selective and to review and emphasize areas of greatest interest and/or debate. Original approaches or perspectives were encouraged; individual chapter authors met this challenge by submitting unique and authoritative reviews.

We hope that the final contents of this text meet the need of those who require a greater understanding of the person undergoing transplantation and that as a result clinical psychiatric work with these patients will be enhanced. Any professional involved in the management of transplant candidates and recipients will benefit from a greater appreciation of the relationship between the procedure and the patient. For investigators interested in the psychiatric aspects of transplantation, this text offers both a synthesis of the currently available literature and an extension of current thinking, thereby providing a direction for future work. It is inevitable that a book of this nature will raise as many questions as it attempts to answer. We look forward to future work and publications which will further our understanding of transplantation and transplant patients.

Toronto   J.C.
January 1992   G.R.

Acknowledgements

The editors would like to thank Ms Debby Proctor and Ms Anne Rydall for preparing the manuscript. The support of the Canadian Psychiatric Research Foundation and the Ontario Mental Health Foundation is gratefully acknowledged.

Contents

Contents

Contributors

Susan Abbey
Assistant Professor of Psychiatry, University of Toronto, Psychiatrist, Psychosomatic Medicine Program, The Toronto Hospital, EN8-219, 200 Elizabeth Street, Toronto, Ontario, Canada M5G 2C4.

Catherine Bart
Research Associate, The Toronto Hospital, CW2-309, 200 Elizabeth Street, Toronto, Ontario, Canada M5G 2C4.

Thomas Beresford
Professor of Psychiatry, Alcohol Research Center, University of Michigan, 400 East Eisenhower Parkway, Ste. A, Ann Arbor, Michigan 48104, USA.

Eduardo Colon
Associate Professor of Psychiatry, University of Minnesota, Associate Director, Consultation-Liaison Service, Box 345, Mayo Bldg., University Hospital, 420 Delaware St., S.E., Minneapolis, Minnesota 50455, USA.

John Craven
Assistant Professor of Psychiatry, University of Toronto, Director, Psychosomatic Medicine Program, The Toronto Hospital, EN8-212, 200 Elizabeth Street, Toronto, Ontario, Canada M5G 2C4

Lori Davis
Resident in Psychiatry, University of Alabama at Birmingham School of Medicine, University Station, Birmingham, Alabama 35294, USA.

Piet de Groen
Fellow in Gastroenterology, Mayo Graduate School of Medicine, Rochester, Minnesota, 55905; Mayo Foundation Extramural Research Fellow in Molecular Biology, Institute of Molecular Biology and Medical Biotechnology, University of Utrecht, Transitorium 3, De Uithof, Padualaan 8, 3584 CH Utrecht, The Netherlands.

David Dixon
Resident in Psychiatry, Graduate Student in Religious Studies, University of Toronto, EN8, 200 Elizabeth Street, Toronto, Ontario, Canada M5G 2C4.

Arthur Freeman III
Professor and Chairman, Department of Psychiatry, Louisiana Medical Center, Shreveport, Louisiana 71130.

Robert Frierson
Associate Professor of Psychiatry, University of Louisville, Director of Consultation Psychiatry, Consultant, Heart and Lung Institute, Jewish Hospital, University of Louisville School of Medicine, 550 South Jackson St., ABC Building, Louisville, Kentucky 40202, USA.

Paul Kelly
Assistant Professor of Behavioural Sciences, University of Toronto, Psychologist, The Toronto Hospital, CW2–309, 200 Elizabeth Street, Toronto, Ontario, Canada M5G 2C4.

Richard Lentz
Clinical Associate Professor of Psychiatry, University of Minnesota Hospital and Clinics, Psychiatrist, Park Nicollet Medical Center, Box 345, Mayo Building, University Hospital, 420 Delaware St., S.E. Minneapolis, Minnesota 50455, USA.

J. Wesley Libb
Professor of Psychiatry, University of Alabama at Birmingham School of Medicine, University Station, Birmingham, Alabama 35294, USA.

Christine Littlefield
Assistant Professor of Psychiatry, University of Toronto, Psychologist, The Toronto Hospital, CW2-329, 200 Elizabeth Street, Toronto, Ontario, Canada M5G 2C4.

Frederick Lowy
Professor of Psychiatry, Director, Center for Bioethics, University of Toronto, Tanz Neuroscience Building, Toronto, Ontario, Canada M5S 1A8.

Douglas Martin
Center for Bioethics, University of Toronto, Cognitive Neurology Laboratory, Sunnybrook Medical Center, University of Toronto, Tanz Neuroscience Building, Toronto, Ontario, Canada M5S 1A8.

Michael Popkin
Professor of Psychiatry and Medicine, University of Minnesota, Chief of Consultation-Liaison Psychiatry Service, University of Minnesota Hospital and Clinics, Box 345, Mayo Building, 420 Delaware St., S.E. Minneapolis, Minnesota 50455, USA.

Gary Rodin
Associate Professor of Psychiatry, University of Toronto, Psychiatrist-in-Chief, The Toronto Hospital, EN8-222, 200 Elizabeth Street, Toronto, Ontario, Canada M5G 2C4.

Jon Rubenow
Fellow, Division of Child and Adolescent Psychiatry, Emory University School of Medicine, 1365 Clifton Rd., N.E., Atlanta, Georgia 30322, USA.

Sandra Sexson
Assistant Professor of Psychiatry and Pediatrics, Director of Training in Child and Adolescent Psychiatry, Emory University School of Medicine, 1365 Clifton Rd., N.E., Atlanta, Georgia 30322, USA.

John G. Soos
Consulting Psychologist, British Columbia Transplant Society, Clinical Health Psychologist, Vancouver General Hospital, Suite 428, 2775 Heather Street, Vancouver, B.C., V5Z 1M9.

Ronald Spears
Transplantation Fellow, Heart and Lung Institute, Jewish Hospital, University of Louisville, School of Medicine, 550 South Jackson St., ABC Bldg., Louisville, Kentucky 40202, USA.

Margaret Stuber
Assistant Professor in Residence, Department of Psychiatry and Bio-behavioural Sciences, University of California Los Angeles, Associate Chief, Pediatric Consultation-Liaison Service, UCLA Neuropsychiatric Institute, 760 Westwood Plaza, Rm. C8-849, Los Angeles, California 90024, USA.

Owen Surman
Associate Professor of Psychiatry, Harvard Medical School, Psychiatrist, Massachusetts General Hospital, Boston, Massachusetts 02114, USA.

David Sutherland
Professor of Surgery, University of Minnesota Medical School, Box 345, Mayo Bldg., University Hospital, 420 Delaware St., S.E. Minneapolis, Minnesota 50455, USA.

James Tabler
Clinical Assistant Professor in Psychiatry, Consultant, Heart and Lung Institute, Jewish Hospital, University of Louisville, School of Medicine, 550 South Jackson St., ABC Bldg., Louisville, Kentucky 40202, USA.

Deane Wolcott
Associate Clinical Professor, Department of Psychiatry and Biobehavioural Sciences, University of California Los Angeles School of Medicine, Director, Psychosocial Services, Cedars, Sinai Comprehensive Cancer Center, 8700 Beverly Blvd., Los Angeles, California 90048, USA.

Stuart Youngner
Associate Professor of Medicine, Psychiatry, and Biomedical Ethics, Case Western Reserve University School of Medicine, 2074 Abington, Cleveland, Ohio 44106, USA.

1 Introduction

J. Craven and G. Rodin

During the past thirty years, technical advances in surgery and intensive care have led to dramatic and increasingly successful attempts at organ transplantion. However, only since the availability of the immunosuppressant cyclosporin has a reliable means been available to inhibit the rejection of a donor organ by the recipient's immune system (Cohen *et al*. 1984). The use of this drug over the past decade has allowed rapid increases in the number and types of successful procedures undertaken. As a result of such scientific advances, many transplant procedures have shifted from being experimental oddities and have become viable treatment options for many patients with end-stage organ disease.

The emotional and psychiatric aspects of organ transplantation have been described in numerous case studies and clinical samples. Some of the most graphic depictions of the personal impact of transplantation have been written by patients themselves (e.g. Squadron 1988). However, the increased frequency of the procedure in recent years has allowed larger samples of candidates and recipients to be studied systematically by means of survey and interview techniques. This research has led to a body of literature regarding the personal aspects of organ transplantation from various perspectives. As the chapters in this book illustrate, our understanding of transplantation has improved greatly in recent years. However, it is also apparent that there are still substantial deficiences in our knowledge of the psychiatric concomitants of these procedures. This text suggests conceptual directions for future research and encourages the application of modern research methodologies which will help to minimize these gaps in our knowledge.

Specific medical and surgical circumstances of patients undergoing transplantation are associated with different psychosocial sequelae. For example, liver transplant recipients appear to be much more susceptible to the neuro-psychiatric side-effects of cyclosporin than are other transplant recipients (Tollemar *et al*. 1988). Anxiety about death is likely to be more common in seriously ill patients awaiting vital organ transplants (e.g. lung, heart) than in patients awaiting kidney transplants, who have the option of continuing with or returning to dialysis. However, the conceptual and clinical issues which arise from a psychosocial perspective on a particular form of transplant are more or less applicable to all types of transplant. For example, while the need for social support varies according to the specific demands of the clinical circumstances, the function and significance of supportive networks apply similarly to individuals with each type of transplant. The value of psychosocial research is optimized when it is approached both conceptually and empirically. The application of biopsychosocial formulations to transplant patients enhances our ability to understand the mechanisms which produce psychiatric complications. For these reasons, the psychiatric aspects of transplantation are reviewed in this book, not only according to the different types of transplant (Part II), but also from the perspective of underlying issues that are not necessarily specific to transplant type (Part I). This organization necessarily involves some duplication of topics that are discussed from different perspectives. However, it was felt that this best suits the needs of the individual reader who may only be interested in certain types of transplant procedures.

Part I begins with a discussion of preoperative assessment. Such assessments are conducted to identify the personal factors that place transplant patients at risk and to help plan specialized management protocols in high risk cases. When alternative management options are not feasible, some have suggested that psychosocial information be used to prioritize candidates for transplants (Frierson and Lippmann 1987). This use of psychosocial criteria to select or prioritize candidates for transplants has generated widespread controversy (Mai *et al.* 1986; Didlake *et al.* 1988; Surman 1989). In fact, differences of opinion in this regard are expressed by various contributors to this book. Questions regarding case selection are complicated with transplantation due to the need to distribute donor organs fairly and to ensure that these scarce resources are utilized in a manner that results in the greatest societal benefit. Unfortunately, a recent American study (Kasiske *et al.* 1991) demonstrated that access to transplantation is affected by racial and socioeconomic factors. Further, our ability to predict compliance behaviour and other outcome variables does not yet approach the degree of accuracy required. Longitudinal studies are needed to identify those variables most predictive of severely problematic compliance or of other maladaptive illness behaviour following transplants. These issues have been widely discussed with regard to liver transplants for alcoholic cirrhosis. This topic is emphasized in Chapter 3 of this text.

Other important psychosocial issues have received far less attention in the transplant literature. Reports of treatment strategies for psychiatric disturbances in these patients are scarce, although presentations at a recent international conference[1] indicated that consultation psychiatrists and psychologists are actively involved in managing transplant patients. The complexities of caring for patients with a chronic illness, a transplanted organ, and concurrent psychiatric disturbance warrant extensive study and discussion. As confidence with the technical aspects of the procedures increases, there will be even less justification to decline the procedure to more vulnerable

[1] First Working Conference on the Psychiatric, Psychosocial and Ethical Aspects of Organ Transplantation, June 8 and 9, 1990, Toronto, Canada.

patients. An inevitable consequence of this widened case selection will be a greater number of transplant patients with significant psychosocial problems. A chapter on psychotherapy with transplant patients and their families is included in Part I. In addition, other selected topics which have received less than adequate attention in the general literature (e.g. social support and transplants in children or adolescents) are reviewed. These chapters present preliminary conceptual formulations and clinical observations which should help to stimulate and guide future study.

A close relationship exists between the psychosocial and the ethical factors that are inherent in the transplant process. For example, clinicians who take part in the selection of candidates find themselves in a position of having divided or conflicting loyalties in relation to the potential candidate, on the one hand, and to the transplant team on the other. The overlapping professional, personal, and ethical aspects of this position may be perplexing and stressful (Murray 1986; Gellman 1986). Transplant patients are confronted with accepting a procedure which may save their life but which is also associated with a high risk of death. The spiritual disciplines offer meaning and comfort for some in the face of a potentially fatal outcome. However, even for the non-devout, traditional religious beliefs are likely to influence attitudes to organ donation, procurement, and to the perception of transplantation. These topics are discussed in a set of chapters on ethical and religious perspectives, and on organ donation and procurement.

The chapters in Part II review, in turn, the psychiatric aspects of kidney, heart, liver, bone marrow, lung, and pancreas transplants. These chapters are each organized roughly according to the clinical progression of patients through the phases of the transplant process. These are the times of application, assessment, waiting for surgery, the early recovery phase, and longer term adjustment and rehabilitation (Brown and Kelly 1976; Allender *et al.* 1983; Kuhn *et al.* 1988). To ensure clarity, we use the terms transplant applicant, candidate, and recipient to indicate respectively, persons being assessed for entry into a transplant programme, those awaiting transplant, and patients who have received a new organ.

It has become evident that each stage of transplantation is associated with unique challenges to psychological integrity. The fear of being rejected from a waiting list contributes to anxiety and apprehension in many applicants. This must be taken into account during the psychosocial assessment, which has become a common component of an applicant's evaluation. Fear of dying prior to the transplant, and efforts to cope with the massive uncertainty and ambiguity inherent in the situation predominate during the time of waiting for a vital organ transplant. Following the immediate postoperative recovery, a seemingly endless list of challenges confront the recipient. These include alterations of body image, adjustment to increased health and autonomy, re-entry into family and vocational roles, coping with intrusive medical protocols, and fear of infection or rejection. Many embark on a search for meaning and satisfaction in life following this experience, which has confronted them with their personal vulnerability and potential mortality. These issues vary in their nature and intensity according to the type of transplant procedure, and the underlying physical illness, but also depending on the individual characteristics of the patient.

This book is designed to synthesize the present state of knowledge in the field and to help provide direction for future work. Our current understanding of the psychiatric aspects of transplantation is still preliminary, and many of the reports in the literature are descriptive in nature. There is a need for studies designed to test hypotheses about such issues as suitability of candidates, prediction of behaviour, the role of psychosocial support services, the causes of delirium, depression, and anxiety. These academic pursuits may be facilitated by interaction and collaboration amongst health care professionals working in the area of transplant psychiatry. We have argued elsewhere (Rodin *et al*. 1991) that research in the psychosocial aspects of physical illness has been too disease-specific and has not adequately taken into consideration findings from research in other illnesses or in the medically well. While the psychological and psychiatric sequelae of transplantation demand very specific study, research will best progress as an integral component of a larger effort to appreciate better the relationships between physical and emotional events. We believe that increased understanding of the psychosocial aspects of transplantation will arise not only from applying the clinical principles of consultation–liaison psychiatry, but also from the conceptual underpinnings and research strategies derived from the fields of psychosomatic and psychological medicine.

References

Allender, J., Shisslak, C., Kaszniak, A., and Copeland, J. (1983). Stages of psychological adjustment associated with heart transplantation. *Journal of Heart Transplantation*, 2, 228–31.

Brown, H. N. and Kelly, M. J. (1976). Stages of bone marrow transplantation: a psychiatric perspective. *Psychosomatic Medicine*, 38, 439–46.

Cohen, D. J., Loertscher, R., Rubin, M. F., Tilney, N. L., Carpenter, C. B., and Strom, T. B. (1984). Cyclosporine: a new immunosuppressive agent for organ transplantation. *Annals of Internal Medicine*, 101, 667–82.

Didlake, R. H., Dreyfus, K., Kerman, R. H., Van Buren, C. T., and Kahan, B. D. (1988). Patient noncompliance: a major cause of late graft failure in cyclosporine-treated renal transplants. *Transplantation Proceedings*, 20 (suppl. 3), 63–9.

Frierson, R. L. and Lippmann, S. B. (1987). Heart transplant candidates rejected on psychiatric indications: Experience in developing criteria for proper patient selection. *Psychosomatics*, 28, 347–55.

Gellman, R. M. (1986). Divided loyalties: a physician's responsibilities in an information age. *Social Science and Medicine*, 23, 817–26.

Kasiske, B. L., Neylan III, J. F., Riggio, R. R., Danovitch, G. M., Kahana, L., Alexander, S. R., *et al.* (1991). The effect of race on access and outcome in transplantation. *New England Journal of Medicine*, 324, 302–7.

Kuhn, W. F., Davis, M. H., and Lippmann, S. B. (1988). Emotional adjustment to cardiac transplantation. *General Hospital Psychiatry*, 10, 108–13.

Mai, F. M., McKenzie, F. N., and Kostuk, W. J. (1986). Psychiatric aspects of heart transplantation: preoperative evaluation and postoperative sequelae. *British Medical Journal*, 292, 311–13.

Murray, T. H. (1986). Divided loyalties for physicians: social context and moral problems. *Social Science and Medicine*, 23, 827–32.

Rodin, G., Craven, J., and Littlefield, C. (1991). *Depression in the medically ill: an integrated approach* (Brunner/Mazel, New York).

Squadron, W. (1988). Two lives on hold. *The New York Times Magazine*, December 18, 39–75.

Surman, O. S. (1989). Psychiatric aspects of organ transplantation. *American Journal of Psychiatry*, 146, 972–82.

Tollemar, J., Ringden, O., Ericzon, B. G., and Tyden, G. (1988). Cyclosporine-associated central nervous system toxicity. *New England Journal of Medicine*, 318, 788–9.

PART I

2 Assessment of transplant candidates and prediction of outcome

A. Freeman III, L. Davies, J. W. Libb, and J. Craven

The number of patients who may potentially benefit from transplantation far exceeds the supply of available donor organs (Kolata 1983; Evans *et al.* 1986). With demand outstripping supply, the selection of recipients becomes a complex task involving ethical, psychosocial, and biomedical factors (Jonsen 1989). Principles of fairness and avoidance of harm must be brought to bear in the application of all criteria. In order for recipients to be selected fairly, a uniform approach to the selection process is needed. However, the psychosocial criteria used by transplant programmes for the selection of candidates vary widely between different centres (Olbrisch and Levenson 1990). Clinicians have described their impressions of what constitutes a 'good' candidate, but for the most part these have not been subjected to rigorous empirical investigation. The Psychosocial Assessment of Candidates for Transplantation rating scale has been proposed as a reliable instrument which could be used for this purpose (Olbrisch *et al.* 1989). In this chapter we argue that with further research, psychosocial criteria may be applied in an ethical manner and, when required by circumstances, may have equal weight to other clinical criteria in the selection of candidates for organ transplant. The ethical aspects of this practice are further discussed in Chapter 8.

Preoperative assessment

The transplant applicant is typically hospitalized for the preoperative assessment. While the medical and surgical evaluation is taking place, the psychosocial group begins its consultation. The preoperative assessment of the transplant applicant is an ongoing evaluation which may take an extended period of time to complete. Each of the patient, family members, and selected professional contacts must be interviewed. The three domains of assessment (medical, psychosocial, and ethical) are intertwined and an interdisciplinary approach is required. This is ideally a collaboration between the psychiatrist, psychologist, social worker, nursing staff, chaplain, internist, and surgeon. Table 2.1 lists the factors which require assessment. The team explores past and present psychiatric conditions, treatment response, alcohol or substance abuse, previous compliance with medical recommendations, personality traits

TABLE 2.1 Preoperative psychosocial assessment

Psychiatric and psychological factors
Assessment of psychiatric disorders
   Type, duration of disorder
   Response to treatment
   Potential for exacerbation or recurrence
   Potential for impairment of outcome
   Openness of patient to psychiatric assistance

Coping abilities
   Range and style
   History of implementation, effectiveness
   Suitability for transplant situation
   Compatibility with social support network

Illness behaviour and adjustment to disability

Ability to provide informed consent

Ability to form working alliance with team

Adherence to medical recommendations

Social factors
Need for emotional and material support

Availability of support person(s)

Ability of social network to provide emotional support

Ability of patient to utilize emotional support

Availability of financial and other material resources

---

and coping style, marital and family harmony, social support, family history of psychiatric illness, attitudes towards surgery, and cognitive function. Self-report symptom inventories may be of adjunctive help in assessing anxiety and depression (Watts *et al.* 1984; Frierson and Lippmann 1987; Craven *et al.* 1990*a*).

In addition to providing the transplant team with detailed information about the applicant, the preoperative consultation serves other functions. During this early stage of involvement with the programme, a relationship is formed between the patient and the psychosocial group, who are perceived ideally as an integral component of the health care team. Supportive interaction is provided during the assessment process and the consultation personnel help to ensure that the patient and their family understand the complex medical data that are being explained to them. Some people may at this point require some further discussion in order to make a final decision about enrolling in the transplant programme. Others benefit from brief counselling to facilitate adjustment to illness or to address obvious marital or family discord. During this time, therapeutic alliances may develop which persist throughout the transplant process.

The assessment group typically makes recommendations to help optimize the mental health of the candidate prior to surgery. Suggestions may be minimal and non-specific for many applicants, or may be extensive and highly individualized, especially for certain patients with pre-existing psychiatric conditions. Some applicants may present with psychiatric disorders (e.g. major depressive episode) that could interfere substantially with their ability to apply themselves to either preoperative or postoperative medical protocols. Treatment may be recommended for these patients prior to their being placed on a waiting list. Other psychiatric conditions may benefit from treatment, but not be problematic enough to defer enrollment. Recommendations for anxiety management or brief counselling for adjustment problems are commonly undertaken while the patient is awaiting surgery. Medical and nursing staff may need to be alerted to persons with potentially problematic personality traits or disorders, and to hear suggestions which would help them work productively with these patients. Any suggestions which will help preserve an amicable working relationship between the patient and the transplant team are beneficial to all involved.

Alternatively, the psychosocial group may be called upon to comment on the suitability of an applicant for transplant. It is crucial that the transplant team and the consultant be aware of the question which is being asked of them. The implications of a request to ensure that patients selected demonstrate at least minimal abilities for treatment compliance are quite different than for a request to help a programme choose the 'best' candidates. Most patients will be accepted to a waiting list with little influence from psychosocial factors. Others may be deferred enrollment while receiving psychiatric treatment, and a small proportion may be declined further consideration by a transplant team (Frierson and Lippmann 1987). Craven *et al.* (1990*a*) found that the few patients who were declined for lung transplant solely on the basis of psycho-social factors had in common multiple psychiatric or psychosocial problems, a lack of a stable personal support network, and an inability or unwillingness to accept professional assistance. These patients were believed to be at very high risk for maladaptive postoperative behaviour and not treatable with the resources available to the team at the time. Although the final decision to accept or defer a patient for transplant typically rests with the programme head, the process will be stressful for all who are involved. This situation maximizes the tensions inherent in the psychosocial consultants' divided loyalties between the best interests of the patient and of the transplant team.

The ethical concerns associated with this decision making process are complex (Jonsen 1989), but demand, at least, that psychosocial assessments be conducted with informed consent. Patients should be informed beforehand whether information provided during the psychosocial assessment may be used in a decision about their suitability for transplantation. Transplant teams who utilize psychosocial exclusion criteria are likely best to be explicit and systematic about the basis for their decisions. This will help ensure that the factors considered in these decisions are fair and justifiable. It is imperative that, whenever possible, these decisions be guided by data with high reliability and validity and that social judgements do not influence the likelihood of transplant (Surman 1989). Loewy (1987) has suggested that social worth criteria should not be applied by physicians, regardless of any higher order goal to allocate organs for the greatest overall benefit. Discrimination on the basis of mentally handicapping conditions must also be avoided. For transplant programmes in the USA, Merrikin and Overcast (1985) have commented on the possible impact of Section 504 of the Rehabilitation Act of 1973. This act prohibits discrimination against persons with handicapping conditions by any programme receiving federal funds. To date, most litigation under this Act has focused on discrimination in access to employment, education, public transportation, or buildings. However, patient selection for medical treatments should likely be considered with reference to this bill.

A list of potential contraindications to transplant surgery is provided in Table 2.2. Items are classified on this table as either absolute or relative. Absolute medical and surgical contraindications to transplant clearly exist. What has been much less clear is whether psychosocial contraindications are best considered as absolute or relative. In the short term, no psychosocial contraindications are absolute, as there is no mental or social disturbance which entirely disallows a person from being anaesthetized and surviving a transplant procedure. However, if longer term medical and functional outcome are taken into consideration, psychosocial factors take on increased relevance. Of greatest clinical importance are conditions or circumstances that predict a

TABLE 2.2 Contraindications to organ transplant

Absolute	Relative
Active infection	Advanced age
Malignancy	Recurrent diseases in the organ
End-stage failure of another vital organ	Diabetes mellitus, or dysfunction in other organ systems
	Non-compliance
	Severe mental illness unresponsive to treatment
	Drug and alcohol abuse
	Inadequate social support

high degree of postoperative noncompliance or maladaptive illness behaviour severe enough to increase morbidity (Marsden 1985). The frequency of this occurrence may vary (Armstrong and Weiner 1981; Didlake *et al.* 1988; Surman 1989). However, predictably severe noncompliance is perhaps the only justifiable psychosocial exclusion criteria.

Psychiatric disorders which have been suggested as absolute contraindications to transplant surgery (e.g. schizophrenia, active substance abuse, severe mental retardation) have in common a high risk of clinically significant noncompliance. However, Didlake *et al.* (1988) recommends psychiatric intervention for the noncompliant or psychiatrically diagnosed rather than denial of transplantation. Psychosis in many patients may be controlled with appropriate treatment. Motivated substance abusers may be deferred enrolment while taking part in an abstinence programme and patients with cognitive impairment could conceivably survive the procedure and manage subsequently if adequate social or professional support is available to compensate for their deficiencies. In fact, kidney transplant may be preferable for some mentally disabled patients who find it difficult to manage dialysis. Surman (1989) has reported successful kidney transplantation in two persons with full-scale intelligence quotients of 50. For a patient with a high risk of noncompliance, the availability of professional support and the willingness or ability of the candidate to accept assistance are factors which greatly influence the likelihood of postoperative complications. These and other considerations suggest that psychosocial exclusion criteria for transplant surgery should be applied in a flexible and individualized manner.

Other variables also determine the weight that psychosocial factors may play in the selection of applicants for transplants. The availability of donor organs indicates that for some procedures (e.g. lung transplant), selection may be more rigorous than for others (e.g. kidney transplant). The viability of a transplant procedure or programme may also be relevant. Programmes which offer experimental procedures or which otherwise are dependent for their continuation upon achieving adequate outcome statistics may try to optimize outcome by selecting highly motivated candidates with greater social and psychological resources. More established programmes may be better able to consider higher risk candidates who are older, with more physical complications and/or psychosocial vulnerabilities (Surman 1989). Further, the resources of an individual team must be taken into account. Some centres have considerable professional support services available for patients in need. However, a team with limited resources may choose to transplant a larger number of uncomplicated cases rather than expend more time and effort on a smaller number of patients with problematic psychiatric disorders. Also, the resources of one team may fluctuate over time and require a variable application of psychosocial contraindications.

The demands of the procedure itself will to some extent define what must be expected of patients. The more that a successful outcome is dependent upon extensive rehabilitation exercises or adherence to an intrusive medical protocol, the greater is the requirement that patients be able to cope with these expectations. Some transplants (e.g. heart, lung, or small bowel transplant) require an extraordinary amount of participation by patients. For these procedures, some patients will be unable to meet the demands that are necessary for an adequate outcome without the availability of massive and protracted supportive measures.

The psychosocial assessment of transplant candidates may be extensive, but the information obtained is nevertheless limited in certain respects. It must be remembered that the assessment is highly dependent upon the information that is provided by the patient and family. Obviously, such individuals usually wish to present themselves in a favourable manner. The situation encourages minimization and denial of psychosocial vulnerabilities. Indeed, patients' awareness that they may be rejected for transplant may encourage dishonesty in their self-reporting. This occurrence is a direct complication of a psychosocial selection process for surgery. However, dissimulation on the part of applicants will compromise the ability of a transplant team to provide optimal care and will interfere with the development of a trusting alliance between the patient and staff. Finally, the time involved in the routine psychosocial assessment of transplant candidates is onerous. As greater numbers of patients are considered for transplantation, it will not be feasible for consultations to be provided on all applicants. Other methods need to be investigated for identifying those patients most at risk and in need of the specialized management skills of mental health professionals.

Prediction of outcome

Inherent in this discussion of preoperative assessment is the assumption that it is desirable to have a detailed understanding of patient variables which may influence outcome. Identification of psychosocial vulnerabilities at an early stage of the transplant process allows intervention to address or compensate for factors which may lead to postoperative complications. However, what constitutes a 'good' outcome is subject to different interpretation. A successful procedure may variously be defined as one in which the patient leaves the operating room alive, is discharged home from hospital, survives for a long period of time, returns to work, or reports a reasonable quality of life. When a new procedure is developed where none was previously available, immediate survival of the patient is of paramount importance. However, as experience increases and the duration of survival lengthens, other outcome variables (e.g. functional outcome, quality of life) need to be addressed. Identifying the components of quality of life constitutes a major task for psychiatrists and others in the evaluation of patients undergoing organ transplantation.

Postoperative illness behaviour and compliance are factors widely believed to influence long term outcome. Predicting which patients may demonstrate poor compliance is useful for two reasons. First, patients who are identified as high risk for problematic behaviours may benefit from education and supportive management strategies designed to optimize self care. Second, when vital resources are in short supply (e.g. donor organs), it may be necessary to distribute them in a manner which has the greatest chance of success. It may be argued that it is undesirable to transplant an organ into a person with a high likelihood of dangerous noncompliance while another person with demonstrated compliant behaviour is unable to obtain a donor organ. However, this prediction depends heavily upon a clear understanding of the factors influencing outcome and the availability of longitudinal data to test hypotheses. It is much less clear whether a person with a greater potential for high quality of life should preferentially receive a donor organ compared to a candidate who is expected to have a less satisfactory outcome. Complicating this question are the problems inherent in defining precisely what is meant by quality of life and the difficulty applying this relatively soft concept to a life and death decision. The remainder of this chapter will discuss the related issues of postoperative outcome, compliance, and quality of life.

Psychiatric disorders and outcome

Freeman *et al.* (1988) and Riether and Stoudemire (1987) suggest that psychiatric disorders play an important role in mediating medical, psychosocial, and quality of life variables. Freeman *et al.* (1988) reported on 70 heart transplant recipients who had been assessed preoperatively. Nineteen patients had been predicted to be at risk due to psychiatric disorder (DSM–III–R Axis I and II disorders). Fourteen of these developed postoperative surgical or psychiatric complications. However, a study by Frierson and Lippmann (1987) found that only 4 of 17 heart transplant recipients with previous psychiatric disorders exhibited clinically significant postoperative noncompliance. Alcoholism is the leading cause of endstage liver disease and is a frequent finding among patients with idiopathic cardiomyopathy. Starzl *et al.* (1988) reported a 73 per cent one year survival in a series of 41 patients who received liver transplants for alcoholic cirrhosis. Recidivism for alcohol dependence was low. These studies represent preliminary attempts to document empirically the outcome of transplants in persons with psychiatric disorders. Better controlled studies which include a larger number of potentially influential variables are required. For example, the nature or extent of support services provided to patients in these studies was not adequately described. Variability in these factors may account for vastly different degrees of association between preoperative psychiatric vulnerability and postoperative complications.

Early studies from the Stanford programme described psychiatric issues that accompanied the heart transplant procedure (Lunde 1969; Christopherson *et al.* 1976). More recent investigations have further documented the psychiatric disorders most likely to occur with transplantation (Mai *et al*. 1984; Freeman *et al*. 1988; Jones *et al*. 1988). These studies indicate that anxiety and depressive symptoms are common in patients awaiting the procedure, while delirium and social complications are prevalent postoperatively. Several investigators have shown that pre-existing psychiatric abnormalities can compound these problems (Freeman *et al*. 1988; Kuhn *et al*. 1988*b*). Kuhn *et al*. (1988*b*) also indicate that following the operation, pre-existing psychopathology tends to worsen or accentuate. In some cases, psychiatric intervention has been required just to ensure the survival of these patients (Kuhn *et al*. 1988*b*).

Craven *et al*. (1990*b*) have reported a study which investigated specifically the risk factors for the development of cyclosporin associated delirium in liver transplant recipients. This group found that a past history of alcohol abuse and preoperative hepatic encephalopathy were more frequent in patients with delirium than in recipients without this complication. These factors were hypothesized to represent pre-existing central nervous system vulnerability to this postoperative complication. In another series of lung transplant recipients, Craven *et al*. (1990*c*) found that organic mental disorders occurred in over half of patients during the first two postoperative weeks, but that a past history of psychiatric disorder was not an associated factor.

Brennan *et al*. (1986) found that lesser elevations on the Minnesota Multiphasic Personality Inventory predicted better medical and quality of life outcomes in heart transplant recipients. However, while patients with certain personality traits or disorders may be at higher risk for maladaptive illness behaviour, treatment noncompliance, or regressive behaviour, the postoperative course of these persons has not been studied adequately. Clinical experience would suggest that manipulative or masochistic tendencies, impulsive behaviour, hostility, pathological dependency, or excessive requirements for reassurance may interfere with self-care or lead to deterioration of professional and personal support relationships. Patients with personality disorders may have difficulty engaging in a trusting therapeutic alliance with the transplant team, may challenge the tolerance of staff and/or may stimulate counter-transference reactions which interfere with the provision of optimal care. In particular, a protracted recovery phase or a sub-optimal outcome may place substantial stress on the ability of these patients to cope.

The diagnosis of borderline or antisocial personality disorder is often regarded as a reason for exclusion (Olbrisch and Levenson 1990). These patients may be unable to isolate self-care behaviour from tendencies to engage in self-destructive or irresponsible behaviour. The psychosocial assessment may be affected by ethical and value judgements by staff who are faced with such a candidate for transplant. Caution should be exercised to ensure that counter-transference reactions do not contribute to these patients being declined for transplant. Research into personality characteristics as determinants of transplant outcome is required to provide an empirical basis for predictions of the ability of these patients to cope adequately with the procedures.

In summary, preliminary reports and common clinical experience suggest that patients with certain psychiatric disorders are at higher than average risk for poorer psychosocial outcome following transplant. Studies are required to identify those disorders or traits which are most predictive of poor outcome and to investigate the mediating mechanisms. Investigations need to be longitudinal in design, and must incorporate other influential variables, most importantly the provision of social and professional support. However, systematic data are difficult to obtain because referral and selection for transplant remains highly selective.

Quality of life

Other than in the case of kidney transplant, early outcome studies dealt almost exclusively with patient survival. Issues of infection, immunosuppression, and rejection were paramount (Jamieson *et al*. 1982). As transplant procedures have been perfected and the rate of survival improved, interest has shifted to include the quality of life after transplantation. From the patient's perspective, quality of life represents a final common denominator of the surgical, medical, and psychosocial interventions which have been undertaken. The challenge for investigators is to measure and predict this outcome variable following transplantation. This will provide useful information for physicians and patients to consider when deciding upon transplantation and will help to define those persons most in need of additional assistance to ensure an adequate quality of postoperative life.

By definition, health-related quality of life refers to the impact of health conditions on the patient's functional status. It is generally agreed that quality of life has both objective and subjective components. Objectively, the ability to maintain self-care, to be engaged in work, and to enjoy relationships with others are of primary importance. Subjectively, the sense of well-being afforded by a transplant, in contrast with the dysphoria caused by ill health prior to surgery, may be the primary value of a transplant.

Numerous measures of quality of life have been proposed in the last 20 years. Kaplan (1988) categorizes these measures into those based on a psychometric approach and a decision theory approach. Proponents of the decision theory approach weight the various dimensions of health status to produce a single measure of quality of life (Bush 1985; Kaplan 1988). Included are such variables as mobility, physical and social activity, and symptoms (e.g. coughing, wheezing, shortness of breath). The aggregate score is used to assess the relative merits of different outcomes. Quality adjusted life years may be derived from these data by multiplying the number of years an individual survives in a given condition by the quality of life score for that period of time.

Recent thinking in the decision theory approach addresses the likelihood that not all factors are weighted equally by individuals. Living just one more year in a wheelchair with frequent visits to the hospital may be highly desirable for a 65 year old 'about-to-be' grandparent, but less satisfactory for a 40 year old business person. Subjective weighting of components has received attention in a recent theoretical article by Miyamoto and Eraker (1988). Their formulation suggests that we must '. . . evaluate the subjective value of both the duration and the quality of life that could result from a treatment of choice'.

As described by Riether and Rubenow (1989), the transplant patient's life has changed dramatically. Many activities, goals, and aspirations which affect quality of life have been altered drastically. The work of several investigators suggests that medical events following surgery, including drug side-effects, rejection episodes, infection, and the necessity for hospitalization can have a deleterious impact on quality of life (Najman and Levine 1981; Allender *et al.* 1983; Lough *et al.* 1987). Observation of heart transplant recipients has revealed that dysphoria occurred with immunosuppressant side-effects and that mood swings were observed in association with rapid shifts in the patient's medical state (Freeman *et al.* 1984; Watts *et al.* 1984; McAleer *et al.* 1985; O'Brien 1985). Lough *et al.* (1985) found that more than 25 per cent of heart transplant recipients felt that life had been less rewarding following heart transplant. Negative percepts were reported most frequently in physical appearance, sexual functioning, and finances. Immunosuppressant associated symptoms and limitations in lifestyle were also associated with poorer quality of life. However, Lough *et al.* (1987) has also noted the lack of conclusive data regarding a relationship between immunosuppressant side-effects and the recipient's perceived quality of life.

Although complications and other factors contribute to an impaired quality of life in some recipients, several studies show that most heart transplant recipients achieve improved physical status following surgery and their quality of life is rated as good to excellent (Lough *et al.* 1985; Jones *et al.* 1988; Freeman *et al.* 1988). A survey of lung transplant recipients who had survived at least six months following the procedure found that life satisfaction was reported as high by over 75 per cent of the sample (Craven *et al.* 1990*a*). Recipients who reported lower satisfaction were much more likely than the others to have had significant postoperative complications or a sub-optimal outcome (Craven *et al.* 1990*b*). The finding that a majority of patients report improved quality of life following a transplant appears to be a testament to their severely impaired state of health prior to surgery and to their ability to adjust following the transplant. Similarly in the context of kidney transplant, it has been repeatedly demonstrated that the quality of life with functioning grafts is clearly superior to that which is achieved with dialysis (Johnson *et al.* 1982; Evans *et al.* 1985). The technical success of kidney transplant, its cost-effectiveness, and demonstrated benefits to quality of life have each contributed to this procedure becoming a routine approach for many persons with endstage renal failure.

Conclusions

The scarcity of donor organs for some types of transplant places the physician in a position of divided loyalty between society, which expects a distribution of organs that is fair and makes the optimal use of this vital resource, and the patient, who expects the doctor to provide whatever care is medically indicated. Psychosocial contraindications to transplant surgery must be considered to be relative to the available resources, including donor organs, social and professional supportive services, and the demands of the procedure. Rather than being considered absolute reasons for exclusion from transplantation, current opinion suggests that while at higher risk for noncompliance, many patients with psychiatric conditions can be transplanted with an adequate outcome (Surman 1989). Noncompliance and other maladaptive illness behaviour is believed to be a common mechanism by which psychosocial variables negatively influence outcome and potentially contribute to graft failure (Didlake *et al.* 1988). Much further work is indicated to develop our predictive ability for those conditions which lead to a suboptimal outcome. This will depend in part upon improved definitions and measurements of outcome itself.

The preoperative psychosocial assessment of the transplant candidate aims to identify the personal strengths and vulnerabilities of candidates. This encourages individually tailored recommendations to minimize the likelihood of maladaptive behaviour and to optimize outcome. Declining transplants on the basis of psychosocial concerns should be the exception rather than the rule, and should be based upon measurable characteristics which are unmanageable by a transplant programme and highly predictive of clinically relevant complications. Greater emphasis should be placed upon the early identification of patients with psychosocial vulnerabilities and the development of management strategies.

References

Allender, J., Shisslak, C., Kaszniak, A., and Copeland, J. (1983). Stages of psychological adjustment associated with heart transplantation. *Heart Transplantation*, 2, 228–31.

Armstrong, S. H. and Weiner, M. F. (1981–2). Noncompliance with post-transplant immunosuppression. *International Journal of Psychiatry in Medicine*, 11, 89–95.

Brennan, A. F., Buccholz, D. J., Kuhn, W., and Davis, M. H. (1986). *Psychological assessment of heart transplantation candidates: Two years experience*. Poster presented at the meeting of the American Psychological Association, Washington, D.C.

Bush, J. W. (1985). General health policy model/Quality of Well-Being (QWB) Scale. In *Assessment of quality of life in clinical trials of cardiovascular therapies* (eds N. K. Wenger, M. E. Mattson, C. D. Furberg, and J. Elinson), pp. 197–289 (Le Jacq, New York).

Christopherson, L. K., Griepp, R. B., and Stinson, E. B. (1976). Rehabilitation after cardiac transplantation. *Journal of the American Medical Association*, 236, 2082–4.

Craven, J., Bright, J., and Dear, C. L. (1990*a*). Psychiatric, psychosocial, and rehabilitative aspects of lung transplant. *Chest Clinics of North America*, 11, 247–57.

Craven, J., Sheinin, L., and The Toronto Liver Transplant Group (1990*b*). Cyclosporine-associated organic mental disorders in liver transplant recipients. Paper presented at The First Working Conference on the Psychiatric, Psychosocial and Ethical Aspects of Organ Transplantation, June 8–9, Toronto, Canada.

Craven, J. and The Toronto Lung Transplant Group (1990*c*). Postoperative organic mental syndromes in lung transplant recipients. *Journal of Heart Transplantation*, 9, 129–32.

Didlake, R. H., Dreyfus, K., Kerman, R. H., Van Buren, C. T., and Kahan, B. D. (1988). Patient noncompliance: a major cause of late graft failure in cyclosporine-treated renal transplants. *Transplantation Proceedings*, 20 (Supplement 3), 63–9.

Evans, R. W., Manninen, D. L., Garrison, L. P. Jr., and Maier, A. M. (1986). Donor availability as the primary determinant of the future of heart transplantation. *Journal of the American Medical Association*, 255, 1892–8.

Evans, R. W., Manninen, D. L., Garrison, L. P. Jr., Hart, L. G., Blagg, C. R., Gutman, R. A., *et al*. (1985). The quality of life of patients with end-stage renal disease. *New England Journal of Medicine*, 312, 553–9.

Freeman, A. M., Folks, D. G., Sokol, R. S., and Fahs, J. J. (1988). Cardiac transplantation: Clinical correlates of psychiatric outcome. *Psychosomatics*, 29, 47–54.

Freeman, A., Watts, D., and Karp, R. (1984). Evaluation of cardiac transplantation candidates: Preliminary observations. *Psychosomatics*, 25, 197–207.

Frierson, R. L. and Lippmann, S. B. (1987). Heart transplantation patients rejected on psychiatric indications. *Psychosomatics*, 28, 347–55.

Jamieson, S. W., Oyer, P. E., and Bieber, C. P. (1982). Transplantation for cardiomyopathy: a review of the results. *Journal of Heart Transplantation*, 2, 28.

Johnson, J. P., McCauley, C. R., and Copley, J. B. (1982). The quality of life of hemodialysis and transplant patients. *Kidney International*, 22, 286–91.

Jones, B. M., Chang, V. P., Esmore, E., Spratt, P., Shanahan, M. X., Farnsworth, A. E., *et al*. (1988). Psychological adjustment after cardiac transplantation. *Medical Journal of Australia*, 149, 118–22.

Jonsen, A. R. (1989). Ethical issues in organ transplantation. In *Medical Ethics* (ed. R. M. Veatch) (Jones and Bartlett, Boston).

Kaplan, R. M. (1988). Health-related quality of life in cardiovascular disease. *Journal of Consulting and Clinical Psychology*, 56, 382–92.

Kolata, G. (1983). Organ shortage clouds new transplant era. *Science*, 221, 32–3.

Kuhn, W. F., Davis, M. H., and Lippmann, S. B. (1988*a*). Emotional adjustment to cardiac transplantation. *General Hospital Psychiatry*, 10, 108–13.

Kuhn, W. F., Myers, B., Brennan, A. F., Davis, M. H., Lippmann, S. B., Gray, L. A., *et al*. (1988*b*). Psychopathology in heart transplant candidates. *Journal of Heart Transplantation*, 7, 223–6.

Loewy, E. H. (1987). Drunks, livers, and values: should social value judgements enter into liver transplant decisions? *Journal of Clinical Gastroenterology*, 9, 436–41.

Lough, M. E., Lindsey, A. M., Shinn, J. A., and Stotts, N. A. (1985). Life satisfaction following heart transplantation. *Journal of Heart Transplantation*, 4, 446–9.

Lough, M. E., Lindsey, A. M., Shinn, J. A., and Stotts, N. A. (1987). Impact of symptom frequency and symptom distress on self-reported quality of life in heart transplant recipients. *Heart and Lung*, 16, 193–200.

Lunde, D. T. (1969). Psychiatric complications of heart transplants. *American Journal of Psychiatry*, 126, 369–73.

Marsden, C. (1985). Ethical issues in heart transplant program. *Heart and Lung*, 14, 495–9.

Mai, F. M., McKenzie, F. N., and Kostuk, W. J. (1984). Liaison psychiatry in heart transplant unit. *Psychosomatic Medicine*, 46, 80–1.

McAleer, M. J., Copeland, J., Fuller, J., and Copeland, J. G. (1985). Psychological aspects of heart transplantation. *Heart Transplantation*, 4, 232–3.

Merrikin, K. J. and Overcast, T. D. (1985). Patient selection for heart transplantation: When is a discriminating choice discrimination? *Journal of Health Politics, Policy and Law*, 10, 7–32.

Miyamoto, J. M. and Eraker, S. A. (1988). A multiplicative model of the utility of survival duration and health quality. *Journal of Experimental Psychology: General*, 117, 3–20.

Najman, J. M. and Levine, S. (1981). Evaluating the impact of medical care and technologies on the quality of life: A review and critique. *Social Science & Medicine — Part F. Medical & Social Ethics*, 15, 107–15.

O'Brien, V. C. (1985). Psychological and social aspects of heart transplantation. *Heart Transplantation*, 4, 229–31.

Olbrisch, M. E., Levenson, J. L., and Hamer, R. (1989). The PACT: A rating scale for the study of clinical decision-making in psychosocial screening of organ transplant candidates. *Clinical Transplantation*, 3, 164–9.

Olbrisch, M. and Levenson, J. (1990). Psychosocial screening procedures and criteria in cardiac transplant: results of an international survey. Presented at The First Working Conference on the Psychiatric, Psychosocial and Ethical Aspects of Organ Transplantation, June 8–9, Toronto, Canada.

Riether, A. M. and Rubenow, J. C. (1989). Psychiatric symptomatology in transplant patients. *Clinical Advances in Psychiatric Disorders*, 3, 8–10.

Riether, A. M. and Stoudemire, A. (1987). Surgery and trauma. In *Principles of medical psychiatry* (eds A. Stoudemire and B. Fogel), pp. 423–33. (Grune & Stratton, Orlando, FL).

Starzl, T. E., Van Thiel, D., Tzakis, A. G., Iwatsuki, S., Todo, S., Marsh, J. W., *et al.* (1988). Orthoptic liver transplantation for alcoholic cirrhosis. *Journal of the American Medical Association*, 260, 2542–4.

Surman, O. S. (1989). Psychiatric aspects of organ transplantation. *American Journal of Psychiatry*, 146, 972–82.

Watts, D., Freeman, A. M., McGiffen, D. G., Kirklin, J. K., McVay, R., and Karp, R. B. (1984). Psychiatric aspects of cardiac transplantation: assessment and management. *Heart Transplantation*, 3, 243–7.

3   Alcohol abuse and liver transplantation

T. Beresford

During 1989, the liver transplant team at the University of Michigan performed 94 orthotopic transplants. In approximately one-third of those cases, liver failure had occurred secondary to alcoholic cirrhosis. Cirrhosis is present in approximately fifteen per cent of those persons who suffer from alcoholism or 'alcohol dependence' as defined by DSM-III-R criteria (American Psychiatric Association 1987). The lifetime prevalence of alcoholism is estimated to be between 7 and 10 per cent of the general population. Using these figures, we estimate that approximately 8000 residents of the state of Michigan, at any given moment, suffer from alcoholic cirrhosis. Clearly, any attempt to provide liver transplantation for a number this large would be impossible. When one further notes that the average cost of the procedure varies from $100 000 to $300 000 (US), it is immediately obvious that the availability of this life-saving procedure is naturally limited by expense, availability of organs, and availability of the surgical procedure itself.

Transplant programmes need to apply this sophisticated technical procedure in a manner that justifies the expense and utilizes organ supply and surgical time optimally. A Michigan court recently declared that any such clinical application must involve persons knowledgeable not only in transplantation but also in alcoholism and other addictive disorders (Beresford *et al.* 1990). There has been an increasing trend to include clinicians experienced in addictive disorders as members of the transplant team, most obviously for alcoholism and liver transplantation. This should be an especially welcome field for physicians expert in consultation–liaison psychiatry, since alcohol abuse is present in 20–40 per cent of patients in general hospitals (Beresford 1979).

Alcohol dependence and liver transplantation

This chapter will review the clinical features of alcohol dependence as it relates to liver transplantation. The issues discussed are also applicable to addicted persons requiring other organ transplants.

Features of alcohol dependence

The natural history of alcoholism has been extensively reviewed in a landmark book by Vaillant (1983). His work is required reading for any clinician involved in understanding alcoholism and especially for those applying current knowledge in the field to diagnostic and prognostic decision making.

For the purposes of this discussion, alcoholism exemplifies four clinical features which form the basis for the diagnosis of substance dependence. The first of these is tolerance: a clinical state in which greater amounts of alcohol are consumed in order to gain an effect originally obtained with lesser amounts. A patient in her early forties might report that at age 18 she felt giddy after only one or two cans of beer, but that the giddy feeling is presently obtained only after five or more drinks. Formal criteria in the DSM-III-R require an increase of 50 per cent over a baseline amount.

With the occurrence of tolerance and continued alcohol use, withdrawal symptoms generally follow. The alcohol withdrawal syndrome consists of symptoms of autonomic discharge occurring some six to twelve hours after a rapid drop in the blood level of alcohol. These include tachycardia, tachypnea, hypertension, hyperpyrexia, tremor, anxiety, nausea with or without vomiting, and diaphoresis. In severe cases, the clinician will find hyperactive reflexes as well as ankle clonus. Patients in severe withdrawal may experience *grand mal* seizures, usually after the first 24 hours. Again, in severe cases, patients may experience delirium tremens, characterized by persistent confusion, visual hallucinations, and profound autonomic discharge, typically occurring on the third day of withdrawal or thereafter. In our experience, most patients presenting for liver transplantation have not undergone the more severe forms of alcohol withdrawal. Clinicians must therefore be alert to the more subtle forms of alcohol withdrawal and should use a standard interview and physical examination to establish the presence of these symptoms.

The third category of symptoms is impaired control of drinking behaviour. This is present when a patient cannot consistently predict his or her drinking behaviour once drinking alcohol has begun. Impaired control is evidenced by multiple attempts to decrease use, repeated instances of drinking more than intended, or being unable to stop alcohol use once a drinking episode has begun. These features are assessed through the clinical history. However, minimization and denial are the rule. It is crucial to explore these symptoms, not only with the patient, but also with the family member or other persons who can corroborate the history.

In contrast, the fourth group of signs is often the most obvious: continued decline in social functioning as a result of alcohol use. Irritation of family members, loss of friends, increasing time spent drinking, to the detriment of social relationships and obligations, are generally the early signs of the social effects of uncontrolled drinking. Loss of job, serious legal problems, and threatened or real breakup of family relationships generally occur later in the process of decline. All of the above signs and symptoms are included in the present standard of diagnosis of alcohol dependence (American Psychiatric Association 1987).

The clinician must be expert in eliciting these symptoms so as to be confident both in their presence as well as their absence. It has been our experience, for example, that approximately 10 per cent of the persons referred for evaluation of alcohol dependence do not merit any psychiatric diagnosis. An additional 10 per cent have shown some evidence of tolerance, but without any of the other symptoms of dependence, and therefore may be considered to have abused alcohol but not yet become dependent on it in the clinical sense. In short, as many as a fifth of the persons likely to be evaluated for alcohol use in the setting of hepatic transplantation will not fulfil the criteria for alcohol dependence. These patients appear to offer a better prognosis than those who fulfil alcohol dependence criteria.

Prediction of course

Once diagnosis has been made, an assessment of prognosis necessarily follows. As a general rule, those patients having social resources which militate toward a structured daily life have a better prognosis than those who do not. In his eight-year prospective study of severe alcoholics, Vaillant noted four factors that were useful prognostically in identifying long-term abstinent subjects (Vaillant 1983, p. 190). These factors all involve providing structure in one's life as a replacement for alcohol use. The first entails finding useful social activities, which Vaillant termed 'substitute dependencies', that fill up the time the subject might otherwise have spent in uncontrolled use of alcohol. These factors were wide-ranging and included attendance at Alcoholics Anonymous meetings, participation in family or work activities, or in organized leisure activities. The common thread for all was the presence of other people and the lack of alcohol use.

The second factor he identified was an improved sense of hope or self-esteem. This was a direct counterbalance to the guilt that alcoholic subjects experience when they consider the damage their drinking has done to their life and the lives of others. Unless balanced by a counterweight of hope, this sense of guilt can itself be a powerful drive to resume drinking. For many, belief in the idea of alcoholism as a disease offers a sense of hope. In the words of one patient, 'it is much easier to think of oneself as an ill person trying to become well than it is to think of oneself as a bad person trying to become good'. The renewed hopefulness or self-esteem can come from many sources. For members of the Alcoholics Anonymous fellowship, it can often be found in the belief in a higher power. For others, it might be found in the religion of their family or upbringing. For those without religious belief, other sources of hope and reliance are necessary.

Vaillant's third factor was the presence of a caring, knowledgeable person in the alcoholic's life. This person could be a spouse, a physician, a psycho-therapist, a friend, a clergy member, or an Alcoholics Anonymous sponsor. Common to all of these significant others, in Vaillant's view, is the clear belief in the alcoholic as a person who could recover and the recognition of the clear limit in the caring person's ability to exert any direct power or force in bringing the alcoholic to recovery. The consistent message from such persons to the alcoholic was that the alcoholic could stay, but that the drinking must go.

The fourth and last of Vaillant's factors is the presence of a physical or social consequence of immediate and noxious import that would occur with certainty the very next time the person drank alcohol. Relevant examples include pancreatic pain, an alcohol–disulfiram reaction, or return to incarceration because of a broken parole agreement. More traditional medical conditions such as liver failure, heart failure, or other more subtle forms of illness did not apply. Because of the strict terms of this negative behavioural consequence, it is generally of limited value in assessing transplant candidates prior to the transplant procedure.

The work of Vaillant and others has demonstrated convincingly that alcohol dependence remits over time for large numbers of affected people. The natural remission rate is thought to be between 30 and 60 per cent, depending on populations studied over appropriately long periods of time. Remission rates may be higher for patients with intact social resources. It is important for the clinician to keep the time course for alcoholism in perspective. Alcoholism is an illness measured in decades rather than in weeks, months, or even a few years. Like diabetes, hypertension, or congestive heart failure, relapses and remissions will occur and should be expected. When assessing prognosis, one must take into account the likelihood of sustained remission and the avail-ability of health care services, such as alcohol rehabilitative services, that promote sustained health and recovery. In Vaillant's sample, those who presented or acquired two or more prognostic factors remained abstinent for three years or more while those with one or none of the factors managed abstinence for only two years or less. In our experience, the great majority of patients seeking a hepatic transplant have presented with the more hopeful prognostic constellation (Beresford *et al.* 1990). This pattern may reflect referral patterns for transplant which are subject to change.

Reflecting the clinical situation of the alcoholic requesting a liver transplant, we have added two additional factors to the preoperative evaluation: acceptance of the alcohol dependence diagnosis when it is pres-ent and a brief index of social stability. The clinician must present the diag-nosis to the applicant and his family or significant other persons and then judge whether this information is taken seriously and worked with as a means of improving the chances of successful postoperative outcome. In specific cases, we have chosen not to offer a transplant when the patient refused to acknowledge the presence of alcohol dependence as a first step in planning for the transplant. This underscores our belief in the importance of developing a therapeutic alliance with these patients. When this is not possible, the possibility of relapse and its risk of maladaptive illness behaviour is likely to increase, depending on the patient's own ability to care for himself. The measurement of alcoholism acknowledgement and its relevance to outcome following transplant is a pivotal question that requires further research.

An additional component of the preoperative evaluation is an assessment of social stability and resources. We require a family interview for each candidate. This allows corroboration of the drinking history, an evaluation of support resources and an opportunity for an alliance to develop between clinician and family. This relationship can serve as an early warning system if relapse occurs or appears imminent. We have used a brief quantification scheme to measure the relative permanence of family, home, and work (Strauss and Bacon 1951).

Polysubstance abuse, usually including alcohol, occurs in approximately 0.5 per cent of the population, a lifetime prevalence which is a tenth that of alcoholism. This condition has a high association with childhood behaviour disturbances, early substance abuses, and dependence on multiple substances by early adulthood. Spontaneous recovery rates prior to the fourth and fifth decade of life are much lower than for the isolated abuse of alcohol.

Features predictive of remission of polysubstance abuse are similar, but not identical to those of alcoholism. Of particular importance for the transplant assessment is that the length of drug- and alcohol-free recovery prior to the transplant is an important predictor of future abstinence. This contrasts to alcoholism in which the length of abstinence prior to transplant appears to be unrelated to the likelihood of subsequent abuse (Beresford *et al.* 1990). Clinicians must be alert to differences between these conditions in order to make valid predictions and recommendations. Our experience has been good with patients who had been in remission well before assessment for a liver transplant. However, polysubstance abusing patients who presented for transplant with recovery periods of less than one year have largely been unable to comply with medical regimens or otherwise to take responsibility of medical self-care. In cases such as this, our centre has decided to not proceed with a liver transplant.

Several of the prognostic factors described have been incorporated into a scale that allows us to compare cohorts of patients over time (Appendix A). This scale is currently under study by our group and is intended for research purposes only. It is not suggested as a substitute for rigorous clinical evaluation.

Outcome following liver transplantation

Our group (Beresford *et al.* 1990) and others (Starzl *et al.* 1988; Van Thiel *et al.* 1989) have published data concerning the medical outcome and rate of returning to uncontrolled drinking, following a liver transplant, of alcohol-dependent patients. These studies all suggest that the medical outcome of alcoholic persons is no worse than that of other liver transplant recipients and it is better than those of some patients with hepatitis B, hepatic or biliary carcinoma, or other forms of cirrhosis. Selected patients with alcoholic liver disease have two-year survival rates from 75 to 85 per cent (Beresford *et al.* 1990). However, it remains uncertain whether benefits will be sustained in recipients who return to heavy alcohol consumption. This subgroup may be at increased long-term risk from noncompliance or from alcohol-induced organ damage.

Follow-up of 22 patients transplanted for alcoholic cirrhosis at our centre (Table 3.1) found that 23 per cent of recipients had consumed alcohol since their transplant. Less than 10 per cent were drinking frequently. It is important to note that most of the patients in this sample were selected for transplantation by having two or more of Vaillant's prognostic factors in their favour. In addition, the belief that death could occur if the resumption of drinking resulted in noncompliance with immunosuppressant drugs appear to have acted as a negative behavioural reinforcer post-transplant. Prospective research is being undertaken by our group to determine whether this influence will be sustained.

TABLE 3.1 Outcome and predictors of continued remission in patients transplanted for alcoholic cirrhosis ($N = 22$; 6–36 months post-transplant).

Outcome	N	percentage
Any alcohol since transplant	5	23
Return to drinking >3 consecutive days or >3 episodes in 30 days	2	9
Substitute activities	8	36
Improved hope/self-esteem	16	72
Supportive relationship	13	59
Negative consequence likely with drinking	17	77

This evidence suggests that patients with endstage alcoholic cirrhosis have an adequate medical outcome and low rate of relapse following liver transplantation. However, patients included in our sample demonstrated favourable prognostic characteristics prior to surgery and the time period for follow-up was limited. Further investigation is required to determine the general reliability of these findings for a less selected group of patients or for a longer time following transplant.

The data depicted in Figs 3.1 and 3.2 indicate that referral patterns to our programme are changing. The social stability index decreased significantly

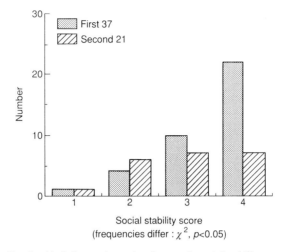

FIG. 1 *Alcohol transplant referral groups by social stability score*

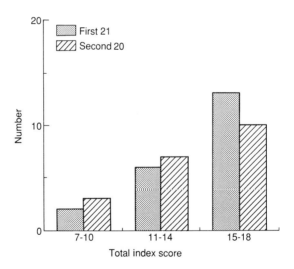

FIG. 2 *Alcohol transplant referral groups by total prognostic index score*

between the first and second cohorts of alcohol-dependent transplant applicants. Interestingly, our aggregate prognostic index scores for the same groups did not vary similarly. This suggests that selection mechanisms in the referring community changed over time, but that prognosis was more determined by Vaillant's factors. The contribution of these individual factors to actual outcome must be investigated in future work.

Alcoholism and transplant priority

Triage is a term coined during the First World War which referred to the classification of casualties into three groups: those who were likely to survive with minimal attention, those who would not survive with available treatment and another group for whom intervention might mean the difference between life and death. The need to triage patients arose from the reality that treatment resources were insufficient to meet the demand. Similarly, a discrepancy exists between current resources and the number of persons with alcoholic cirrhosis who might be medically suitable for a liver transplant. It has been our practice to identify three groups of such patients. These include candidates who will tolerate the procedure well despite a diagnosis of alcoholism, those with little hope of remission, and a third group who fall in between. The transplant team's decision whether to accept a patient for a liver transplant depends in part upon this determination.

The largest and most challenging group of patients is that which falls between the two extremes. Such patients present with some evidence of acceptance of their alcoholism, varying degrees of family recognition of the condition, and a reasonably stable living environment, but without clear evidence of the predictive factors for long-term abstinence as defined by Vaillant (1983). In many such instances, referral for alcoholism treatment has proven beneficial in beginning the process of change that constitutes recovery from alcoholism. When the physical condition does not permit referral, we have typically elected to proceed with the transplant and to encourage treatment for alcohol dependence following surgery. Our experience has been favourable with this approach. However, systematic follow-up studies are needed to confirm this impression.

Others have argued that since alcohol dependence is in part a self-induced condition, these candidates should be granted lesser priority for transplant as long as resources are limited (Moss and Siegler 1991). Our approach has been to prioritize all candidates solely on the basis of medical need and our best ability to predict postoperative illness behaviour and outcome. It may be that even with this assessment, a larger number of patients are found suitable for transplant than there are resources available. Society may be forced to incorporate factors other than the predicted risks and benefits of a transplant for an individual patient. However, in the emotionally charged situation of the alcoholic or other substance abusing patient requesting a transplant, improved longitudinal research will clarify these decisions by optimizing our predictive ability.

Conclusions

The number of persons with endstage alcoholic cirrhosis currently far surpasses the resources available to provide liver transplants for all. Society may be forced to make decisions regarding the allocation of these resources. However, many applicants for liver transplants who suffer from alcohol dependence have potential for an adequate medical outcome and are able to refrain from alcohol abuse immediately following the transplant. Long-term follow up studies are not available. Unless further evidence demonstrates otherwise, there appears to be no psychiatric reason to reject alcoholic patients categorically or to place spurious roadblocks between them and liver transplants.

Acknowledgements

This work was supported in part by grants R01-AA-07236 and P50-AA-07378 from the United States National Institute on Alcohol Abuse and Alcoholism.

References

American Psychiatric Association (1987). *Diagnostic and statistical manual of mental disorders, third edition, revised*. (American Psychiatric Press, Washington, DC).

Beresford, T. P., Turcotte, J. G., Merion, R., Burtch, G., Blow, F. C., Campbell, D., *et al*. (1990). A rational approach to liver transplantation for the alcoholic patient. *Psychosomatics*, 31, 241–54.

Beresford, T. P. (1979). Alcohol consultation and general hospital psychiatry. *General Hospital Psychiatry*, 1, 293–300.

Moss, A. H. and Siegler, M. (1991). Should alcoholics compete equally for liver transplantation? *Journal of the American Medical Association*, 265, 1295–8.

Starzl, T. E., Van Thiel, D., Tzakis, A. G., Iwatsuki, S., Todo, S., Marsh, J. W. *et al*. (1988). Orthotopic liver transplantation for alcoholic cirrhosis. *Journal of the American Medical Association*, 260, 2542–5.

Strauss, R. and Bacon, S. D. (1951). Alcoholism and social stability. *Quarterly Journal of Studies in Alcohol*, 12, 231–60.

Vaillant, G. E. (1983). *The natural history of alcoholism* (Harvard University Press, Cambridge, MA).

Van Thiel, D. H., Gavaler, J. S., Tarter, R. E., Dindzans, V. J., Gordon, R. D., Iwatsuki, S., *et al*. (1989). Liver transplantation for alcoholic liver disease: a consideration of reasons for and against. *Alcoholism*, 13, 181–4.

Appendix A: Alcoholism prognosis scale for major organ transplant candidates

University of Michigan Alcohol Research Center
400 E. Eisenhower Parkway, Suite A
Ann Arbor, Michigan 48104

Instructions

This scale is intended for comparative purposes only. Its use presupposes that the clinician has made a diagnosis of 'alcohol dependence', as described in the *Diagnostic and statistical manual of mental disorders, third edition, revised* (American Psychiatric Association: Washington, DC, American Psychiatric Press Inc., 1987), for any patient under study. The scoring system offers a method of quantifying clinical impressions for the purposes of statistical comparison. Neither the scale nor any part thereof should be used in isolation as a means of offering or declining to offer medical or surgical assistance (Beresford *et al.* 1990).

1. Acceptance of alcoholism Yes: patient and family, 4 points
patient alone, 3 points
family alone, 2 points
No: 1 point (neither pt. nor fam.)
(The patient *and* a family member or another person with a strong personal commitment to the patient's welfare clearly acknowledge the patient's alcoholism as a condition beyond the patient's control.)

2. Substitute activities   Yes: 3 points; No: 1 point
(The patient engages in time-consuming, constructive activities during the time he or she would otherwise have been drinking. Examples include extensive involvement with Alcoholics Anonymous, community volunteer activities, gainful employment, or educational pursuits. They must make up a major portion of the patient's average day. For severely debilitated patients, use appropriate historical data from when he or she last felt well.)

3. Behavioural consequences   Yes: 3 points; No: 1 point
(The patient understands that by resuming drinking he or she will incur specific and unpleasant consequences that will significantly alter the ability to function. Examples include being asked to leave the home by his or her family, immediate and severe medical consequences such as severe pain or imminent death or immediate incarceration (relatively subtle or non-immediate consequences

such as kidney or liver failure do not count, nor do the results of failing to care for the transplanted organ).)

4. Hope/self-esteem   Yes: 3 points; No: 1 point
(The patient describes spontaneously a new or renewed interest in an activity from which he or she derives a personal sense of hope for his or her own future or an improved sense of personal worth irrespective of the future. Examples include active participation in a religion or religious organization or in the spiritual programme of the Twelve Steps of Alcoholics Anonymous.)

5. Social relationship   Yes: 3 points; No: 1 point
(The patient reports, and the object of his or her affection confirms, the existence of a new or renewed relationship involving the patient's affection that has existed with the knowledge and understanding of the patient's alcoholism on the part of both parties and in the specific absence of active addictive drinking by either party. Examples include a spouse, a mentor, a close friend, or a psychotherapist.)

6. Social stability   0–4 points
The patient had a steady job for the past three years to which he or
she may return following surgery. For women, this may include
household or child-rearing duties and tasks.   1 point
The patient had a stable residence for the two years prior to the
evaluation for surgery.   1 point
The patient does not live alone.   1 point
The patient is currently married or lives with a spouse.   1 point

Maximum score   20 points
Minimum score   5 points

4 Transplants in children and adolescents

S. Sexson and J. Rubenow

New developments in transplantation have generally proceeded first in adults and have then been applied to children and adolescents. Obstacles to paediatric transplant have included the relative lack of appropriately sized donor organs, intricate surgical techniques, and the need for specific immuno-suppressant regimens (Lum *et al*. 1985; Sheldon *et al*. 1985; Paradis *et al*. 1988). Transplantation of youths is not uncommon. One in four liver transplant candidates are under 18 years of age as are one in ten kidney, heart, and pancreas candidates (Sexson *et al*. 1990). Unfortunately, with the exception of renal transplants, the child and adolescent research literature remains limited in terms of systematic outcome studies.

The option of organ transplantation has raised expectations for patients, families, and health care providers. Bernstein (1977, p. 145) emphasized that the dramatic possibilities of transplantation represent '... an instance in medicine when a child returns from a terminally ill state to an active state of health'. Paradis *et al*. (1988, p. 409) even imply that transplantation represents a '... cure ... obtainable because the surgeons have overcome major technical obstacles ... and cyclosporine A has made the management of rejection easier'. More realistically, transplantation represents the exchange of one chronic condition for another. Improvement in the quality of life following paediatric transplants has been demonstrated, particularly as related to activity level and autonomous functioning (Korsch *et al*. 1973; Bernstein 1977; Parness and Nadas 1988; Zitelli *et al*. 1988). However, concerns about adaptation to transplants exist. These include the impact on developmental progression and the occurrence of risk-taking behaviours by the adolescent recipient.

Developmental considerations

Chronically ill children and adolescents must try to negotiate similar develop-mental stages to healthy children. Garrison and McQuiston (1989) have reviewed some important aspects of chronic illness in childhood. The manage-ment of organ transplant recipients must be guided by the impact of chronic illness upon the developmental tasks of childhood and adolescence and the child's cognitive ability to form health concepts. The first may offer strategies to facilitate developmental progression in transplant recipients and the second must be taken into account in educating the child about the transplantation process. Table 4.1 summarizes the potential impact that chronic illness and organ transplant may have on the achievement of developmental tasks during childhood and adolescence. Table 4.2 summarizes the developmental progression of children's concepts of health and illness.

Longitudinal studies

Bernstein (1977) concluded from a study of 100 children and adolescents who had undergone kidney transplant that the ability to adjust following surgery was significantly influenced by developmental stage. Pre-school children demonstrated rapid gains in physical growth and social development following transplant. The most complicated adjustment was found during adolescence. Adolescents undergoing renal transplant were particularly bothered by steroid-induced cushingoid appearance and growth failure due to the combined effect of kidney disease and immunosuppressant drugs. For some of the adolescents, these physical changes had considerable negative impact on their self-image. Psychiatric disturbances, including suicidal ideation, occurred in some. Bernstein (1971) suggested that adolescent conflicts over identity, dependency, and authority heightened the risk of psychosocial and behavioural complications with transplants. Korsch *et al.* (1978) also identified adolescents as most susceptible to psychiatric symptomatology as well as to noncompliance. Adolescent girls showed increased vulnerability over boys. However, Korsch *et al.* (1978) also found that adolescents most at risk for noncompliant behaviour were those with psychiatric disturbances antedating both renal failure and transplantation. Studies are needed to define which paediatric candidates are most vulnerable to psychosocial decompensation so that preventative measures may be implemented.

　　Later studies have investigated cognitive and motor development in children with endstage renal or liver disease, both before and after transplant (Rasbury *et al.* 1983; Fennell *et al.* 1984; Stewart *et al.* 1987, Stewart *et al.* 1988; Stewart *et al.* 1989). Rasbury *et al.* (1983) assessed the impact of chronic renal failure on the cognitive functioning of 14 paediatric patients with endstage renal disease at two points: prior to institution of renal dialysis and one month after kidney transplant. Their findings indicated that renal disease itself impairs cognition and learning. Improved problem-solving abilities were demonstrated post-transplant as reflected in performance tasks on the Weschler Intelligence Scale for Children—Revised and the Halstead–Reitan Category Test. Patients with endstage renal disease demonstrated improvement on the Peabody Individual Achievement Tests in mathematics and reading post-transplant. However, Fennell *et al.* (1984) reported on a larger cohort (20 patients) which included the patients described by Rasbury *et al.* (1983). They found that one year after kidney transplant, the improvements in performance intelligence quotient and mathematics achievement had not been sustained.

TABLE 4.1 Effects of chronic illness on development

Stage	Developmental tasks	Impact of chronic illness
Infancy	Biobehavioural organization	Major interruption of bio-behavioural organization
	Parent–infant attachment	Compromise of attachment because of vulnerability and multiple separations
Toddler	Psychological separation	Separation process compromised by multiple separation stresses and parental overprotectiveness
	Emerging autonomy	Interruption of consistent, predictable environment which helps establish developmental equilibrium
		Limitation on physical methods of coping
Pre-school	Continued separation	Magical explanations of illness lead to maladjustment
	Body image	Threats to body integrity compromise body image development
	Initiative	Initiative compromised by limits
School-aged child	School mastery	Irregular school attendance Potential cognitive impairment related to disease
	Peer acceptance	Immunosuppression may limit peer interaction
		Abnormalities of appearance may threaten peer relationships
		Activity restrictions limit peer interactions
	Continued movement toward independence	Forced dependency compromises moves toward independence
Adolescence	Independence	Independence may be expressed in risk-taking behaviours (noncompliance)
	Establishing sense of personal identity	Physical abnormalities compromise identity formation, lower self esteem increase emotional difficulties
	Identification with peers	Differentness may impair peer relationships
	Preparation for sexual roles	Sexual roles may be delayed or alternatively acted out in life-threatening ways

TABLE 4.2 Developmental concepts of illness and transplantation

Stage	Illness concept	Potential impact on coping
Infancy	Anxiety caused by separation	Increased developmental vulnerability
		Impaired attachment between parents and child
		Failure to progress developmentally
Toddler/ Pre-school	Magical, non-logical view	Difficulty understanding need for and process of transplantation
	Illness is punishment	Development of guilt related to assigning causality to self
School-aged	Contamination causality theory	Understanding of process limited to very concrete explanations
		Actual conceptualization of illness may lag behind ability to repeat rote knowledge
	Threat to establishing competence with peers	Difficulty in maintaining peer relationships
		Peer response to patient influenced by own contamination theory of illness
Adolescence	Physiological explanation	Capable of understanding transplant process
	Denial of own illness	Denial may interfere with treatment and/or compliance

Stewart *et al.* (1987) studied development in young patients awaiting liver transplants. Their findings suggest that infants and children with endstage liver disease secondary to biliary atresia were subject to both mental and motor developmental delays. In a subsequent paper, Stewart *et al.* (1988) demonstrated further that intellectual delays occurred most in the children who had early onset of liver disease or who had a longer duration of illness. Poor nutritional status and growth delays were also more common in those children with cognitive impairment. Intellectual delays were correlated significantly with vitamin E deficiency, particularly in infants. They suggested that the metabolic abnormalities associated with chronic liver disease may be more deleterious to the developing brain of the infant and toddler than to the more mature brain of later childhood. They raise the question of whether earlier transplantation might improve developmental outcome.

Stewart *et al.* (1989) described the cognitive, motor, and social functioning in 29 children with endstage liver disease prior to and one year following transplantation. They found a non-significant increase in intellectual and motor scores in patients at one year follow-up. From the group data, it appeared that the development of children with early onset liver disease would probably remain delayed, at least for the first postoperative year. However, a subgroup of children with significant delays prior to transplant was within the normal range when tested one year later. Variables predicting which children would improve could not be differentiated with this small sample.

In the domain of social functioning, Stewart *et al.* (1989) found that children greater than four years of age at the time of transplantation demonstrated significant improvement. Children younger than four did not show this gain. The authors posit that early deprivation of opportunities for social development may lead to more persistent impairment in social functioning. Continued parental overprotection, which was observed more frequently in earlier onset children, may foster extreme dependency and decreased opportunities for normal peer contact, thus limiting the development of social skills.

These preliminary studies of both paediatric kidney and liver transplant patients suggest that cognitive, social, and motor development may in some children be impaired by the chronic illness that necessitates transplantation. Although the specific findings may not be identical, there is a trend in both populations for children with earlier onset disease, either renal or liver, and/or with longer periods of endstage organ disease, to be at higher risk for developmental morbidity. Improvement following transplantation may occur, but these characteristics which distinguish those who improve are unclear, as is the duration of recovery. Vulnerability to developmental morbidity may also be influenced by preoperative and postoperative rehabilitative efforts.

The infant

Developmental tasks of infancy involve the integration and regulation of several systems, leading to a higher level of biobehavioural organization. These activities are very much compromised by chronic illness in early infancy, or potentially by transplantation itself. However, when the transplant is followed by improved health, developmental progression may be facilitated. Of special concern in early infancy is the impact of the illness on the parent–child relationship. The potential appears high for the development of overprotectiveness and other characteristics of the vulnerable child syndrome (Green and Solnit 1964).

The toddler and pre-schooler

Lewandowski (1984) has suggested that hospitalization between ages one and three years has great potential for negative effect due to the developmental tasks of the period. The toddler is negotiating separation and developing a sense of autonomy, while remaining dependent on care-givers. Limitation of movement, exploration, and opportunities to master the environment may compromise the ability to work through these tasks. Further, toddlers require a consistent and predictable environment in order to feel secure while experimenting with increased independence. This is disrupted by illness and hospitalization.

The pre-school child demonstrates increased verbal competency, but lacks logical skills. Therefore, they will have difficulty appreciating the need for limitations in physical activity and procedural interventions. They may misunderstand aspects of their illness or treatment. For example, young children typically view illness as punishment and may need to be reassured repeatedly (Garrison and McQuiston 1989). The limited ability of pre-schoolers to conceptualize illness in abstract terms makes it particularly difficult for them to understand internal or unobservable disease processes and body parts. Additionally, their tendency to use illogical explanations for events will impair their ability to integrate educational information. Educational efforts must be repeated, encouraging pre-school children to express their beliefs and to question family members and the treatment team. Interventions have also been suggested to facilitate developmental progression in chronically ill hospitalized toddlers and pre-schoolers (Garrison and McQuiston 1989, p. 66). These are applicable to the transplant candidate and may be summarized as follows:

1. Limit separation from primary care-givers by encouraging rooming-in or frequent and predictable visiting during hospitalization.

2. Ensure consistency and continuity of care by minimizing the number of medical care-givers.

3. Maintain familiar routines during hospitalization and provide familiar objects from home for the hospitalized child.

4. Provide play opportunities with as little restriction as feasible.

The school-aged child

The school-aged child has progressed cognitively and is able to understand and reason, albeit in a concrete manner. These capabilities make it easier for the child to cope with illness. However, restrictions on physical activity, special diets, and absences from school compromise their ability to develop peer relationships. Lewandowski (1984) has offered some suggestions to transplant teams concerning the management of the school-aged child with chronic illness. Explanations are essential in language which is appropriate for the child's cognitive–developmental level. Typically, adult explanations exceed the child's level of conceptual understanding. Adults may miscalculate a child's understanding, as actual conceptualization of illness may lag behind the child's ability to repeat the information presented. Further, the age of the child does not necessarily indicate developmental level, particularly in some transplant patients, in whom development may have been delayed by chronic illness. Thus, the cognitive level of the child should be assessed specifically prior to engaging in any educational endeavours.

The school-aged child needs to be prepared for medical treatments as well as for hospitalization. Assessment of the coping style of the child is helpful in determining the approach. Some children may need intensive preparation while others become anxious with more information. Videotapes, therapeutic play, and an opportunity to visit the operating room, handle equipment, and to rehearse procedures may be helpful with children of this age group. Such interventions allow the child to perceive some control over what may otherwise be a chaotic environment. Finally, it is important to keep both the school and the child's friends involved during the absences from school. Return to school is a priority when medically feasible. Parents may resist recommendations to return the child to the school by reporting that their child is doing better academically with a home-bound teacher. This tendency is aggravated in parents of transplant recipients who may fear increased risk of infection in their immunosuppressed child. Reassurance is indicated. Much of the developmental progression of middle childhood occurs with peers in the school setting, and may be hampered markedly if the child is restricted to the home.

Adolescence

Two of the primary developmental tasks of adolescence, increasing independence from the family, and the establishment of a sense of personal identity in relation to a peer group, may be impaired by both chronic illness and the process of transplantation. School attendance may be interrupted, reducing involvement with peers and limiting participation in activities such as sports. Delayed or abnormal physical development may contribute to decreased self-esteem and to discomfort with body image. Adolescents may deny the fact that they even have an illness, thus increasing the potential for noncompliance. Further, dangerous risk-taking behaviour may occur (Korsch *et al.* 1978; Garrison and McQuiston 1989). 'Forgetting' to take medications, failing to observe dietary restrictions, neglecting to use barrier methods of birth control, etc., may place the adolescent transplant recipient at risk for life-threatening complications. Adolescent renal transplant patients are also more vulnerable to emotional problems of various sorts (Bernstein 1977). These patients are much more likely to be suicidal and dissatisfied with their appearance than either younger or older kidney transplant recipients. Adolescent girls appear to be more disturbed by the surgical scars than boys. Boys may attempt to explain their scars with fantasized stories of accidents, knife fights, etc. However, preliminary observations of a small cohort of female adolescent liver transplant recipients have not shown overt preoccupation with surgical scars (Sexson *et al.* 1990).

Adjustment to transplantation

Although the literature on adults has addressed the psychological adjustment to transplantation, only a small number of reports address this topic in the paediatric transplant recipient (Bernstein 1977; Gulledge *et al.* 1983; Lawrence and Fricker 1987). Emotional complications which may arise in the paediatric transplant group include (Gardner *et al.* 1977): death anxiety; dependent behaviour; guilt due to perceived and real burdens on the family; survival guilt when other transplant patients have died; changes in family dynamics; and body image concerns. Survivor guilt may, in particular, first become evident following hospital discharge and upon recovery towards normal functioning (Patenaude and Rappeport 1982).

Bernstein (1977) reported that immediately after the transplant, paediatric kidney transplant recipients perceived their new kidney as if it were a foreign body. During the first three months, children described preoccupation with the kidney and its function, but by one year most children experienced the kidney as their own, and were not preoccupied with its function. Younger children frequently expressed feeling overpowered or alternatively being more powerful after receiving an adult kidney. Occasionally, questions about potential impact on sexual identity may be expressed about an opposite-sexed donor kidney (Bernstein 1977).

In general, transplant recipients experience a much improved physical status subsequent to recovery from the transplantation process (Korsch *et al.* 1973; Zarinsky 1975; Bernstein 1977; Gartner *et al.* 1984; Klein *et al.* 1984; Samuelsson *et al.* 1984; Freund and Siegel 1986; Fine and Tejani 1987; Lawrence and Fricker 1987; Colonna *et al.* 1988; Parness and Nadas 1988; Shaw *et al.* 1988; Zitelli *et al.* 1988). Most of the literature reports that children generally return to school after transplantation, although the social and academic success of their return may be limited, at least at first (Khan *et al.* 1971; Zarinsky 1975; Lawrence and Fricker 1987). Younger children with kidney transplants have been reported to have fewer problems readjusting to peers and school than adolescent recipients (Bernstein 1977). Younger children reported that their peers were intrigued by physical evidence of the transplantation whereas adolescents attempted to conceal evidence of operative scarring. While younger children were protected by their peers, adolescents were often subjected to teasing.

Return to school is considered an indicator of positive outcome following paediatric liver and heart transplantation (Lawrence and Fricker 1987; Stewart *et al.* 1987; Colonna *et al.* 1988; Zitelli *et al.* 1988; Stewart *et al.* 1989). Colonna *et al.* (1988) reported that all school-aged children with liver transplants in their cohort had returned to school. No report of school performance or adjustment was included. Zitelli *et al.* (1988) reported in their follow-up study of liver transplant recipients that all but one child was attending school and that approximately 77 per cent of the sample were either at an age-appropriate grade level or, at most, one year behind in school. Lawrence and Fricker (1987) reported that all seven paediatric heart transplant recipients studied were able to attend school regularly. van der Wal *et al.* (1988) raised the issue that bone marrow transplant recipients may be especially vulnerable to school avoidance problems because of prolonged school absences and/or neurological complications of the bone marrow transplant procedure.

Other authors have addressed the effect of paediatric organ transplantation on family functioning (Korsch *et al.* 1972; Korsch *et al.* 1973; Patenaude *et al.* 1979; Gold *et al.* 1986; Freund and Siegel 1986; Serrano *et al.* 1987; Weichler 1988; Zitelli *et al.* 1988; Uzark and Crowley 1989). Throughout the transplant process, maintenance of functional family relationships is almost impossible because of conflicting demands (work, spouse, other children). Role strain is common because parental or spousal demands often exceed the parent's personal resources (Uzark and Crowley 1989). Social isolation is ubiquitous. Gold *et al.* (1986) reported their experiences with a support group for families of children undergoing liver transplantation.

Although essentially anecdotal, a number of important family issues have been identified. It is essential that the family be involved with the child in the decision for transplant (Serrano *et al.* 1987). Weichler (1988) reports that the information needs of parents are very high throughout the transplant process. However, Gold *et al.* (1986) commented on the severe anxiety which occurs prior to and around the time of surgery, and suggested that coping with practical issues (e.g. finances, transportation) is complicated by the emotional intensity of the situation. Parental capabilities for processing information during this time are limited (Weichler 1988). Patenaude *et al.* (1979) report that latent problems in family dynamics may be exacerbated during the transplant process. They encourage families to focus on current tasks and to postpone attempts to resolve long-standing emotional problems unless relevant to medical concerns.

Following surgery, parents typically experience some realignment of their roles with the child and the staff, assuming a more traditional parenting role while relinquishing some of their preoperative medical care responsibilities. Although ecstatic about a successful implantation, families are confronted with the realization that a complete cure has not occurred (Uzark and Crowley 1989). Parents struggle to maintain a balance between hope and the constant fear of organ rejection or infection. Bernstein (1977) states that these episodes precipitate the bulk of emotional disturbances found in her cohort of kidney transplant patients. Additional organ-specific studies have also emphasized the increased emotional vulnerability of the family when postoperative complications occur (Korsch *et al.* 1973; Gold *et al.* 1986; van der Wal *et al.* 1988).

As the patient recovers, the prospect of discharge may stimulate additional concerns. While excitement about discharge is common, prolonged periods of enforced dependency often makes going home appear risky and frightening (Patenaude *et al.* 1979; Gold *et al.* 1986; Freund and Siegel 1986; Atkins and Patenaude 1987). Parents may become concerned about their ability to ensure their child's safety. This may be a time when the information and counselling needs are the greatest for the family of the transplant patient (Weichler 1988). Parents may find themselves thinking of reasons the child cannot go home or considering the possibility of moving the family closer to the hospital.

Once discharge occurs, parents are likely to be overprotective of the child, and siblings may feel competitive. Coping with the child who is no longer acutely ill requires major adjustment. However, the possibility of recurrent infection or rejection may contribute to a perception that the child is physically fragile and vulnerable. This may impede parental reconceptualization of their child as a relatively healthy survivor. Gold *et al.* (1986) suggest the preoccupation with the risk of rejection and infection constitutes a syndrome which occurs following transplant and is similar to that referred to by Koocher and O'Malley (1981) as the 'Damocles Syndrome'.

Little has been written about problems of compliance in paediatric transplant recipients (Korsch *et al.* 1973; Korsch *et al.* 1978; Gulledge *et al.* 1983). Korsch *et al.* (1978) described 14 paediatric patients (including 12 adolescent females) who interrupted immunosuppressive treatment subsequent to kidney transplant. Compared to compliant patients, these patients tended to demonstrate poor self-esteem and poor social adaptation.

The use of living related donors for paediatric organ transplantation is controversial from the point of view of both the recipient and the donor (Starkman 1980; Blohme *et al.* 1981; Ogden 1983; Wiley *et al.* 1984; Smith *et al.* 1986; Steele and Altholz 1987; Liounis *et al.* 1988; Singer *et al.* 1989). Ethical issues, particularly those involving children as donors, are discussed later in this chapter. Most follow-up studies of living donors report positive outcome with little identified morbidity for the donor (Ogden 1983; Smith *et al.* 1986; Liounis *et al.* 1988). However, financial as well as psychosocial stressors have been identified (Blohme *et al.* 1981; Wiley *et al.* 1984; Smith *et al.* 1986; Steele and Altholz 1987). Starkman (1980) describes interference in the separation/individuation process of adolescents who receive a kidney transplant from a parent. Ambivalence toward the donor may result in noncompliance. An adolescent who receives an organ from an opposite sex parent may experience this as a threat to their sexual identity (Delmar-McClure 1985; Starkman 1980). Although not necessarily pathological, changes in the family system are inevitable (Wiley *et al.* 1984).

There may be some emotional differences encountered with the various transplant types. However, the similarities between the more recent preliminary data from heart and liver transplants and the older kidney and bone marrow experience suggest that there are common psychological issues across organ subgroups (Korsch *et al.* 1973; Bernstein 1977; Patenaude *et al.* 1979). Although long-term studies are especially sparse regarding paediatric heart and liver transplant outcome, no studies thus far demonstrate distinct psychiatric issues which correspond to a particular type of paediatric transplant procedure.

Preoperative assessment

Assessment of the transplant candidate has received considerable attention in literature on adults (Frierson and Lippmann 1987; Freeman *et al.* 1988) and in some of the studies of renal transplantation in adolescents (Bernstein 1977; Korsch *et al.* 1978). Two approaches can be taken to the preoperative assessment: a disqualifying or selection process, or a means of identifying those most in need of support and psychiatric intervention. The selection process view of the preoperative assessment is frequently taken by the medical and surgical team. Their question centres upon who will comply with the long-term treatment recommendations. Regardless of the purpose of the preoperative assessment, evaluation of the family of the paediatric transplant recipient is a necessary component.

A few studies have looked at outcome in an effort to correlate pre-transplant risk factors with post-transplant psychiatric outcome (Korsch *et al.* 1973; Bernstein 1977; Korsch *et al.* 1978; Zitelli *et al.* 1986). Table 4.3 summarizes the risk factors highlighted by these studies. A group at highest risk for post-transplant complications are adolescent females from disrupted homes and with poor social support systems. Pre-existing psychiatric difficulties complicate adjustment further. However, predictive factors have not been identified that would suggest a particular emphasis for the assessment of families.

Atkins and Patenaude (1987) view the assessment process as a time of observing the reactions to stress while facilitating appropriate parenting. Direct support of the patient and the medical team may also be a preventive strategy. Serrano *et al.* (1987) include several psychometric measures to assess developmental factors which could promote appropriate coping in patients and families. Their interventional style is described anecdotally, but no data are offered to identify those patients at increased risk for complications.

Until more clear-cut psychosocial predictors of poor outcome can be determined, psychiatric assessment of potential transplant recipients must focus more on identification of risk factors. Therapeutic interventions to address these factors must be studied objectively before specific risk factors are designated as reasons for exclusion from transplant.

TABLE 4.3 Predictors of negative outcome in paediatric transplant

Author	Outcome	Risk Factors
Korsch *et al.* (1973) Korsch *et al.* (1978)	Noncompliance	Adolescence Female Absent father Poor family support Poor community support Pre-existing psychiatric disorders Cosmetic side effects
Bernstein (1977)	Vulnerability to complications post-transplant	Disrupted families Poor body image Continued health problems Parental ambivalence Adolescence Female

Ethical considerations in children and adolescents

Ethical considerations in the field of organ transplantation in children are the source of much controversy, mostly unresolved (Fost 1977; Hollenberg 1977; Caplan 1983; Delmar-McClure 1985; Holzgreve *et al.* 1987; Moskop 1987; Erikson and Mitchell 1988). The ethical principles of beneficence, autonomy, and justice are frequently used to assess ethical issues in organ transplantation of children (Moskop 1987).

Beneficence demands that the act benefit the person involved, in this case, the paediatric organ recipient. Kidney transplantation in children has been an established treatment choice for endstage renal disease for a number of years and more recently liver transplantation has been demonstrated to be of benefit to children. Heart transplant is increasingly available and lung, heart–lung, and pancreas transplants are being offered. Since these interventions can save children's lives, the principle of beneficence may be satisfied. However, the death with dignity movement reminds us that prolonging life may not always be a benefit to a patient. This may be relevant when paediatric patients are subjected to life-prolonging measures with slim hope of receiving a transplant, potentially decreasing their opportunity to die with dignity. There remains a diversity of opinion as to the beneficence of organ transplantation in certain, high-risk cases.

The second principle, autonomy, is even more confusing in the paediatric population than in adults (Moskop 1987; Parness and Nadas 1988). Autonomy in health care is usually expressed as the concept of informed consent. With minors, this is a substituted judgment by the parent or guardian. Once provided with information needed to make a considered treatment decision, parents should be allowed to make their decision without coercion. However, such decisions may be influenced greatly by the way in which medical staff present information (Fost 1977; Moskop 1987). Additionally, our society does not give parents unlimited power in relation to their children. Thus, medical care providers can assume the role of the child advocate when parental consent is not forthcoming in cases where there is a disagreement regarding the best interests of the child. The courts may be petitioned to override parental refusal of organ transplants.

Additional concerns have been raised for paediatric transplant teams relative to the minor status of the paediatric patient (Parness and Nadas 1988). The question arises as to whether the inability of the parental figure to provide adequate support and care after a transplant should be a consideration in the acceptance of a child for a transplant. If transplantation becomes the standard of care, will the medical profession need to seek foster care for such children to optimize the likelihood of an adequate outcome? Can people be found who can make such a demanding commitment? As transplantation becomes more an accepted mode of care, these decisions will become more complicated when looked at from both the ethical perspective of autonomy and the distribution of resources.

Another ethical issue concerns children as living–related organ donors, primarily for bone marrow and kidney transplant candidates. Informed consent of the child is questionable, as the potential for parental influence is great. However, Fost (1977) has proposed that ethical standards could be met in certain cases. The substituted judgement for a child donor may be valid if such a donation is morally sound, if the child overtly acquiesces and thirdly, if such a donation is in the best interests of the donating child. He suggests that informed consent is a false issue since the emotional implications of such a decision prevent true informed consent even in adults. However, in a response to this proposal, Hollenberg (1977) cautions against covert coercion in order to satisfy Fost's criteria.

The bone marrow transplant field depends frequently on sibling donors because of the increased likelihood for a compatible match. Many of these donors are minors who may potentially experience psychological complications should the recipient have a poor medical outcome (Wiley *et al.* 1984). More study on the psychological effects of organ donation is necessary before the ethical questions concerning acceptable organ donation criteria for minor donors can be adequately addressed.

More recently, liver transplants have become possible using living–related donors (Singer *et al.* 1989). The risk of perioperative morbidity and mortality for the donor appears to be greater than that for more established living–related donor programmes such as kidney and bone marrow. The appeal lies in the fact that cadaveric liver donors for children and particularly infants, are extremely scarce. However, some might question whether donor parents can make an autonomous judgment in the face of the impending death of their child. Singer *et al.* (1989) have proposed that in selected cases, parent donors can give consent despite considerable internal and external pressure. They suggest specific elements in their protocol to minimize coercion, including psychiatric evaluation of the donor and provision for an unrelated advocate for the donor.

Conclusions

Transplant of the child or adolescent with endstage organ disease is an increasingly viable option. Patients and their families require extensive information and assistance in order to make appropriate decisions regarding the procedures and to cope well with the child recipient. Developmental delay associated with chronic childhood illness may be ameliorated in some, but not in all, children following a transplant. Illness and transplant may contribute to psychological and behavioural disturbances which vary according to the developmental level of the child. The involvement of families in the process of transplant is necessary with paediatric patients. However, decision-making processes, interactions with team members, and appreciation of the child's motivation for surgery are complicated by the multiple parties involved.

References

Atkins, D. M. and Patenaude, A. F. (1987). Psychosocial preparation and follow-up for pediatric bone marrow transplant patients. *American Journal of Orthopsychiatry*, 57, 246–52.

Bernstein, D. M. (1971). After transplantation—the child's emotional reactions. *American Journal of Psychiatry*, 127, 1189–93.

Bernstein, D. M. (1977). Psychiatric assessment of the adjustment of transplanted children. In *Gift of life: the social and psychological impact of organ transplantation* (eds R. G. Simmons, S. D. Klein, R. L. Simmons), pp. 119–47 (Wiley, New York).

Blohme, I., Gabel, H., and Brynger, H. (1981). The living donor in renal transplantation. *Scandanavian Journal of Urology and Nephrology*, 64, Supplement, 143–51.

Caplan, A. L. (1983). Organ transplants: the costs of success. *The Hastings Center Report*, 13, 23–32.

Colonna, J. O. II., Brems, J. J., Hiatt, J. R., Millis, J. M., Ament, M. E., Baldrich-Quinones, W. J., *et al.* (1988). The quality of survival after liver transplantation. *Transplantation Proceedings*, 20, Supplement 1, 594–7.

Delmar-McClure, N. (1985). When organs match and health beliefs don't: Bioethical challenges. *Journal of Adolescent Health Care*, 6, 233–7.

Erikson, I. and Mitchell, C. (1988). Which child gets the transplant? *American Journal of Nursing*, 88, 287–8.

Fennell, R. S. III, Rasbury, W. C., Fennell, E. B., and Morris, M. K. (1984). Effects of kidney transplantation on cognitive performance in a pediatric population. *Pediatrics*, 74, 273–8.

Fine, R. N. and Tejani, A. (1987). Renal transplantation in children. *Nephron*, 46, 81–6.

Fost, N. (1977). Children as renal donors. *New England Journal of Medicine*, 296, 363–67.

Freeman, A. M. III, Folks, D. G., Sokol, R. S., and Fahs, J. J. (1988). Cardiac transplantation: clinical correlates of psychiatric outcome. *Psychosomatics*, 29, 47–54.

Freund, B. L. and Siegel, K. (1986). Problems in transition following bone marrow transplantation: psychosocial aspects. *American Journal of Orthopsychiatry*, 56, 244–52.

Frierson, R. L. and Lippmann, S. B. (1987). Heart transplant candidates rejected on psychiatric indications. *Psychosomatics*, 28, 347–55.

Gardner, G. G., August, C. S., and Githens, J. (1977). Psychological issues in bone marrow transplantation. *Pediatrics*, 60, 625–31.

Garrison, W. T. and McQuiston, S. (1989). *Chronic Illness during childhood and adolescence: psychological aspects.* Developmental Clinical Psychology and Psychiatry Series, No. 19 (Sage, Newbury Park).

Gartner, J. C., Zitelli, B. J., Malatack, J., Shaw, B. W., Iwatsuki, S., and Starzl, T. E. (1984). Orthotopic liver transplantation in children: two-year experience with 47 patients. *Pediatrics*, 74, 140–5.

Gold, L. M., Kirkpatrick, B. S., Fricker, F. J., and Zitelli, B. J. (1986). Psychosocial issues in pediatric organ transplantation: the parents' perspective. *Pediatrics*, 77, 738–44.

Green, M. and Solnit, A. J. (1964). Reactions to the threatened loss of a child: a vulnerable child syndrome. *Pediatrics*, 34, 58.

Gulledge, A. D., Busztu, C., and Montague, D. K. (1983). Psychosocial aspects of renal transplantation. *Urologic Clinics of North America*, 10, 327–35.

Hollenberg, N. K. (1977). Altruism and coercion: should children serve as kidney donors? *New England Journal of Medicine*, 296, 390–1.

Holzgreve, W., Beller, F. K., Buchholz, B., Hansmann, M., and Kohler, K. (1987). Kidney transplantation from anencephalic donors. *New England Journal of Medicine*, 316, 1069–70.

Khan, A. U., Herndin, M. A., and Ahmadian, S. Y. (1971). Social and emotional adaptations of children with transplanted kidneys and chronic hemodialysis. *American Journal of Psychiatry*, 127, 1194–8.

Klein, S. D., Simmons, R. G., and Anderson, C. R. (1984). Chronic kidney disease and transplantation in childhood and adolescence. In *Chronic illness and disabilities in childhood and adolescence* (ed. R. W. Blum), pp. 429–57 (Grune & Stratton, Orlando).

Koocher, G. P. and O'Malley, J. E. (1981). *The Damocles Syndrome: psychosocial consequences of surviving childhood cancer*, pp. xvii–xx, 1–30 (McGraw-Hill, New York).

Korsch, B. M., Gardner, J. E., Fine, R. N., and Negrete, V. F. (1972). Long-term follow up on kidney transplant patients and their families. *Proceedings of the European Dialysis and Transplant Association*, pp. 359–63.

Korsch, B. M., Negrete, V. F., Gardner, J. E., Weinstock, C. L., Mercer, A. S., Grushkin, C. M., *et al.* (1973). Kidney transplantation in children: psychosocial follow-up study on child and family. *Journal of Pediatrics*, 83, 399–408.

Korsch, B. M., Fine, R. N., and Negrete, V. F. (1978). Noncompliance in children with renal transplants. *Pediatrics*, 61, 872–6.

Lawrence, K. S. and Fricker, F. J. (1987). Pediatric heart transplantation: quality of life. *Journal of Heart Transplantation*, 6, 329–33.

Lewandowski, L. A. (1984). Psychosocial aspects of pediatric critical care. In *Nursing care of the critically ill child* (ed. M. F. Hazinski) (C. V. Mosby, St Louis).

Liounis, B., Roy, L. P., Thompson, J. F., May, J., and Sheil, A. G. R. (1988). The living related kidney donor: a follow-up study. *Medical Journal of Australia*, 148, 436–44.

Lum, C. T., Wassner, S. J., and Martin, D. E. (1985). Current thinking in transplantation in infants and children. *Pediatric Clinics of North America*, 32, 1203–32.

Moskop, J. C. (1987). Organ transplantation in children: ethical issues. *Journal of Pediatrics*, 110, 175–80.

Ogden, D. A. (1983). Consequences of renal donation in man. *American Journal of Kidney Disease*, II, 501–11.

Paradis, K. J. G., Freese, D. K., and Sharp, H. (1988). A pediatric perspective on liver transplantation. *Pediatric Clinics of North America*, 35, 409–33.

Parness, I. A. and Nadas, A. S. (1988). Cardiac transplantation in children. *Pediatrics in Review*, 10, 111–18.

Patenaude, A. F. and Rappeport, J. M. (1982). Surviving bone marrow transplantation: the patient in the other bed. *Annals of Internal Medicine*, 97, 915–18.

Patenaude, A. F., Szymanski, L., and Rappeport, J. (1979). Psychological costs of bone marrow transplantation in children. *American Journal of Orthopsychiatry*, 49, 409–22.

Rasbury, W. C., Fennell, R. S., and Morris, M. K. (1983). Cognitive functioning of children with end-stage renal disease before and after successful transplantation. *Journal of Pediatrics*, 102, 589–92.

Samuelsson, R. G., Hunt, S. A., and Schroeder, J. S. (1984). Functional and social rehabilitation of heart transplant recipients under age thirty. *Scandinavian Journal of Thoracic and Cardiovascular Surgery*, 18, 97–103.

Serrano, J. A., Verougstraete, C., and Ghislain, T. (1987). Psychological evaluation and support of pediatric patients and their parents. *Transplantation Proceedings*, 19, 3358–62.

Sexson, S., Rubenow, J., and Buchanan, C. (1990). Psychiatric morbidity in adolescent liver transplant patients: a preliminary report. Presented at the First Working Conference on The Psychiatric, Psychosocial and Ethical Aspects of Organ Transplantation, Toronto, Canada, June 1990.

Shaw, B. W., Wood, R. P., Kaufman, S. S., Williams, L., Antonson, D. L., Kelly, D. A., *et al.* (1988). Liver transplantation therapy for children: Part II. *Journal of Pediatric Gastroenterology and Nutrition*, 7, 797–815.

Sheldon, C. A., Najarian, J. S., and Mauer, S. M. (1985). Pediatric renal transplantation. *Surgical Clinics of North America*, 65, 1589–621.

Singer, P. A., Siegler, M., Whittington, P. F., Lantos, J. D., Emond, J. C., Thistlethwaite, J. R., *et al.* (1989). Ethics of liver transplantation with living donors. *New England Journal of Medicine*, 321, 620–2.

Smith, M. D., Kappell, D. F., Province, M. A., Hong, B. A., Robson, A. M., Dutton, S., *et al.* (1986). Living-related kidney donors: a multicenter study of donor education, socioeconomic adjustment, and rehabilitation. *American Journal of Kidney Diseases*, 8, 223–33.

Starkman, M. N. (1980). Psychological problems resulting from parent-to-adolescent renal transplantation. *General Hospital Psychiatry*, 2, 289–93.

Steele, C. I. and Altholz, J. A. (1987). Donor ambivalence: a key issue in families of children with end-stage renal disease. *Social Work in Health Care*, 13, 47–57.

Stewart, S. M., Uauy, R., Waller, D. A., Kennard, B. D., and Andrews, W. S. (1987). Mental and motor development correlates in patients with end-stage biliary atresia awaiting liver transplantation. *Pediatrics*, 79, 882–8.

Stewart, S. M., Uauy, R., Kennard, B. D., Waller, D. A., Benser, M., and Andrews, W. S. (1988). Mental development and growth in children with chronic liver disease of early and late onset. *Pediatrics*, 82, 167–72.

Stewart, S. M., Uauy, R, Waller, D. A., Kennard, B. D., Benser, M., and Andrews, W. S. (1989). Mental and motor development, social competence, and growth one year after successful pediatric liver transplantation. *Journal of Pediatrics*, 114, 574–81.

Uzark, K. and Crowley, D. (1989). Family stress after pediatric heart transplantation. *Progress in Cardiovascular Nursing*, 4, 23–7.

van der Wal, R., Nims, J., and Davies, B. (1988). Bone marrow transplantation in children: Nursing management of late effects. *Cancer Nursing*, 11, 132–43.

Weichler, N. K. (1988). Assessment of the information needs of mothers of children after liver transplantation. *Transplantation Proceedings*, 20, 598–9.

Wiley, F. M., Lindamood, M. M., and Pfefferbaum-Levine, B. (1984). Donor–patient relationship in pediatric bone marrow transplantation. *Journal of the Association of Pediatric Oncology Nurses*, 1, 8–14.

Zarinsky, I. (1975). Psychological problems of kidney transplanted adolescents. *Adolescence*, 10, 101–9.

Zitelli, B. J., Malatack, J. J., Gartner, J. C., Urbach, A. H., Williams, L., Miller, J. W., *et al*. (1986). Evaluation of the pediatric patient for liver transplantation. *Pediatrics*, 78, 559–65.

Zitelli, B. J., Miller, J. W., Gartner, J. C., Malatack, J. J., Urbach, A. H., Belle, S. H., *et al*. (1988). Changes in life-style after liver transplantation. *Pediatrics*, 82, 173–80.

5 Social support and organ transplantation

C. Littlefield

The serious deterioration of a vital organ creates unique needs for help and support from others in society. The gravity of their situation makes transplant patients extremely vulnerable both within their own social network, and also with respect to the larger health care system. When the heart, lungs, or liver fail, survival itself depends upon the altruistic donation of an organ by an anonymous, grieving family. In the case of kidneys or bone marrow, a close family member is often called upon to make a donation. Throughout the transplant process, and typically for an extended time prior to surgery, patients are in need of strong emotional support and practical assistance to cope with the demands of their illness. When personal and professional social structures work in concert with the available technical advances, many patients with endstage organ failure have the support necessary to survive a catastrophic illness.

This chapter discusses the importance of the social network to the transplant patient's emotional and physical well-being. At present, the absence of a support person is a relative contraindication to acceptance in heart transplant programmes in 67 per cent of US and 43 per cent of non-US centres and is an absolute contraindication in 9 per cent and 3 per cent respectively (Olbrisch and Levenson 1990). Yet the validity of this criterion with respect to patient outcome (either medically or psychologically) has not been established. Research on social support and transplantation remains in its infancy. Much of what we currently know about social support comes from mental health and epidemiological research conducted in clinical areas other than transplantation. Evidence from these sources is converging to indicate that perceived support from others and integration within a social network protects individuals from depression (Barnett and Gotlib 1988; Krause *et al*. 1989) and from physical morbidity and mortality (House *et al*. 1988). By extrapolation, a better understanding of the particular social support needs and problems of transplant candidates and their families could well have implications not only for emotional well-being, but also for the survival of many transplant patients.

How social support has been investigated in non-transplant populations is described here, and the findings applied to the transplant experience. Clearly, the contribution of social support to the mental and physical health of transplant patients is an area that cries out for its own research agenda. An important objective of this chapter is to attempt to illuminate the directions that a social support research initiative might take among these patients.

The concept and measurement of social support

Social support has been described variously as the presence of social ties (Berkman and Syme 1979); the perception that support is available from others (Schaefer et al. 1981; Procidano and Heller 1983; Sarason et al. 1983; Turner et al. 1983); the comfort, assistance, and information provided by others (Wallston et al. 1983); the functions performed for an individual by others (Cohen et al. 1985; Thoits 1986); and the adequacy of the support provided (Barrera 1981). In a survey of 60 social support researchers, O'Reilly (1988) concluded that definitions of the concept typically include three elements: 'Support is seen as (a) an interactive process in which (b) particular actions or behaviors (c) can have a positive effect on an individual's social, psychological, or physical wellbeing' (p. 863).

Models

Two conceptual models have been used most commonly to describe how social support may protect people from ill health (Cohen and Wills 1985). The main effect model predicts that persons with adequate social support will be healthier and happier than those without social support, regardless of their life circumstances. In other words, according to this model, social support is thought to have a blanketing positive effect that protects persons from ill health. In the second model, called the buffering model, the protective effect of social support is predicted to be apparent specifically in the face of adversity. According to this model, social support is expected to interact with stress such that persons experiencing high stress and who have good support will have better health outcomes than those whose support is inadequate. In this model, social support is not expected to influence the well-being of persons who are not experiencing stress.

Both the main effect and the buffering models have received empirical support. To some extent, which model has the strongest explanatory power depends on the circumstances and the measure used. In an important review, Cohen and Wills (1985) drew a number of conclusions about the relationship between models of social support and well-being. They reported that evidence for the main effect model is found when the support measure assesses a person's degree of integration in a large community social network. This is done by aggregating a variety of structural measures such as marital status, close friends, group participation, social contacts, etc. Although embeddedness in a social network is beneficial to general well-being, it is not necessarily helpful in the face of stress. Thus, social integration does not necessarily influence a person's ability to cope with stressful events. They concluded that evidence for the buffering model is found when the social support measure assesses inter-personal resources that are responsive to the needs elicited by stressful events (i.e. functional measures such as degree of support from a confidant, perceived availability of support relating to self-esteem, companionship, information). The authors suggested that specific support functions (such as esteem enhancement, the provision of information, help with concrete needs, or companionship) are helpful in reducing distress because they are responsive to stressful events. On the other hand, social network integration is beneficial because it promotes feelings of stability and well-being, regardless of stress level.

A third model of social support is the person–environment fit model proposed by Broadhead *et al.* (1983). According to this model, well-being is dependent upon the 'goodness of fit' between the demands of the environment and the social resources of the individual. Cohen and Wills (1985) alluded to this model when they suggested that support should function best as a buffer when it provides stressor-specific coping resources. However, there is no direct evidence in the literature that this is true. Rather, the available research suggests that the perception of being emotionally supported has a diffuse positive effect (Sarason *et al.* 1987). Investigation of the person–environment fit model would appear to be a fruitful area for further research, especially among transplant patients whose needs for support from others are both intense and very specific. The applicability of this model to the transplant situation is explored in greater detail later in this chapter.

Measurement

There are as many measures of social support as there are definitions. It is beyond the scope of this chapter to describe each instrument; however, the interested reader is directed to McColl and Skinner (1988) for a review of 12 measures of social support and an evaluation of their appropriateness for use in rehabilitation settings. I briefly discuss here some general approaches to the measurement of social support.

Indicators of social support fall into two main categories: structural and functional measures (Cohen and Wills 1985; Wortman and Conway 1985; Orth-Gomer and Unden 1987; Ganster and Victor 1988). Structural measures document the existence, but not the quality, of social relationships. Specific measures can include network size or other quantitative aspects of the social environment, such as marital status, number of contacts with others, or amount of participation in clubs or religious involvement. Several of these factors may be aggregated to form a global structural measure. Functional measures reflect the perceptions of the recipient and indicate the extent to which existing relationships provide particular functions. Four functions are assessed most commonly in the literature: (a) esteem support, or the sense that one is esteemed and accepted by others (also known as emotional support and expressive support); (b) informational support; (c) social companionship; and (d) instrumental support, or help with concrete needs such as finances, material resources, or services.

Structural measures tend to be used in large epidemiological studies. A number of such studies have demonstrated that the relative risk for mortality is increased when social support is lacking. For instance, in both the Alameda County study (Berkman and Syme 1979) and the Tecumseh study (House *et al.* 1982), persons with fewer social ties had a significantly greater relative risk for mortality over 9–12 years than persons who were more integrated within their social network. This was true even controlling for medical illness and other standard physical risk factors such as weight, smoking, exercise level, etc. Being single, in particular, has been associated with increased mortality (Kitigawa and Hauser 1973). In terms of psychological morbidity, counting the size of the social network or the frequency of social contacts alone typically does not predict mental health and well-being (Cohen and Wills 1985). However, a few studies that have assessed social support by aggregating across several structural measures that tap into degree of social integration (e.g. marital status, living close to family and friends, belonging to clubs, church, or organizations) have found an association with well-being (Lin *et al.* 1979; Miller and Ingham 1979; Schaefer *et al.* 1981; Williams *et al.* 1981; Bell *et al.* 1982).

Functional measures of social support have proven to be more informative than structural ones, on balance, when it comes to predicting mental health and well-being. Several reviews of population studies have noted a consistent association between psychological distress and poor social support when functional measures are used (Barnett and Gotlib 1988; Bloom 1990; Cohen and Wills 1985). However, because they are subjective judgments, there has been some question about whether low ratings of social support truly reflect the individual's social reality or rather reflect a demoralized perception. This potentially confounding issue was addressed in a recent prospective study which found that changes in satisfaction with social support temporally preceded symptoms of depression in a community sample of older adults (Krause *et al.* 1989). In addition, poor social support has been found to distinguish remitted depressed patients from normal controls (Barnett and Gotlib 1988). These studies suggest that inadequate social support is a risk factor for depression, rather than an artefact of it.

Social support in the physically ill

From the perspective of the main effect model, poor social support can be thought of as a vulnerability factor. Persons in need of a vital organ transplant who also have limited social resources would be expected to be at higher risk for morbidity, mortality, and psychological distress. Research on patients with a variety of medical conditions supports this view. A number of studies that have investigated the relevance of different types of support to a variety of clinical situations and outcomes are discussed below.

Structural measures

Measures of the structural components of support (e.g., the size or composition of the social network) have limited usefulness in the prediction of patient adjustment to illness. For example, the effect of marital status on depression in the medically ill has been commonly investigated, with mixed results. About as many studies do not find an association between marital status and depressive symptoms as do. Interestingly, no studies have found that single persons who become ill do better than those who are married, suggesting that in its effect on depression, marriage is at worst neutral, and at best positive (Rodin *et al*. 1991). However, the magnitude of the effect that marital status has on depressive symptoms is generally quite small, usually accounting for very little of the variance in depression. This is likely because patient satisfaction with the marital relationship, a measure of its functional adequacy, is an overriding factor (Gove *et al*. 1983).

When marital status has been used to predict survival from disease, the findings, although not completely uniform, have been more positive. Several studies have examined the effect of marital status on survival from cancer. In the largest of these, Goodwin *et al*. (1987) examined 27 779 cases of cancer listed in the New Mexico Tumor Registry from 1969 to 1982. Unmarried persons had poorer survival than those who were married, after adjusting for age and sex. The unmarried also tended to be diagnosed at a more advanced stage of cancer and to receive less treatment. The authors noted that being married was associated with an increase in five year survival that was equivalent to being in an age category 10 years younger. The risk for divorced persons was greater than for those who were widowed or never married. In another population study, Neale *et al*. (1986) found that between 1949 and 1968, the 10 year survival from breast cancer was greater for 910 married women than for 351 widowed women, after adjusting for age, socio-economic status, stage of disease, and delay in seeking treatment for symptoms. On the other hand, two studies did not find an association between marital status and survival from either lung (Stavraky *et al*. 1988) or breast cancer (Funch and Marshall 1983). These studies had much smaller samples and in one case, followed patients for a substantially shorter period of time, factors that may have obviated the population trends that emerged in the other studies. On balance, it appears that being unmarried increases a person's vulnerability to mortality from cancer. However, because they are based on population data, the applicability of these findings to the individual case is highly limited.

For patients in need of a vital organ transplant, specific structural measures such as marital status and network size may be much better individual predictors of both emotional well-being and survival than they are in other patient groups. Family size can influence the likelihood that a living–related donor will be found for a bone marrow or kidney transplant. This has implications for survival in a very concrete sense. In addition, depending on the type of transplant, the presence or absence of a support person may increase the likelihood that a patient will overcome the challenges inherent in the process of referral to a transplant programme. It may also influence their accessibility to the waiting list of some programmes. For many adult patients, the likelihood of having such a support person available is greatly influenced by marital status. If relocation to another city or country is necessary in order to procure the transplant, only a spouse may be willing or able to make a move for a prolonged period of time. This is also an instance where the size of the family network can be an important factor. Large families have been known to set up a rotating support schedule (Bright *et al*. 1990).

In terms of recovery from the transplant surgery itself, married patients and/ or those with large support networks may again have a distinct advantage. Kulik and Mahler (1989) reported that among 72 men undergoing coronary-bypass surgery, none of the 16 patients who were unmarried were visited more than twice during their entire stay in hospital. Among married patients, those whose wives visited more often tended to take less post-operative pain medication and be released faster from the surgical intensive care unit than those whose spouses visited less frequently. In the immediate post-transplant phase, the presence of a supportive spouse or other family member could be a major factor in facilitating recovery.

Functional measures

Due to the demands of both their illness and the transplant situation, these patients would be expected to have a strong need for expressive support from significant others. In other medical samples, there is no question that deficiencies in the functional aspects of social support are associated with depressive symptoms. Among women with breast cancer, for example, dissatisfaction with support from significant others and from care-givers has been related to increased depression (Funch and Mettlin 1982; Neuling and Winefield 1988). In addition, Bloom (1982) found that breast cancer patients who felt more supported reported using fewer negative coping behaviours such as smoking, overeating, and drinking alcohol than those who felt less supported. Studies of patients on renal dialysis (Siegal *et al*. 1987) and persons with paraplegia and quadraplegia (Schulz and Decker 1985), have found that psychological distress was negatively associated with (respectively) the perceived helpfulness of, and satisfaction with, support from significant others. Also, negative interactions with family and friends have been found to be significantly related to poorer morale and depressive symptoms among elderly stroke patients following their discharge from hospital (Stephens *et al*. 1987).

It is not common for functional measures of social support to be used to predict mortality among medical patients. One study that did so found that among 224 patients with lung cancer, those who reported a higher need for 'sympathy and devotion' had almost a three-fold risk of death one year later compared with those who rated their need as average to low (Stavraky *et al.* 1988). In addition, patients in this study who were classified as 'reserved' according to a standard personality inventory were nearly four times as likely to die in the subsequent year as those who were found to be average or outgoing. The authors did not examine the social need and personality factors together, so it is not clear whether or not they were related. However, the findings raise the interesting possibility that patients with poorer social skills were more in need of support from others and that this in some way influenced their survival rate. Alternatively, persons with poor social skills who become ill may have fewer social resources and less ability to develop a therapeutic alliance with available personal or professional support networks.

Two studies have compared the structural and functional aspects of social support, one with respect to depression and the other to physical illness. Goodenow *et al.* (1990) examined the relative impact of structural and functional measures of social support on depressive symptoms among women with rheumatoid arthritis. They reported that degree of perceived support, with respect to functions such as information, task assistance, ego support, affection, and opportunity for confiding, accounted for a significant amount of the variance in depression even after degree of network integration had been accounted for. Seeman and Syme (1987) examined the relationship between structural and functional social factors and the extent of coronary athero-sclerosis found among patients undergoing diagnostic angiography. Size of the social network was unrelated to coronary disease, whereas instrumental support and feelings of being loved predicted disease independent of standard risk factors including age, sex, complications, smoking, family history, and Type A behaviour pattern. Clearly, the perception on the part of medical patients that their social support needs are being met is related to their physical and emotional well-being.

The functional support needs of transplant patients would be expected to be at least as strong as those of other medical patients, if not stronger. In other words, poor social support is probably an important vulnerability factor for patients experiencing the endstages of disease of a vital organ. If they are required to move to another city or country to await a transplant, candidates must adjust to a strange place without the full availability of family and friends. As a consequence, they may begin to feel marginalized and left out of ongoing family life, as they miss important events such as birthdays and holidays. Once a transplant occurs, further adjustment is required. If successful, the patient must move back into the family and perhaps be faced with changes in family dynamics and roles that occurred as a consequence of their illness or separation. Re-integration within both the family and the larger social network may be complicated.

Buffering model

Only a few studies have tested the buffering model as it relates either to illness onset, or to the adjustment of patients once illness has been diagnosed. In a study of the factors related to the onset of illness among a group of naval students, Sarason *et al.* (1985) found that although social support alone was not related to illness, in subjects with low social support, the relationship between negative life events and illness was stronger than it was in persons with high social support. This suggests that in the face of adversity, the perception of being supported by others protects against the subsequent development of illness. In a study of persons already diagnosed with an illness, Littlefield *et al.* (1990) used the patients' degree of disability as an indicator of illness severity. Among these patients with diabetes (some of whom also had complications including endstage renal failure), social support was found to buffer the effect of physical impairment on depressive symptoms. In other words, patients who were more physically impaired, but had adequate social support, had lower depression scores than impaired patients with inadequate social support. Consistent with the buffering model, the adequacy of their social support did not influence the depression scores of patients who were less physically impaired.

The buffering model could be tested in patients in need of different types of organ transplant. The study by Littlefield *et al.* (1990) suggests that social support may protect from depression those patients who are experiencing more severe illness or who are closer to death. However, a caveat with respect to testing this model among transplant patients is that these patients may be too uniformly ill for the buffering effect to be evident. The buffering model assumes a wide range of variability in the stressor variable in order for the buffering effect to be demonstrated. Because most patients with endstage organ disease are already at the high end of the stress continuum, this could mask the moderating effect of social support.

Social support for transplant patients

When considering how social support may contribute to the well-being and survival of transplant patients, a theoretical approach with a great deal of intuitive appeal is the person–environment fit model (Broadhead *et al.* 1983). This approach has considerable potential for identifying specific patient needs with respect to social support, and in pointing the way towards interventions that may improve patient outcome. In addition to its utility in predicting outcome, the person–environment fit model may have its greatest applicability in identifying directions for the provision of support to transplant and other physically ill persons. The final section of this chapter will emphasize this model and discuss how it might be used to organize a social support research agenda in patients awaiting organ transplants.

According to this model, the adequacy of social support is defined by the 'person–environment fit' (Broadhead *et al*. 1983). Goodness of fit is thought to depend upon the match between the demands of the environment, the person's abilities to meet those demands, the needs of the individual, and the resources from the environment available to satisfy those needs. Although these elements have both objective and subjective components, it is a person's subjective perception of goodness of fit that is thought to influence most directly their responses to the situation. The social support needs of patients may be thought of as those specific needs that remain after the situational demands and personal resources are matched. Alternatively, some needs may be general to all patients facing a particular type of transplant or attending a particular centre. To apply this model to patients awaiting a vital organ transplant, each of its elements are examined in turn.

Demands of the transplant process

The first step in assessing the goodness of fit of the patient's support system is to identify what the stressors are. In fact, much of the emphasis of this text is to help the reader appreciate the type and enormity of the challenges facing transplant patients and their families. These demands may be classified by a number of parameters, a few of which are illustrated in the following brief discussion.

Different demands may occur with different types of transplants. For example, renal failure is not usually life-threatening because most patients can be maintained on dialysis until an organ can be found. However, if a relative (usually a sibling) turns out to be a suitable donor, the patient may be faced with the mixed feelings associated with requesting and receiving such a fundamental gift. Worse, the patient may have to come to terms with the knowledge that his or her sibling refused to donate their kidney. Although unusual, Kemph *et al*. (1969) described a situation in which four of five siblings withdrew after initially agreeing to be a kidney donor.

Patients awaiting heart, lung, or liver transplants, on the other hand, are in a life-threatening situation. This poses different and additional challenges for the patient and their support network. The patient is typically quite ill, must face the transplant selection process and then wait their turn for a scarce resource. From her experience working with patients awaiting a cardiac transplant, Christopherson (1976) described the precarious balance that must be maintained between hope and grief, as patients and families simultaneously anticipate both life and death. Patients in need of a bone marrow transplant are also in a life-threatening situation. They are often limited in their range of possible donors due to the necessity of a close histological match between donor and recipient. A sibling is typically the donor of choice. In a well-publicized recent case, the mother of an 18 year old patient in need of a bone marrow transplant conceived another child in the hope that the baby would be a suitable match. Fortunately, this dramatic example of a support person attempting to meet the very specific demands of a transplant situation produced a suitable donor sibling (Morrow 1991).

In addition to the type of graft, each transplant programme has its own specific demands. An important part of the assessment process is for centres to identify how the structural demands of the programme influence the patient's social support network. For example, due to the short survival time of donor organs, the Toronto Lung Transplant Program expects that patients move with a support person to within $1\frac{1}{2}$ hours of the hospital, from the time of acceptance into the programme until three months post-transplant (Craven *et al.* 1990). Obviously, this involves a major disruption of the patient's family and social network and can have an enormous impact on the patient's social support needs. Indeed, such an extreme disruption may be impossible for some families to negotiate or may have negative effects on the ultimate success of the transplant. Keegan *et al.* (1983), reporting on a study with a relatively small number of kidney transplant patients, found that patients who had been required to move to another city for their transplant had significantly poorer adjustment and survival than persons who did not have to relocate. This is not to suggest that transplant programmes stop accepting patients who are non-residents of their cities, but simply to underscore the need to assess the impact of relocation on the patient's social support system. Other programme demands, such as the need for a support person to move with the patient to the transplant centre, are also important to consider.

Supporting a loved one in need of a vital organ transplant places a tremendous burden on the support network, particularly parents and spouses. In an article tellingly titled 'Two lives on hold', Squadron (1988) poignantly described the couple's wait for a heart–lung transplant for his wife. Helplessness and frustration, alternating grief and hope, the paralysis of waiting—all appear to take a tremendous toll on the support person. The needs of the family members must take a back seat to those of the patient. But at what cost to everyone involved? Spouses are typically each other's primary source of comfort, advice, and support. What happens when one spouse is too ill to serve this function any longer? Rideout *et al.* (1990) reported that the perception that they were unsupported by their ill partner was strongly related to feelings of depression among the well spouses of patients on renal dialysis. In the case of transplantation, increased demand for support on the part of the ill partner together with a curtailment of their own role as a support person, may cause the well spouse to feel overburdened. Consequent emotional withdrawal in the well spouse could have serious implications for the patient's well-being. Assessing the resources of the support person is thus an important component in considering the overall demands of the situation.

Social resources

The next step in the assessment of the person–environment fit of social support is to gauge the existing resources of the patient. A patient's life circumstances, particularly financial resources, can have a profound effect on the demands placed on the social support network. For example, the ability to pay for domestic help or nursing care can relieve the burden on family and friends. The size, availability, and composition of the patient's social network can influence the burden of care placed on any one individual. In addition, involvement in organizations, such as a strong religious affiliation, provides potential access to social resources that go beyond the patient's personal network. For instance, a church affiliation can provide ready access to a social network for patients who relocate.

The availability of resources to fulfil the various support functions is clearly an important factor. What are the patient's existing resources with respect to emotional support, access to information, companionship, and help with everyday and illness-related tasks? Are people available to transport the patient to and from the hospital, for example? If not, is there access to public transportation for the disabled? Does the transplant centre provide ready access to information or counselling for patients when needed? Do the patient's family members and friends feel comfortable discussing concerns among themselves?

It is clear that medical patients look to different people for different kinds of support. Dakof and Taylor (1990) reported that among cancer patients, 'intimate others' were most valued for the esteem/emotional support that they provided. However, misguided emotional support from these persons was also perceived to be most unhelpful. Other cancer patients and physicians were more valued for informational support, although emotional support from other patients was somewhat important. Absent or misguided emotional support from physicians was perceived to be uniformly unhelpful by these patients. The findings for nurses paralleled those of intimate others. The most helpful and unhelpful actions from nurses fell into the esteem/emotional support category, rather than in the informational or tangible aid categories, as was expected. An important question to assess among transplant patients is whether or not they are receiving the most helpful type of support from the right person.

The patient's own abilities and experience both in dealing with adversity and with respect to getting their own needs met are important internal resources to consider. For example, the more difficult it is for patients to be enrolled in a transplant programme (e.g. a newly developed procedure available in only a few centres), the more likely that patients may be selected in terms of assertiveness and potential for active intervention. In these cases, the rigours of the transplant selection process mean that only the most determined patients reach the stage where they 'make it' to the transplant waiting list, that is, of being accepted into the programme. However, this very quality of single-minded assertiveness could present difficulties in the social milieu of the ward. Thus, what was a strength in terms of getting access to life-sustaining treatment could become a liability when it comes to eliciting social support once in the programme. Assessment of patient coping style is thus important, from the point of view of both strengths and weaknesses.

Person–environment fit

The match between the demands of the situation and the individual's personal resources defines the goodness of fit of the transplant patient's social support system. A poor fit can cause increased distress and potentially interfere with the patient's emotional and physical well-being. The person–environment fit model places no absolute value on the amount of social support needed or provided, but rather emphasizes the balance between the two. Thus, while clearly the source of enormous comfort during the transplant process, social relationships also can have limitations and at times may lead to complications. Some patients may have trouble accepting the offer of support from others. At the same time, support persons may find it difficult to attune themselves to the specific needs of the patient. The goodness of fit model provides a framework for understanding problems that may arise in relation to social support. This model may be most applicable in circumstances where there is conflict regarding the nature and/or amount of support best provided. As exemplified by the following case, this may be particularly evident in circumstances that are especially demanding, such as relocation to another city.

Case history   Mr B., a 27 year old single man, was awaiting a lung transplant for cystic fibrosis. An older brother had died at an early age from the same disease. In compliance with the requirements of the transplant programme, Mr B. had moved from a distant city to live with his sister near the hospital where the transplant would take place. Within one month of being listed, the patient approached the transplant coordinator and asked if it was possible to be on the list without an identified support person. Questioning elicited a variety of difficulties which had arisen since moving in with his sister.

Mr B.'s sister had moved out of the family home several years earlier to attend nursing college. She and her brother had maintained an amicable relationship over the years, even though they had not been able to visit often. When the need arose, the sister offered, without hesitation, her home and support for Mr B. while he was awaiting transplant. However, Mr B. felt that his sister was treating him like an invalid. At his own home he had been used to looking after himself around the house, but his sister now made all his meals for him and even made his bed before he had a chance to do it on his own. She demanded that he go to bed much earlier than he was used to and repeatedly checked to see if he was following his prescribed rehabilitative exercises. Mr B. had gently tried to let her know that he was able to do more for himself, but stated that his sister responded that she wanted him to save his strength for the transplant.

Rather than perceiving his sister as helpful and supportive, Mr B. began to resent his dependence on her for accommodation. Living a life as independently and normally as possible had previously been a major source of self-esteem. Losing this freedom left the patient feeling frustrated and demoralized. In addition, the patient stated that he was used to 'looking on the bright side' when faced with health problems. He reported with pride that he had 'beaten the odds' placed against him by cystic fibrosis and attributed this in no small part to his positive attitude towards the illness and his life in general. Alternatively, his sister, while voicing optimism, persistently asked questions that reminded Mr B. of his severe illness and often stated her hopes that he would 'make it to surgery'. The patient found this 'negative' thinking unbearable and feared that it would compromise his attitude towards surgery.

A counselling meeting was arranged with Mr B. and his sister. Mr B. was encouraged to express his concerns, along with his gratitude for all that his sister was offering to him. He acknowledged that he would be unable to manage until the transplant without her support. The sister expressed surprise that he was unhappy with her help. She mentioned that before her other brother had died from cystic fibrosis, she had helped her mother to look after him. With this statement it immediately became apparent that she was equating the present circumstance with the palliative care given her other brother years earlier. With encouragement, she was able to describe the guilt that she had felt as a youth when her brother had died 'even though' she had tried to look after him well. She showed clear evidence of unresolved grief about this brother's death and was terrified that she was now going to see her second brother asphyxiate. She recognized that the support she had been offering him in her home was motivated in part by her desire to protect him from the fate which she feared would occur. Mr B. was able to explain that while he did not want to die, he feared invalidism much more than death itself. The sister continued with periodic individual counselling and the two were able to agree upon a more satisfactory supportive relationship thereafter.

This case illustrates the difficulties that can occur when the available support is incompatible with the needs of the patient. In this instance, the patient's sister was being overly supportive, behaviour that was interpreted by Mr B. as an affront to his hard-won independence. Social support problems are usually thought of in terms of a deficit. Although little has been written about the effects of excess or poorly attuned support, it may not be an uncommon phenomenon. Littlefield *et al.* (1990) reported that 70 per cent of a sample of 158 persons with diabetes reported receiving as much or *more* support as they needed from other people. Whereas insufficient social support may cause patients to feel isolated and alone with their illness, excess or inappropriately applied support can potentially undermine independence and autonomy.

Conclusions

That integration within a pre-existing supportive network and the perception of being cared for helps patients to cope with the various stressors associated with an organ transplant is self-evident. This hypothesis is supported by research in many settings. Simple demonstrations of this effect among transplant candidates seem unnecessary. A more fruitful area for research within the transplant population may be to identify more specific mechanisms by which social support influences the health, well-being, and survival of patients.

Needs that are general to many patients on the basis of transplant type or centre may be best met institutionally. It may be that the programme could be altered either to eliminate or meet certain needs. For example, the institution of groups that meet regularly to provide information to patients and support persons could fulfil a number of functional support needs. If implemented, the efficacy of such groups should be assessed and the therapeutically 'active ingredient' identified. Because they were charting unknown territory, structural decisions were made by many programmes on the basis of best judgment rather than on any empirical evidence. The time has come to test the necessity of programme demands that impact on the patient's social network (for example, placing a strong emphasis on the availability of a support person when assessing candidates for the programme). It is also important to test the efficacy of any structural changes that are made to meet social support needs.

References

Barnett, P. A. and Gotlib, I. H. (1988). Psychosocial functioning and depression: distinguishing among antecedents, concomitants, and consequences. *Psychological Bulletin*, 104, 97–126.

Barrera, M. Jr. (1981). Social support in the adjustment of pregnant adolescents: assessment issues. In *Social networks and social support* (ed. B. H. Gottlieb), pp. 69–96 (Sage, Beverly Hills).

Bell, R. A., LeRoy, J. B., and Stephenson, J. J. (1982). Evaluating the mediating effects of social supports upon life events and depressive symptoms. *Journal of Community Psychology*, 10, 325–40.

Berkman, L. F. and Syme, S. L. (1979). Social networks, host resistance, and mortality: a nine year follow-up study of Alameda County residents. *American Journal of Epidemiology*, 109, 186–204.

Bloom, J. R. (1982). Social support, accommodation to stress and adjustment to breast cancer. *Social Science and Medicine*, 16, 1329–38.

Bloom, J. R. (1990). The relationship of social support and health. *Social Science and Medicine*, 30, 635–7.

Bright, J., Craven, J., Kelly, P., and The Toronto Lung Transplant Group (1990). Psychosocial stress in lung transplant candidates. *Health and Social Work*, 15, 125–32.

Broadhead, W. E., Kaplan, B. H., James, S. A., Wagner, E. H., Schoenbach, V. J., Grimson, R., *et al.* (1983). The epidemiologic evidence for a relationship between social support and health. *American Journal of Epidemiology*, 117, 521–37.

Christopherson, L. K. (1976). Cardiac transplant: preparation for dying or for living. *Health and Social Work*, 1, 58–72.

Cohen, S. and Wills, T. A. (1985). Stress, social support, and the buffering hypothesis. *Psychological Bulletin*, 98, 310–57.

Cohen, S., Mermelstein, R., Kamarck, T., and Hoberman, H. M. (1985). Measuring the functional components of social support. In *Social support: theory, research and applications* (eds. I. G. Sarason and B. R. Sarason), pp. 73–94 (Martinus Nijhoff, Boston).

Craven, J., Bright, J., and Dear, C. L. (1990). Psychiatric, psychosocial, and re-habilitative aspects of lung transplantation. *Clinics in Chest Medicine*, 11, 247–57.

Dakof, G. A. and Taylor, S. E. (1990). Victims' perceptions of social support: what is helpful from whom? *Journal of Personality and Social Psychology*, 58, 80–9.

Funch, D. P. and Marshall, J. (1983). The role of stress, social support and age in survival from breast cancer. *Journal of Psychosomatic Research*, 27, 77–83.

Funch, D. P. and Mettlin, C. (1982). The role of support in relation to recovery from breast surgery. *Social Science and Medicine*, 16, 91–8.

Ganster, D. C. and Victor, B. (1988). The impact of social support on mental and physical health. *British Journal of Medical Psychology*, 61, 17–36.

Goodenow, C., Reisine, S. T., and Grady, K. E. (1990). Quality of social support and associated social and psychological functioning in women with rheumatoid arthritis. *Health Psychology*, 9, 266–84.

Goodwin, J. S., Hunt, W. C., Key, C. R., and Samet, J. M. (1987). The effect of marital status on stage, treatment, and survival of cancer patients. *Journal of the American Medical Association*, 258, 3125–30.

Gove, W. R., Hughes, M., and Style, C. B. (1983). Does marriage have positive effects on the psychological well-being of the individual? *Journal of Health and Social Behavior*, 24, 122–31.

House, J. S., Robbins, C., and Metzner, H. L. (1982). The association of social relation-ships and activities with mortality: prospective evidence from the Tecumseh Community Health Study. *American Journal of Epidemiology*, 116, 123–40.

House, J. S., Landis, K. R., and Umberson, D. (1988). Social relationships and health. *Science*, 241, 540–5.

Keegan, D. L., Shipley, C., Dineen, T., and Steiger, M. (1983). Adjustment to renal transplantation. *Psychosomatics*, 24, 25–31.

Kemph, J. P., Bermann, E. A., and Coppolillo, H. P. (1969). Kidney transplant and shifts in family dynamics. *American Journal of Psychiatry*, 125, 1485–90.

Kitigawa, E. M. and Hauser, P. M. (1973). *Differential mortality in the United States: a study in socio-economic epidemiology* (Harvard University Press, Cambridge MA).

Krause, N., Liang, J., and Yatomi, N. (1989). Satisfaction with social support and depressive symptoms: a panel analysis. *Psychology and Aging*, 4, 88–97.

Kulik, J. A. and Mahler, H. I. M. (1989). Social support and recovery from surgery. *Health Psychology*, 8, 221–38.

Lin, N., Ensel, W. M., Simeone, R. S., and Kou, W. (1979). Social support, stressful life events, and illness: a model and an empirical test. *Journal of Health and Social Behavior*, 20, 108–19.

Littlefield, C. H., Rodin, G. M., Murray, M. A., and Craven, J. L. (1990). The influence of functional impairment and social support on depressive symptoms in persons with diabetes. *Health Psychology*, 9, 739–51.

McColl, M. A. and Skinner, H. A. (1988). Concepts and measurement of social support in a rehabilitation setting. *Canadian Journal of Rehabilitation*, 2, 93–107.

Miller, P. M. and Ingham, J. G. (1979). Reflections on the life-events-to-illness link with some preliminary findings. In *Stress and anxiety* Vol. 6 (eds. I. G. Sarason and C. D. Spielberger), pp. 313–36 (Wiley, New York).

Morrow, L. (1991). When one body can save another. *Time*, 17 June, 1991, pp. 38–42.

Neale, A. V., Tilley, B. C., and Vernon, S. W. (1986). Marital status, delay in seeking treatment and survival from breast cancer. *Social Science and Medicine*, 23, 305–12.

Neuling, S. J. and Winefield, H. R. (1988). Social support and recovery after surgery for breast cancer: frequency and correlates of supportive behaviours by family, friends and surgeon. *Social Science and Medicine*, 27, 385–92.

Olbrisch, M. E. and Levenson, J. L. (1990). *International cardiac transplantation study*. Presented at the First Working Conference on the Psychiatric, Psychosocial, and Ethical Aspects of Organ Transplantation, Toronto, June 8, 1990.

O'Reilly, P. (1988). Methodological issues in social support and social network research. *Social Science and Medicine*, 26, 863–73.

Orth-Gomer, K. and Unden, A. L. (1987). The measurement of social support in population surveys. *Social Science and Medicine*, 24, 83–94.

Procidano, M. E. and Heller, K. (1983). Measures of perceived social support from friends and from family: three validation studies. *American Journal of Community Psychology*, 11, 1–24.

Rideout, E. M., Rodin, G. M., and Littlefield, C. H. (1990). Stress, social support, and symptoms of depression in spouses of the medically ill. *International Journal of Psychiatry in Medicine*, 20, 37–48.

Rodin, G., Craven, J. L., and Littlefield, C. (1991). *Depression in the medically ill: an integrated approach* (Brunner/Mazel, New York).

Sarason, I. G., Levine, H. M., Basham, R. B., and Sarason, B. R. (1983). Assessing social support: The Social Support Questionnaire. *Journal of Personality and Social Psychology*, 44, 127–39.

Sarason, I. G., Sarason, B. R., Potter, E. H. III, and Antoni, M. H. (1985). Life events, social support, and illness. *Psychosomatic Medicine*, 47, 156–63.

Sarason, B. R., Shearin, E. M., Pierce, G. R., and Sarason, I. G. (1987). Interrelations of social support measures: theoretical and practical implications. *Journal of Personality and Social Psychology*, 52, 813–32.

Schaefer, C., Coyne, J. C., and Lazarus, R. S. (1981). The health-related functions of social support. *Journal of Behavioral Medicine*, 4, 381–406.

Schulz, R. and Decker, S. (1985). Long-term adjustment to physical disability: the role of social support, perceived control, and self-blame. *Journal of Personality and Social Psychology*, 48, 1162–72.

Seeman, T. E. and Syme, S. L. (1987). Social networks and coronary artery disease: a comparison of the structure and function of social relations as predictors of disease. *Psychosomatic Medicine*, 49, 341–54.

Siegal, B. R., Calsyn, R. J., and Cuddihee, R. M. (1987). The relationship of social support to psychological adjustment in endstage renal disease patients. *Journal of Chronic Diseases*, 40, 337–44.

Squadron, W. (1988). Two lives on hold. *The New York Times Magazine*, December, 39–75.

Stavraky, K. M., Donner, A. P., Kincade, J. E., and Stewart, M. A. (1988). The effect of psychosocial factors on lung cancer mortality at one year. *Journal of Clinical Epidemiology*, 41, 75–82.

Stephens, M. A. P., Kinney, J. M., Norris, V. K., and Ritchie, S. W. (1987). Social networks as assets and liabilities in recovery from stroke by geriatric patients. *Psychology and Aging*, 2, 125–9.

Thoits, P. A. (1986). Social support as coping assistance. *Journal of Consulting and Clinical Psychology*, 54, 416–23.

Turner, R. J., Frankel, B. G., and Levin, D. M. (1983). Social support: conceptualization, measurement, and implications for mental health. *Research in Community and Mental Health*, 3, 67–111.

Wallston, B. S., Alagna, S. W., DeVellis, B. M., and DeVellis, R. F. (1983). Social support and physical health. *Health Psychology*, 2, 367–91.

Williams, A. W., Ware, J. E. Jr., and Donald, C. A. (1981). A model of mental health, life events, and social supports applicable to general populations. *Journal of Health and Social Behavior*, 22, 324–36.

Wortman, C. B. and Conway, T. L. (1985). The role of social support in adaptation and recovery from physical illness. In *Social support and health* (eds S. Cohen and S. L. Syme), pp. 281–301 (Academic Press, New York).

6 Organic brain syndromes in transplant patients

P. de Groen and J. Craven

Postoperative delirium and other organic brain syndromes have been reported following kidney (Fricchione 1989), heart (Mai *et al.* 1986), and bone marrow transplants (de Fronzo *et al.* 1973; Sullivan *et al.* 1982). Liver transplant recipients appear particularly prone, with postoperative delirium and other organic brain syndromes occurring in up to one-third of patients (de Groen *et al et al.* 1987; Tollemar *et al.* 1988). Craven *et al.* (1990*a*) have reported that over 50 per cent of the first 30 lung transplant recipients at their centre demonstrated delirium during the first two postoperative weeks. Delirium also occurred in later cohorts from this centre, but at a decreased frequency (Craven *et al.* 1990*b*, *c*).

Some transplant candidates are at risk for impaired orientation and decreased level of consciousness prior to surgery. Episodes of clinical hepatic encephalopathy are common in liver transplant candidates (Tarter *et al.* 1984) and high carbon dioxide pressures may cause impaired mentation in certain candidates for lung transplant (Craven *et al.* 1990*b*). In both of these instances, brain function can recover rapidly following transplant of a well functioning organ. Some patients who have been treated with dialysis for an extended period of time may show evidence of cognitive impairment (Nissenson *et al.* 1977; Stewart and Stewart 1979). The clinical or subclinical abnormalities of dialysis encephalopathy may persist in some patients following kidney transplant (Waniek *et al.* 1977; Nordal *et al.* 1985), but have been documented to improve in other patients (Morales-Otero *et al.* 1988).

The neurological functioning of a transplant recipient may be compromised owing to the cardiopulmonary bypass used during the transplant of certain organs, drugs prescribed postoperatively, graft failure, or other postoperative complications or phenomena associated with the complex surgical procedures. A single aetiological agent which explains all abnormalities may not be defined in the individual patient. Rather, most of these patients are exposed to multiple factors with potential to influence brain function. However, this chapter will emphasize the various agents which may cause organic brain syndromes in transplant patients. For purposes of clarity we will discuss these individually. As cyclosporin is an immunosuppressant drug which frequently has been implicated in the development of neurological and psychiatric abnormalities, this drug will be discussed in greater detail.

Drug-induced neurotoxicity

Cyclosporin

Cyclosporin is commonly prescribed to prevent organ rejection following allogeneic transplantation. In addition to its desired immunosuppressant activity, it has been associated with a variety of central nervous system side-effects. Neurological symptoms include headache, flushing, sleep disturbance, tremors, cortical blindness, quadriplegia, seizures, and coma (Noll and Kulkarni 1984; Atkinson *et al*. 1984; Wilczek *et al*. 1985; Adams *et al*. 1987; Urase *et al*. 1987; Lane *et al*. 1988; Deierhoi *et al*. 1988; Wilson *et al*. 1988; Vogt *et al*. 1988; Appleton *et al*. 1989; Gharpure *et al*. 1990). A reversible white matter disorder has been observed in several cases (Shah *et al*. 1984; Berden *et al*. 1985; Rubin and Kang 1987; de Groen *et al*. 1987; Scheinman *et al*. 1990; Hughes 1990). A wide range of neuropsychiatric effects has also been described. These include: disorientation and altered level of consciousness (Wilczek *et al*. 1985; Atkinson *et al*. 1984; Berden *et al*. 1985; de Groen *et al*. 1987; Adams *et al*. 1987; Bhatt *et al*. 1988; Davenport *et al*. 1988); visual hallucinations (Noll and Kulkarni 1984; Katirji 1987); persecutory delusions (de Groen *et al*. 1987); anxiety, agitation, racing thoughts, and insomnia (Wamboldt *et al*. 1984; de Groen *et al*. 1987); and depression, apathy, inactivity, flattened affect, loss of energy, and anorexia (Morgenstern 1980; Powles *et al*. 1980; Hows *et al*. 1982; de Groen *et al*. 1987; Craven 1989). Patients in whom mental state changes occur often also demonstrate other neurological side effects such as tremulousness or headache (de Groen *et al*. 1987; Surman *et al*. 1987). In addition, case reports suggest that the more lethal, neurotoxic complications of this drug appear to be frequently preceded by mental state changes, and in particular by persistent drowsiness or somnolence (Craven 1991).

 Very high whole blood cyclosporin levels in the absence of hyperlipidaemia are a frequent cause of neurotoxicity (Beaman *et al*. 1985; Labar *et al*. 1986). However, many patients have developed neurotoxicity with cyclosporin levels within the desired range for immunosuppression. Many of these patients presented with concurrent conditions thought to predispose to the toxic CNS side-effects of cyclosporin. These include: pre-existing liver disease with hepatic encephalopathy; a disturbance in the function of the blood brain barrier; cerebrovascular ischaemia; allograft rejection; concurrent high-dose methylprednisolone treatment; hypertension; hypomagnesaemia; aluminium overload and hypocholesterolaemia. These conditions are discussed individually in this chapter. Others have suggested that subclinical or partial complex seizures may occur with cyclosporin and account for the mental status changes which occur in some transplant recipients (Famiglio *et al*. 1989; Surman 1989). Anticonvulsants may be indicated when electroencephalographic evidence of such activity is present (Surman 1989).

Several mechanisms have been postulated to explain the side-effects of cyclosporin. First, cyclosporin itself may interfere with normal membrane function. Second, cyclosporin may inhibit DNA and RNA synthesis, possibly via inhibition of the peptidyl-prolyl *cis-trans* isomerase activity of cyclophilin (Fischer *et al.* 1989; Kahan 1989; Takahashi *et al.* 1989), the intracellular, cyclosporin-binding protein (Handschumacher *et al.* 1984). Third, cyclosporin metabolites may be the cause of the observed neurotoxicity (Kunzendorf *et al.* 1988, 1989). Fourth, an abnormal or inactive hepatic cytochrome P-450 isoenzyme may impair normal cyclosporin metabolism (Lucey *et al.* 1990). Fifth, endothelial toxicity of cyclosporin or its metabolites due to inhibition of prosta-glandin synthesis may result in a dysfunction of the blood brain barrier (Sloane *et al.* 1985; Lane *et al.* 1988) or in development of focal haemorrhages (Zaal *et al.* 1988). Sixth, Hoefnagels *et al.* (1988) have suggested that fat embolism induced by the solvent of cyclosporin (polyoxyethylated castor oil) may have contributed to encephalopathy in a patient who required long-term intravenous infusion of cyclosporin. However, when one adheres to the recommended instructions for the preparation of intravenous cyclosporin, fat embolism seems an unlikely cause of CNS symptoms (Krupp *et al.* 1989). Seventh, free, rather than bound, plasma levels of cyclosporin may be a more appropriate indicator of tissue exposure. As cyclosporin is predominantly bound to red blood cells and lipo-proteins, low haematocrit or low lipid levels may be associated with increased levels of free cyclosporin and concomitant clinical toxicity (Legg and Rowland 1987; Lindholm and Henricsson 1989). However, the methods to measure free cyclosporin levels are of unproven value and the clinical significance of increases in the free fraction has yet to be determined. Eighth, hepatotoxicity may result in the formation of neurotoxic substances. Cyclosporin-induced inhibition of the mitochondrial steroid 26-hydroxylase, an enzyme involved in the formation of bile acids from cholesterol and deficient in cerebrotendinous xanthomatosis, has been hypothesized to cause, or contribute to the observed CNS toxicity (de Groen 1988). However, preliminary results do not support this hypothesis (de Groen, unpublished data).

Cyclosporin-associated neurotoxicity has been studied *in vivo* and *in vitro*. Famiglio *et al.* (1989) described abnormal behaviour and electroencephalo-grams in rats exposed to high doses of parenteral cyclosporin. Brain histology, however, was essentially normal. In subsequent work it was shown that cyclosporin also lowered the seizure threshold for electroshock-induced seizures (Racusen *et al.* 1990). Intravenous cyclosporin reduces cerebral vasospasm after subarachnoid haemorrhage in dogs (Peterson *et al.* 1990). Intracarotid infusion of cyclosporin with concomitant opening of the blood brain barrier resulted in acute neurotoxicity in dogs (de Groen *et al.* 1990). We have also examined the effects of intravenous cyclosporin on rat dorsal root ganglion neurons in cell culture (Blexrud *et al.* 1990). Dorsal root ganglion neurons exposed to the intravenous cyclosporin preparation exhibited axonal swelling and degeneration. When individual components were tested, no isolated effect of cyclosporin was seen. However, the polyoxyethylated castor oil produced axonal swelling, degeneration, and demyelination.

Liver transplant recipients appear to develop central nervous system abnormalities, including cyclosporin-induced side-effects, more frequently than recipients of other types of allograft (Tollemar *et al.* 1988). The Toronto Liver Transplant Group has found that neurological complications account for one third of all deaths during the first three months following transplant (P. Greig, personal communication). A survey of the first 75 liver transplant recipients at this centre has shown that one third of neurological abnormalities following liver transplant are temporally associated with the administration of cyclosporin (Craven *et al.* 1990*c*). To explain this increased risk, Tollemar *et al.* (1988) have suggested that previous liver failure may have damaged the blood brain barrier and facilitated cyclosporin-induced neurotoxicity. Indeed, hepatic encephalopathy, a sign of endstage liver disease, is associated with an increase in the permeability of the blood brain barrier for medium-sized molecules (1000–5000 Daltons; Opolon 1984) such as cyclosporin (1202 Daltons: Petcher *et al.* 1976). Furthermore, it has been estimated that up to 60 per cent of cirrhotic patients without clinical evidence of encephalopathy have latent or covert hepatic encephalopathy (Capocaccia *et al.* 1984). Trzepacz *et al.* (1988) diagnosed delirium in 18 (17 per cent) of 108 consecutive liver transplantation candidates. Of the 90 patients without delirium, 38 (42 per cent) displayed abnormalities on either a psychometric test or on an electroencephalogram.

In a retrospective analysis of 48 liver transplant recipients, 54 per cent of patients with cyclosporin-related neurotoxicity experienced at least one clinical episode of hepatic encephalopathy preoperatively, as compared to only 23 per cent of patients without CNS side effects (de Groen *et al.* 1988). In addition, patients with cyclosporin neurotoxicity also had low preoperative cholesterol, albumin and pseudocholinesterase levels, further evidence of endstage liver disease. Craven *et al.* (1990*c*) reported evidence that suggested that pre-existing central nervous system vulnerability (including preoperative hepatic encephalopathy or a history of significant alcohol abuse) was a risk factor for postoperative cyclosporin-associated delirium in liver transplant recipients.

An increased risk for the development of cyclosporin-associated neurotoxicity was observed in patients with low total serum cholesterol levels in the immediate postoperative period (de Groen *et al.* 1987). Subsequently these observations have been confirmed by others (Bhatt *et al.* 1988; Cooper *et al.* 1989). However, three cases of delayed cyclosporin-induced neurotoxicity have been described with rising (Hughes 1990), normal (Scheinman *et al.* 1990), and high serum cholesterol levels (de Bruijn *et al.* 1989).

Low serum cholesterol levels may only be a non-specific marker of advanced liver failure and not be related to the development of neurotoxicity (Hughes 1990). However, several mechanisms possibly relate low cholesterol levels to neurotoxicity (de Groen *et al.* 1987). Cyclosporin may interfere with the transport of cholesterol and other lipids into the brain, and low cholesterol levels could magnify this effect. Alternatively, low cholesterol levels may lead to increased concentrations of cyclosporin and its polyoxyethylated vehicle (castor oil in the intravenous solution, oleic glycerides in the oral solution, and glycolysed glycerides in the capsules) in lipoprotein particles, especially low-density lipoproteins, thereby increasing the uptake of cyclosporin and the vehicle by the brain (de Groen 1988; Blexrud *et al.* 1990). Finally, low total serum cholesterol levels may be associated with relatively high levels of free plasma cyclosporin.

General principles for the management of delirium may be applied to patients who are delirious secondary to cyclosporin, but particular consideration is required for certain aspects of their treatment. Toxic levels should be strictly avoided, and the drug should be administered in the lowest dose required to provide adequate immunosuppression. Severe neurotoxicity in liver transplant recipients has been successfully managed by temporarily withholding cyclosporin, adding azathioprine to prednisone, and later restarting cyclosporin at a lower dose (de Groen *et al.* 1987; Craven 1991). This may be required when there is evidence of structural damage, *status epilepticus*, or coma, and should be considered when imminent deterioration is suggested by a persistent decrease in the level of consciousness. Neurotoxic symptoms may in some patients return rapidly with re-administration of cyclosporin (Wilczek *et al.* 1985). However, in others it is often possible to reintroduce the drug gradually without catastrophic effects.

If necessary, haloperidol may be prescribed in low doses to control symptoms of agitation, aggressiveness, hallucinations, or delusions. This drug has minimal cardiorespiratory effects (Settle and Ayd 1983) and is a preferred drug for treating delirium secondary to physical illness (Tesar *et al.* 1985; Adams 1988). Compared with other types of sedatives, it has less potential for over-sedation if used sparingly, and exerts more specific action on psychotic symptoms. Compared with other neuroleptics, it has less potential for the autonomic side-effects associated with these drugs. However, iatrogenic over-sedation must be strictly avoided in patients with cyclosporin-induced delirium, as this may interfere with the early recognition of clinical deterioration. Kast (1989) has suggested a potential competitive interaction of neuroleptics and cyclosporin at the lymphocyte binding site. He has suggested that neuroleptics be avoided in these patients until it is documented that the immunosuppressant action of cyclosporin is not interfered with. However, despite the frequent use of neuroleptic drugs (e.g. metoclopramide, perchlorperazine) in these patients, there is at present no published evidence to support a clinically relevant interaction. Systematic research is required to test this hypothesis, but at present the transient use of low dose haloperidol appears to be warranted by the potential severity of the complications which may result from psychosis in these patients.

Other immunosuppressants

Most transplant recipients receive corticosteroids during the immediate postoperative period. Bolus dosages of these drugs are administered at times of allograft rejection. The neuropsychiatric manifestations of prednisone and related agents are well described (Ling *et al.* 1981). Restlessness, insomnia, emotional lability and hypersensitivity, organic mood, and delusional syndromes due to corticosteroids can be expected in a subset of transplant recipients. Seizures have been reported after high dose methyl-prednisolone treatment for allograft rejection (Williams and Doak 1977; el Dahr *et al.* 1987). Others have suggested an interaction between corticosteroids and cyclosporin in the aetiology of generalized seizures (Durrant *et al.* 1982; Boogaerts *et al.* 1982; Powell-Jackson *et al.* 1984). Much less common is the development of corticosteroid-induced spinal lipomatosis (Zampella *et al.* 1987; Vazquez *et al.* 1988).

Several new immunosuppressants have been tested for use following transplant. Although clinical experience with the macrolide-derived immunosuppressive drug FK 506 is limited, neurological side-effects similar to cyclosporin-related side-effects have recently been reported (Starzl *et al.* 1990; Van Thiel *et al.* 1990). Murine monoclonal antibodies directed against the CD3 molecule of the human T-cell, muromonab-CD3, have become widely accepted in the treatment of allograft rejection. Fever, headache, confusion, seizures, and aseptic meningitis after treatment with muromonab-CD3 have been observed (Emmons *et al.* 1986; MMWR 1986; Thistlethwaite *et al.* 1988; Kormos *et al.* 1990; Richards *et al.* 1990).

Anti-infectious and chemotherapeutic agents

Trimethoprim-sulfamethoxazole or co-trimoxazole is used in allograft recipients at risk for *Pneumocystis carinii* infection or in the treatment of active infection with this or certain other micro-organisms. Although not yet reported in a transplant recipient, headaches, confusion, fever, and aseptic meningitis are recognized side-effects related to the use of trimethoprim-sulfamethoxazole (Kremer *et al.* 1983; Derbes 1984; Haas 1984; Joffe *et al.* 1989; Tunkel and Starr 1990).

In many transplant programmes, acyclovir is used for the treatment and prophylaxis of herpes simplex and varicella zoster infections. Neurological symptoms associated with parenteral use include lethargy, agitation, tremor, disorientation, and transient hemiparaesthesias (Wade and Meyers 1983). Gancyclovir is an intravenously administered anti-viral agent which is associated with delirium (Davis *et al.* 1990).

Delirium following bone marrow transplantation is commonly associated with either chemotherapeutic agents or irradiation used to destroy the patient's bone marrow. This occurs most frequently when intrathecal methotrexate is given in combination with high dose intravenous methotrexate and cranial irradiation (Wade and Meyers 1983; Davis and Patchell 1988). The risk of delirium is increased with higher doses of methotrexate given during or after, as compared to before cranial irradiation (Bleyer 1981). Intravenous and intrathecal administration of cytosine arabinoside is also known to be associated with CNS toxicity (Grossman *et al.* 1983; Sloane *et al.* 1985; Johnson *et al.* 1987). As with methotrexate, the CNS toxicity of cytosine arabinoside is dose-dependent. The alkylating agent mechlorethamine, an antineoplastic nitrogen mustard, has been associated with confusion, disorientation, head-ache, hallucinations, lethargy, tremors, paraplegia, and seizure. The likelihood of these symptoms appears to be heightened with increased age of the patient, higher total mechlorethamine dose, and the administration of additional cytostatic agents (Hartmann *et al.* 1981; Sullivan *et al.* 1982).

Infection

Because, primarily, of the immunosuppressant drugs used to prevent allograft rejection, transplant recipients are predisposed to certain bacterial, protozoan, fungal, and viral infections. Organisms that depend on cellular defence mechanisms are most frequently observed. These include listeria; myco-bacteria; nocardia; toxoplasma; candida; aspergillus; histoplasma; *P. carinii*; herpes; cytomegalovirus; and Epstein–Barr virus. Several of these organisms can penetrate the central nervous system and cause meningitis, cerebritis, and brain abscesses. The clinical presentation of these conditions is highly variable, but includes headache, fever, confusion, lethargy, and seizures. Infectious cerebritis should be included in the differential of any transplant recipient presenting with delirium, especially when fever is present. In addition, the systemic effects of Gram-negative organisms in particular can lead to hypotension and cerebral hypoperfusion, further impairing brain function. In fact, a change in mental state may be the presenting feature of sepsis in some patients.

Despite the use of selective bowel decontamination and prophylactic antibiotics, bacterial sepsis may be encountered after any type of trans-plantation. In some cases, meningitis, cerebritis, or brain abscesses develop in association with the septic episode. Bacteria most commonly found to cause meningitis after transplantation includes *Listeria monocytogenes* (Niklasson *et al.* 1978), nocardia (Raby *et al.* 1990), *Pseudomonas aeruginosa*, *Staphyloccus aureus*, *Streptococcus pneumonia*, and Gram-negative enteric bacilli (Wiznitzer *et al.* 1984). Brain abscesses and cerebritis can develop due to infection with a variety of aerobe and anaerobe bacteria.

Protozoan infections after transplantation are not frequently seen. The main parasite known to cause meningoencephalitis and cerebral abscesses is

Toxoplasma gondii (Ackerman *et al*. 1986; Tsanaclis and de Morais 1986). Other parasites, such as cysticercosis (Gordillo-Paniagua *et al*. 1987), are only rarely found.

In one series, fungal infections were the most frequent cause of cerebromeningitis after kidney transplant (Tilney *et al*. 1982). *P. carinii, Candida albicans*, and *Aspergillus fumigatus* (Boon *et al*. 1990) are the predominant fungi causing cerebral infections. Others include mucormyces (Schober and Herman 1973; Morduchowicz *et al*. 1986), *Cryptococcus neoformans* (Duston *et al*. 1981; van den Elshout *et al*. 1987), sporotrichosis (Gullberg *et al*. 1987), histoplasma (Karalakulasingam *et al*. 1976) and *Torulopsis glabrata* (Van Cutsem *et al*. 1986).

Many viral infections can involve the central nervous system. Cytomegalovirus (Cordonnier *et al*. 1983; Ang *et al*. 1989; Donaghy *et al*. 1989) and herpes simplex virus (Patchell *et al*. 1985) are among the most frequently observed. Epstein–Barr virus may not only affect brain function due to direct infection (Randhawa *et al*. 1990), but also via the formation of central nervous system lymphoma (van Diemen-Steenvoorde *et al*. 1986). Rarely reported conditions include progressive multifocal leukoencephalopathy due to JC virus infection (Reznick *et al*. 1981; Saxton *et al*. 1984; Embrey *et al*. 1988; Aksamit *et al*. 1990), and infections with adenovirus (Davis *et al*. 1988), varicella zoster virus (Peterson and Ferguson 1984) and measles virus (Agamanolis *et al*. 1979). Lastly, because of the need for blood transfusions, transplant recipients are at increased risk for developing an infection with the human immunodeficiency virus (Dummer *et al*. 1989). The neuropsychiatric manifestations of this infection are well characterized (Holland and Tross 1985; Catalan 1988).

Other aetiologic agents

Electrolyte abnormalities

Electrolyte and fluid abnormalities may cause drowsiness, confusion, stupor, coma, and seizures. Transplant recipients are exposed to abnormal electrolyte concentrations for a variety of reasons. These may be due to their underlying disease or to large volume losses and replacements during transplantation. Furthermore, electrolyte concentrations may fluctuate in accordance with the function of the allograft and due to the effects of specific drugs (e.g. cyclosporin, amphotericin) on the kidney. Preoperative treatment of oedema or ascites in heart and liver allograft recipients is often associated with hyponatraemia. In renal allograft recipients the situation is even more complex. Both rejection as well as cyclosporin nephrotoxicity can result in a rapid deterioration of allograft function and multiple electrolyte abnormalities. Other electrolyte changes associated with neurological dysfunction include hyperchloraemia (Zazgornik *et al.* 1988) and hypophosphataemia (Tyden *et al.* 1988).

Low serum magnesium concentrations were initially reported to predispose to central nervous system side effects, especially cyclosporin-induced seizure activity (Thompson *et al.* 1984). However, more recent investigations have shown, that cyclosporin has a direct effect on the proximal renal tubule and markedly decreases magnesium re-absorption. Thus, a low magnesium level probably is not a separate risk factor for the development of CNS symptoms but rather a concomitant, renal side effect of the use of cyclosporin. Furthermore, several authors have observed cyclosporin-induced CNS symptoms in the absence of decreased magnesium levels (Allen *et al.* 1985; de Groen *et al.* 1987).

Low sodium levels are frequently seen in transplant candidates with endstage heart or liver disease. The administration of diuretics further exacerbates the problem. Large volume losses and replacements during and after surgery may cause rapid changes in serum and cerebral sodium concentrations. These changes may result in functional abnormalities, including encephalopathy and seizure activity, which regress with stabilization of sodium levels. However, structural lesions may occur in some patients, resulting in central pontine and extrapontine myelinolysis (Estol *et al.* 1989*a,b*; Wszolek *et al.* 1989). Severe hyponatraemia has also been observed after combined pancreatic and renal transplantation (Rabb *et al.* 1989).

Hypertensive encephalopathy

Hypertension may develop following transplantation. Several factors contribute to this occurrence including enhanced cardiac function after heart transplantation, improved maintenance of intravascular volume after liver and kidney transplantation, and the administration of corticosteroids and cyclosporin. True hypertensive encephalopathy can develop as a result of renal artery stenosis after renal transplantation (McGonigle *et al.* 1984). In one study (McEnery *et al.* 1989), hypertension was the most important aetiological factor explaining seizures in children following kidney transplants.

Several reports have suggested that hypertension associated with cyclosporin may predispose to seizure activity (Joss *et al.* 1982; Vellodi *et al.* 1987). However, many authors did not observe hypertension at the time of neurotoxic symptoms (Atkinson *et al.* 1984; Powell-Jackson *et al.* 1984; Lavenstein *et al.* 1988). Others have suggested that hypertension and neurotoxicity are concurrent side-effects of this drug (Noll and Kulkarni 1984; de Groen *et al.* 1987). The absence of arteriolar spasm or papilloedema and blood pressure readings lower than typically associated with hypertensive encephalopathy support the hypothesis of concomitant side-effects (Lopez Messa *et al.* 1986; de Groen *et al.* 1987). Therefore it is likely that many recipients demonstrate mild to moderate postoperative hypertension, but that hypertension rarely contributes directly to encephalopathy.

Cerebrovascular events

Cerebral haemorrhages and infarcts are seen at increased frequency in liver and bone marrow recipients (Wiznitzer *et al*. 1984; Patchell *et al*. 1985; Mawk *et al*. 1988; Rothfus *et al*. 1988; Ang *et al*. 1989). Low concentrations of coagulation factors, low lipoprotein levels causing hypoaggregability of platelets (Desai *et al*. 1989*a,b*; de Groen *et al*. 1989) and low total platelet counts probably contribute to this increased frequency. Occasionally isolated angiitis of the brain may present as depression and dementia (Rothenberg 1985).

Baulac *et al*. (1989) reported seizures in eight of 129 heart transplant recipients receiving cyclosporin therapy. Infectious or acute cerebrovascular causes were absent. Four of the patients were known to have ischaemic cerebrovascular disease prior to transplantation. Thus, the authors suggested that ischaemic brain damage due to cerebrovascular disease prior to transplantation may predispose heart transplant recipients to cyclosporin-induced seizures after transplantation.

Rejection encephalopathy

Gross *et al*. (1982) described episodes of encephalopathy in association with severe kidney allograft rejection. Symptoms and signs consisted of seizures, headache, confusion, disorientation, irritability, and papilloedema. Encephalopathy was related to the severity of the rejection episode and not to other features such as blood pressure, fever, corticosteroid administration, or electrolyte imbalance. Treatment of rejection and correction of blood pressure and electrolytes resulted in reversal of the encephalopathy. Prognosis was excellent with no long-term sequelae. However, the existence of 'rejection encephalopathy' or 'transplant encephalopathy' as a distinct entity is controversial (Gross *et al*. 1985). It remains unclear whether allograft rejection contributes directly to the development of central nervous system toxicity.

Central nervous system tumours

Long term use of immunosuppressant drugs, such as cyclosporin and azathioprine, is uncommonly associated with the growth of malignant lesions. The most commonly found malignant tumour is a B-cell lymphoma (Cockburn 1987; Penn 1987). More intensive immunosuppressive treatment and prior Epstein–Barr virus infection are two predisposing factors for the development of lymphoma (Ho *et al*. 1988; Nalesnik *et al*. 1988). Several patients have developed Epstein–Barr virus-induced central nervous system lymphoma (van Diemen-Steenvoorde *et al*. 1986). Fortunately, most polyclonal and some monoclonal lymphomas regress after withdrawal or dose reduction of the immunosuppressants (Peest *et al*. 1988; Wilkinson *et al*. 1989). These tumours may present with characteristics of abnormal mental functioning. In addition, neurologic symptoms due to recurrence of leukaemia is not uncommon (Wiznitzer *et al*. 1984). A history of central nervous system involvement prior to bone marrow transplant may predispose to this condition.

Vitamin E deficiency

Chronic fat malabsorption is a known feature of cholestatic liver diseases. Severe and prolonged malabsorption of the fat-soluble vitamin E may cause a syndrome of spinocerebellar degeneration (Harding *et al*. 1985). Symptoms consist of weakness, ataxia, proprioceptive loss, areflexia, opthalmoplegia, retinal pigmentation, and myopathy (Satya-Murti *et al*. 1986). Although no cases of vitamin E deficiency after liver transplantation have been described, transplant recipients with chronic cholestatic liver diseases probably are at increased risk for the development of this disorder (Sokol *et al*. 1985). At the Mayo Clinic, some patients with chronic cholestatic liver disease receive a vitamin E supplement before liver transplantation and all patients receive vitamin E after transplantation (de Groen, unpublished observations).

Graft versus host disease

Although the central nervous system may be a potential site for graft versus host disease, we are not aware of any reported cases (Patchell *et al*. 1985; Nelson and McQuillen 1988). In patients with neurologic abnormalities and graft versus host disease, electrolyte disturbances and infection are the most likely causes. However, myasthenia gravis may develop as a rare complication of graft versus host disease (Bolger *et al*. 1986; Nelson and McQuillen 1988).

Cerebral radiation

Total body or craniospinal irradiation is frequently employed in an attempt to eradicate residual leukaemia prior to bone marrow transplantation. Development of encephalopathy is a well recognized complication of cranial radiation, especially when radiation is combined with the use of neurotoxic drugs or with intrathecal cytotoxic therapy (Atkinson *et al*. 1977; Wiznitzer *et al*. 1984; Devinsky *et al*. 1987; Davis and Patchell 1988).

Uraemia and aluminium overload

It is well recognized that chronic renal failure as well as maintenance dialysis may predispose to cognitive impairment, possibly secondary to aluminium overload (Nissenson *et al*. 1977; Stewart and Stewart 1979). Nordal *et al*. (1985) suggested that in some patients, aluminium overload prior to transplantation may lead to subclinical encephalopathy, which predisposes these patients to cyclosporin-induced neurotoxicity after transplantation. Hawley *et al.* (1990) observed a syndrome characteristic of dialysis encephalopathy in three renal transplant recipients. All were receiving cyclosporin at the time of onset of neurological disease. In two of the three patients, evidence for increased body stores of aluminium was found. Lastly, a 31 year old renal transplant recipient with a history of poliomyelitis at age three and a known abnormal electro-encephalogram developed irreversible dementia following cyclosporin therapy (Bertoli *et al.* 1988). The author suggested that the pre-existence of an abnormal electroencephalogram together with clinical evidence of an alumin-ium overload may have enhanced the neurotoxic side-effects of cyclosporin, thereby creating an irreversible lesion. Waniek *et al.* (1977) found more psychometric abnormalities after kidney transplant in patients with a previous history of prolonged and complicated dialysis. However, Morales-Otero *et al.* (1988) found that in their group of transplant recipients, dialysis encephalo-pathy reversed gradually following the implantation of a well functioning graft.

Conclusions

Organic brain syndromes and other central nervous system complications are not uncommon in transplant candidates and recipients. The numerous factors which must be considered as potential aetiologic agents are reviewed in this chapter. The immunosuppressant cyclosporin has been associated with organic brain syndromes and other neurotoxic effects. This compound alone likely manifests a low to moderate propensity for neurotoxic effects, but their likelihood of occurrence appears to be increased substantially by the presence of other factors. Liver transplant recipients are at greatest risk for central nervous system complications. The reasons for this remain unclear, but may be due in part to an increased prevalence of multiple pre-existing vulnerabilities including changes associated with chronic liver disease, the blood–brain barrier, hypocholesterolaemia, hepatic encephalopathy, or in other currently unrecognized factors.

References

Ackerman, Z., Or, R., and Maayan, S. (1986). Cerebral toxoplasmosis complicating bone marrow transplantation. *Israel Journal of Medical Sciences*, 22, 582–6.

Adams, F. (1988). Emergency intravenous sedation of the delirious, medically ill patient. *Journal of Clinical Psychiatry*, 49, 22–7.

Adams, D. H., Ponsford, S., Gunson, B., Boon, A., Honigsberger, L., Williams, A., *et al.* (1987). Neurological complications following liver transplantation. *Lancet*, 1, 949–51.

Agamanolis, D. P., Tan, J. S., and Parker, D. L. (1979). Immunosuppressive measles encephalitis in a patient with a renal transplant. *Archives of Neurology*, 36, 686–90.

Aksamit, A. J., Okazaki, H., Proper, J., and de Groen, P. C. (1990). Cyclosporine-induced leukoencephalopathy and progressive multifocal leukoencephalopathy (PML) in a liver transplant recipient (abstract). *Neurology*, 40(suppl 1), 456.

Allen, R. D., Hunnisett, A. G., and Morris, P. J. (1985). Cyclosporin and magnesium (letter). *Lancet*, 1, 1283–4.

Ang, L. C., Gillett, J. M., and Kaufmann, J. C. (1989). Neuropathology of heart transplantation. *Canadian Journal of Neurological Sciences*, 16, 291–8.

Appleton, R. E., Farrell, K., Teal, P., Hashimoto, S. A., and Wong, P. K. H. (1989). Complex partial *status epilepticus* associated with cyclosporin A therapy. *Journal of Neurology, Neurosurgery and Psychiatry*, 52, 1068–71.

Atkinson, K., Clink, H., Lawler, S., Lawson, D. N., McElwain, T. J., Thomas, P., *et al.* (1977). Encephalopathy following bone marrow transplantation. *European Journal of Cancer*, 13, 623–5.

Atkinson, K., Biggs, J., Darveniza, P., Boland, J., Concannon, A., and Dodds, A. (1984). Cyclosporine-associated central nervous system toxicity after allogeneic bone marrow transplantation. *Transplantation*, 38, 34–7.

Baulac, M., Smadja, D., Cabrol, A., Cabrol, C., and Laplane, D. (1989). Cyclosporin and convulsions after cardiac transplantation. *Revue Neurologique*, 145, 393–7.

Beaman, M., Parvin, S., Veitch, P. S., and Walls, J. (1985). Convulsions associated with cyclosporin A in renal transplant recipients. *British Medical Journal*, 290, 139–40.

Berden, J. H., Hoitsma, A. J., Merx, J. L., and Keyser, A. (1985). Severe central-nervous-system toxicity associated with cyclosporin (letter). *Lancet*, 1, 219–20.

Bertoli, M., Romagnoli, G. F., and Margreiter, R. (1988). Irreversible dementia following cyclosporin therapy in a renal transplant patient. *Nephron*, 49, 333–4.

Bhatt, B. D., Meriano, F. V., and Buchwald, D. (1988). Cyclosporine-associated central nervous system toxicity. *New England Journal of Medicine*, 318, 788–9.

Blexrud, M. D., Windebank, A. J., and de Groen, P. C. (1990). Potential neurotoxicity of the solvent vehicle in which intravenous cyclosporin is formulated (abstract). *Neurology*, 40(suppl 1), 344.

Bleyer, W. A. (1981). Neurologic sequelae of methotrexate and ionizing radiation: a new classification. *Cancer Treatment Report*, 65, 89–98.

Bolger, G. B., Sullivan, K. M., Spence, A. M., Appelbaum, F. R., Johnston, R., Sanders, J. E., *et al.* (1986). Myasthenia gravis after allogeneic bone marrow transplantation: relationship to chronic graft-versus-host disease. *Neurology*, 36, 1087–91.

Boogaerts, M. A., Zachee, P., and Verwilghen, R. L. (1982). Cyclosporin, methyl-prednisolone, and convulsions (letter). *Lancet*, 2, 1216–17.

Boon, A. P., Adams, D. H., Buckels, J., and McMaster, P. (1990). Cerebral aspergillosis in liver transplantation. *Journal of Clinical Pathology*, 43, 114–18.

de Bruijn, K. M., Klompmaker, I. J., Slooff, M. J. H., Fockens, P., and Hillen, P. H. (1989). Cyclosporine neurotoxicity late after liver transplantation (letter). *Transplantation*, 47, 575–6.

Capocaccia, L., Fischer, J. E., and Rossi-Fanelli, F. (1984). Assessment and evaluation of hepatic encephalopathy. In *Hepatic encephalopathy and chronic liver failure* (eds L. Capocaccia, J. E. Fischer, and F. Rossi-Fanelli), pp. 239–44 (Plenum, New York).

Catalan, J. (1988). Psychosocial and neuropsychiatric aspects of HIV infection: review of their extent and implications for psychiatry. *Journal of Psychosomatic Research*, 32, 237–48.

Cockburn, I. (1987). Assessment of the risks of malignancy and lymphomas developing in patients using Sandimmune. *Transplantation Proceedings*, 19, 1804–7.

Cooper, D. K. C., Novitzky, D., Davis, L., Huff, J. E., Parker, D., Schlesinger, R., *et al.* (1989). Does central nervous system toxicity occur in transplant patients with hypocholesterolemia receiving cyclosporine? *Journal of Heart Transplantation*, 8, 221–4.

Cordonnier, C., Feuilhade, F., Vernant, J. P., Marsault, C., Rodet, M., and Rochant, H. (1983). Cytomegalovirus encephalitis occurring after bone marrow transplantation. *Scandinavian Journal of Haematology*, 31, 248–52.

Craven, J. L. (1989). Methylphenidate for cyclosporine-associated organic mood disorder (letter). *American Journal of Psychiatry*, 146, 553.

Craven, J. L. (1991). Cyclosporine-associated organic mental disorders in liver transplant recipients. *Psychosomatics*, 32, 94–102.

Craven, J. and the Toronto Lung Transplant Group. (1990*a*). Postoperative organic mental syndromes in lung transplant recipients. *Journal of Heart Transplantation*, 9, 129–32.

Craven, J. and the Toronto Lung Transplant Group (1990*b*). Psychiatric aspects of lung transplant. *Canadian Journal of Psychiatry*, 35, 759–64.

Craven, J. L., Bright, J., and Lougheed Dear, C. L. (1990). Psychiatric, psychosocial and rehabilitative aspects of lung transplantation. *Clinics in Chest Medicine*, 11, 247–57.

Craven, J., Sheinin, L., and the Toronto Liver Transplant Group (1990*c*). Cyclosporine-associated organic mental disorders in liver transplant recipients. Paper presented at The First Working Conference on the Psychiatric, Psychosocial and Ethical Aspects of Organ Transplantation, June 8–9, Toronto, Canada.

Van Cutsem, E., Boogaerts, M. A., Tricot, G., and Verwilghen, R. L. (1986). Multiple brain abscesses caused by *Torulopsis glabrata* in an immunocompromised patient. *Mykosen*, 29, 306–8.

el Dahr, S., Chevalier, R. L., Gomez, R. A., and Campbell, F. G. (1987). Seizures and blindness following intravenous pulse methylprednisolone in a renal transplant patient. *International Journal of Pediatric Nephrology*, 8, 87–90.

Davenport, A., Will, E. J., Davison, A. M., and Ironside, J. W. (1988). Toxicity of cyclosporine metabolites. *Lancet*, 2, 333.

Davis, D. G. and Patchell, R. (1988). Neurological complications of bone marrow transplantation. *Neurologic Clinics*, 6, 377–87.

Davis, D., Henslee, P. J., and Markesbery, W. R. (1988). Fatal adenovirus meningoencephalitis in a bone marrow transplant patient. *Annals of Neurology*, 23, 385–9.

Davis, C. L., Springmeyer, S., and Gmerek, B. J. (1990). Central nervous system side effects of gancyclovir (letter). *New England Journal of Medicine*, 322, 933–4.

Deierhoi, M. H., Kalayoglu, M., Sollinger, H. W., and Belzer, F. O. (1988). Cyclosporine neurotoxicity in liver transplant recipients: report of three cases. *Transplantation Proceedings*, 20, 116–18.

Derbes, S. J. (1984). Trimethoprim-induced aseptic meningitis. *Journal of the American Medical Association*, 252, 2865–6.

Desai, K., Bruckdorfer, R., Hutton, R. A., and Owen, J. S. (1989*a*). Binding of apoE-rich high density lipoprotein particles by saturable sites on human blood platelets inhibits agonist-induced platelet aggregation. *Journal of Lipid Research*, 30, 831–40.

Desai, K., Mistry, P., Bagget, C., Burroughs, A. K., Bellamy, M. F., and Owen, J S.

(1989*b*). Inhibition of platelet aggregation by abnormal high density lipoprotein particles in plasma from patients with hepatic cirrhosis. *Lancet*, 1, 693–5.

Devinsky, O., Lemann, W., Evans, A. C., Moeller, J. R., and Rottenberg, D. A. (1987). Akinetic mutism in a bone marrow transplant recipient following total-body irradiation and amphotericin B chemoprophylaxis. A positron emission tomographic and neuropathologic study. *Archives of Neurology*, 44, 414–17.

van Diemen-Steenvoorde, R., Donckerwolcke, R. A., Kluin, P. M., Kapsenberg, J. G., Lepoutre, J. M., Fleer, A., *et al*. (1986). Epstein–Barr virus related central nervous system lymphoma in a child after renal transplantation. *International Journal of Pediatric Nephrology*, 7, 55–8.

Donaghy, M., Gray, J. A., Squier, W., Kurtz, J. B., Higgins, R. M., Richardson, A. J., *et al*. (1989). Recurrent Guillain–Barre syndrome after multiple exposures to cytomegalovirus. *American Journal of Medicine*, 87, 339–41.

Dummer, J. S., Erb, S., Breinig, M. K., Ho, M., Rinaldo, C. R. Jr., Gupta, P., *et al*. (1989). Infection with human immunodeficiency virus in the Pittsburgh transplant population: A study of 583 donors and 1043 recipients, 1981–1986. *Transplantation*, 47, 134–9.

Durrant, S., Chipping, P. M., Palmer, S., and Gordon-Smith, E. C. (1982). Cyclosporin A, methylprednisolone, and convulsions (letter). *Lancet*, 2, 829–30.

Duston, M., McHenry, M. C., Braun, W. F., Fieker, D. H., Gavan, T. L., and Novick, A. C. (1981). Cryptococcal meningitis causing fever of unknown origin in renal transplant recipients: report of two cases initially diagnosed by urine cultures. *Transplantation*, 32, 334–6.

van den Elshout, F. J., Huysmans, F. T., Muytjens, H. L., and Koene, R. A. (1987). *Cryptococcus neoformans* meningitis following renal transplantation. *Netherlands Journal of Medicine*, 31, 183–90.

Embrey, J. R., Silva, F. G., Helderman, J. H., Peters, P. C., and Sagalowsky, A. I. (1988). Long-term survival and late development of bladder cancer in renal transplant patient with progressive multifocal leukoencephalopathy. *Journal of Urology*, 139, 580–1.

Emmons, C., Smith, J., and Flanigan, M. (1986). Cerebrospinal fluid inflammation during OKT_3 therapy (letter). *Lancet*, 2, 510–11.

Estol, C. J., Faris, A. A., Martinez, A. J., and Ahdab-Barmada, M. (1989*a*). Central pontine myelinolysis after liver transplantation. *Neurology*, 39, 493–8.

Estol, C. J., Lopez, O., Brenner, R. P., and Martinez, A. J. (1989*b*). Seizures after liver transplantation: a clinicopathologic study. *Neurology*, 39, 1297–301.

Famiglio, L., Racusen, L., Fivush, B., Solez, K., and Fisher, R. (1989). Central nervous system toxicity of cyclosporine in a rat model. *Transplantation*, 48, 316–21.

Fischer, G., Wittmann-Liebold, B., Lang, K., Kiefhaber, T., and Schmid, F. X. (1989). Cyclophilin and peptidyl-prolyl *cis-trans* isomerase are probably identical proteins. *Nature*, 337, 476–8.

Fricchione, G. L. (1989). Psychiatric aspects of renal transplantation. *Australian and New Zealand Journal of Psychiatry*, 23, 407–17.

de Fronzo, R. A., Braine, H., Colvin, O. M., and Davis, P. J. (1973). Water intoxication in man after cyclophosphamide therapy: Time course and relation to drug activation. *Annals of Internal Medicine*, 78, 861–9.

Gharpure, V. S., Hutchinson, R. M., and Durrant, S. T. S. (1990). Migraine after bone-marrow transplantation (letter). *Lancet*, 335, 57.

Gordillo-Paniagua, G., Munoz-Arizpe, R., and Ponsa-Molina, R. (1987). Unusual complication in a patient with renal transplantation: cerebral cysticercosis. *Nephron*, 45, 65–7.

de Groen, P. C. (1988). Cyclosporine, low density lipoprotein and cholesterol. *Mayo Clinic Proceedings*, 63, 1012–21.

de Groen, P. C., Aksamit, A. J., Rakela, J., Forbes, G. S., and Krom, R. A. F. (1987). Central nervous system toxicity after liver transplantation: the role of cyclosporine and cholesterol. *New England Journal of Medicine*, 317, 861–6.

de Groen, P. C., Aksamit, A. J., Rakela, J., and Krom, R. A. F. (1988). Cyclosporine associated central nervous system toxicity (letter). *New England Journal of Medicine*, 318, 789.

de Groen, P. C., Aksamit, A. J., Westmoreland, B. F., Kottke, B. A., and Krom, R. A. F. (1989). Serum cholesterol levels and stroke mortality (letter). *New England Journal of Medicine*, 321, 1340–1.

de Groen, P. C., Janssen, H. L. A., Jardine, I., and Steffen, R. (1990). Cyclosporine neurotoxicity and blood brain barrier function (abstract). *Hepatology*, 12, 991.

Gross, M. L. P., Sweny, P., Pearson, R. M., Kennedy, J., Fernando, O. N., and Moorhead, J. F. (1982). Rejection encephalopathy. An acute neurological syndrome complicating renal transplantation. *Journal of Neurological Sciences*, 56, 23–34.

Gross, M. L. P., Pearson, R. M., Sweny, P., and Moorhead, J. F. (1985). Convulsions associated with cyclosporin A in renal transplant recipients (letter). *British Medical Journal*, 290, 555.

Grossman, L., Baker, M. A., Sutton, D. M. C., and Deck, J. H. (1983). Central nervous system toxicity of high-dose cytosine arabinoside. *Medical & Pediatric Oncology*, 11, 246–50.

Gullberg, R. M., Quintanilla, A., Levin, M. L., Williams, J., and Phair, J. P. (1987). Sporotrichosis: recurrent cutaneous, articular, and central nervous system infection in a renal transplant recipient. *Review of Infectious Diseases*, 9, 369–75.

Haas, E. J. (1984). Trimethoprim-sulfamethoxazole: another cause of recurrent meningitis (letter). *Journal of the American Medical Association*, 252, 346.

Handschumacher, R. E., Harding, M. W., Rice, J., Drugge, R. J., and Speicher, D. W. (1984). Cyclophilin: a specific cytosolic binding protein for cyclosporin A. *Science*, 226, 544–7.

Harding, A. E., Matthews, S., Jones, S., Ellis, C. J. K., Booth, I. W., and Muller, D. P. R. (1985). Spinocerebellar degeneration associated with a selective defect of vitamin E absorption. *New England Journal of Medicine*, 313, 32–5.

Hartmann, D. W., Robinson, W. A., Morton, N. J., Mangalik, A., and Glode, L. M. (1981). High-dose nitrogen mustard (HN_2) with autologous nonfrozen bone marrow transplantation in advanced malignant melanoma. A phase I trial. *Blut*, 42, 209–20.

Hawley, C. M., Rigby, R. J., Boyle, R. S., and Petrie, J. J. (1990). Onset of dialysis encephalopathy in cyclosporine-treated renal allograft recipients. *American Journal of Kidney Diseases*, 15, 364–8.

Ho, M., Jaffe, R., Miller, G., Breinig, M. K., Dummer, J. S., Makowka, L., *et al.* (1988). The frequency of Epstein–Barr virus infection and associated lymphoproliferative syndrome after transplantation and its manifestations in children. *Transplantation*, 45, 719–27.

Hoefnagels, W. A. J., Gerritsen, E. J., Brouwer, O. F., and Souverijn, J. H. (1988). Cyclosporin encephalopathy associated with fat embolism induced by the drug's solvent (letter). *Lancet*, 2, 901.

Holland, J. C. and Tross, S. (1985). The psychosocial and neuropsychiatric sequelae of the acquired immunodeficiency syndrome and related disorders. *Annals of Internal Medicine*, 103, 760–4.

Hows, J. M., Palmer, S., and Gordon-Smith, E. C. (1982). Use of cyclosporine A in allogeneic bone marrow transplantation for severe aplastic anemia. *Transplantation*, 33, 382–6.

Hughes, R. L. (1990). Cyclosporine-related central nervous system toxicity in cardiac transplantation (letter). *New England Journal of Medicine*, 323, 420–1.

Joffe, A. M., Farley, J. D., Linden, D., and Goldsand, G. (1989). Trimethoprim-sulfamethoxazole-associated aseptic meningitis: case reports and review of the literature. *American Journal of Medicine*, 87, 332–8.

Johnson, N. T., Crawford, S. W., and Sargur, M. (1987). Acute acquired de-myelinating polyneuropathy with respiratory failure following high-dose systemic cytosine arabinoside and marrow transplantation. *Bone Marrow Transplantation*, 2, 203–7.

Joss, D. V., Barrett, A. J., Kendra, J. R., Lucas, C. F., and Desai, S. (1982). Hypertension and convulsions in children receiving cyclosporin A (letter). *Lancet*, 1, 906.

Kahan, B. D. (1989). Drug Therapy. Cyclosporine. *New England Journal of Medicine*, 321, 1725–38.

Karalakulasingam, R., Arora, K. K., Adams, G., Serratoni, F., and Martin, D. G. (1976). Meningoencephalitis caused by *Histoplasma capsulatum*: occurrence in a renal transplant recipient and a review of the literature. *Archives of Internal Medicine*, 136, 217–20.

Kast, R. (1989). Blocking of cyclosporine immunosuppression by neuroleptics. *Transplantation*, 47, 1095–6.

Katirji, M. B. (1987). Visual hallucinations and cyclosporine. *Transplantation*, 43, 768–9.

Kormos, R. L., Armitage, J. M., Dummer, J. S., Miyamoto, Y., Griffith, B. P., and Hardesty, R. L. (1990). Optimal perioperative immunosuppression in cardiac transplantation using rabbit antithymocyte globulin. *Transplantation*, 49, 306–11.

Kremer, I., Ritz, R., and Brunner, F. (1983). Aseptic meningitis as an adverse effect of co-trimoxazole (letter). *New England Journal of Medicine*, 308, 1481.

Krupp, P., Busch, M., Cockburn, I., and Schreiber, B. (1989). Encephalopathy associated with fat embolism induced by solvent for cyclosporin (letter). *Lancet*, 1, 168–9.

Kunzendorf, U., Brockmoller, J., Jochimsen, F., Keller, F., Walz, G., and Offermann, G. (1988). Cyclosporin metabolites and central-nervous-system toxicity (letter). *Lancet*, 1, 1223.

Kunzendorf, U., Brockmoller, J., Jochimsen, F., Roots, I., and Offermann, G. (1989). Neurotoxicity caused by a high cyclosporine metabolite level. *Transplantation*, 48, 531–2.

Labar, B., Bogdanic, V., Plavsic, F., Francetic, E., Dobric, I., Kastelan, A., *et al.* (1986). Cyclosporin neurotoxicity in patients treated with allogeneic bone marrow transplantation. *Biomedicine & Pharmacotherapy*, 40, 148–50.

Lane, R. J., Roche, S. W., Leung, A. A., Greco, A., and Lange, L. S. (1988). Cyclosporin neurotoxicity in cardiac transplant recipients. *Journal of Neurology, Neurosurgery & Psychiatry*, 51, 1434–7.

Lavenstein, B., Stewart, C., and Tina, L. U. (1988). Cyclosporine-associated encephalopathy in childhood transplant patients. *Transplantation Proceedings*, 20(suppl 3), 285–7.

Legg, B. and Rowland, M. (1987). Cyclosporin: measurement of fraction unbound in plasma. *Journal of Pharmacy and Pharmacology*, 39, 599–603.

Lindholm, A. and Henricsson, S. (1989). Intra- and interindividual variability in the free fraction of cyclosporine in plasma in recipients of renal transplants. *Therapeutic Drug Monitoring*, 11, 623–30.

Ling, M. H. M., Perry, P., and Tsuang, M. T. (1981). Side effects of corticosteroid therapy: psychiatric aspects. *Archives of General Psychiatry*, 38, 471–7.

Lopez Messa, J. B., Gonzalez Gomez, N., Alonso Alonso, R., Arranz Saez, R., Sanchez Garcia, M., Montalvo, M., *et al.* (1986). Convulsions and arterial hypertension in three bone marrow transplant patients and cyclosporine A treatment. *Revista Clinica Espanola*, 178, 186–8.

Lucey, M. R., Kolars, J. C., Merion, R. M., Campbell, D. A., Aldrich, M., and Watkins, P. B. (1990). Cyclosporin toxicity at therapeutic blood levels and cytochrome P-450 IIIA. *Lancet*, 335, 11–15.

McEnery, P. T., Nathan, J., Bates, S. R., and Daniels, S. R. (1989). Convulsions in children undergoing renal transplantation. *Journal of Pediatrics*, 115, 532–6.

McGonigle, R. J., Bewick, M., Trafford, J. A., and Parsons, V. (1984). Hypertensive encephalopathy complicating transplant renal artery stenosis. *Postgraduate Medical Journal*, 60, 356–8.

Mai, F., Mckenzie, N., and Kostuk, W. (1986). Psychiatric aspects of cardiac transplantation: preoperative evaluation and postoperative sequelae. *British Medical Journal*, 292, 311–13.

Mawk, J. R., Shaw, B. W., Wood, R. P., and Williams, L. (1988). Neurosurgical complications of paediatric orthotopic liver transplantation. *Childs Nervous System*, 4, 26–9.

MMWR (1986). Aseptic meningitis among kidney transplant recipients receiving a newly marketed murine monoclonal antibody preparation. *Journal of the American Medical Association*, 256, 1873.

Morales-Otero, L. A., Gonzalez, Z. A., and Santiago-Delpin, E. A. (1988). Neurological complications after kidney transplantation. *Transplantation Proceedings*, 20, 443–5.

Morduchowicz, G., Shmueli, D., Shapira, Z., Cohen, S. L., Yussim, A., Block, C. S., *et al.* (1986). Rhinocerebral mucormycosis in renal transplant recipients: report of three cases and review of the literature. *Review of Infectious Diseases*, 8, 441–6.

Morgenstern, G. R. (1980). Cyclosporine A for the prevention of graft-versus-host disease following allogeneic bone marrow transplantation in man. *Blut*, 41, 177–9.

Nalesnik, M. A., Jaffe, R., Starzl, T. E., Demetris, A. J., Porter, K., Burnham, J. A., *et al.* (1988). The pathology of posttransplant lymphoproliferative disorders occurring in the setting of cyclosporine A-prednisone immunosuppression. *American Journal of Pathology*, 133, 173–92.

Nelson, K. R. and McQuillen, M. P. (1988). Neurologic complications of graft-versus-host disease. *Neurologic Clinics*, 6, 389–403.

Niklasson, P. M., Hambraeus, A., Lundgren, G., Magnusson, G., Sundelin, P., and Groth, C. G. (1978). Listeria encephalitis in five renal transplant recipients. *Acta Medica Scandinavica*, 203, 181–5.

Nissenson, A. R., Levin, M. L., Klawans, H. L., and Nausieda, P.L. (1977). Neurological sequelae of end stage renal disease (ESRD). *Journal of Chronic Diseases*, 30, 705–33.

Noll, R. B. and Kulkarni, R. (1984). Complex visual hallucinations and cyclosporine. *Archives of Neurology*, 41, 329–30.

Nordal, K. P., Talseth, T., Dahl, E., Attramadal, A., Albrechtsen, D., Halse, J., *et al.* (1985). Aluminium overload, a predisposing condition for epileptic seizures in renal-transplant patients treated with cyclosporine? (letter) *Lancet*, 2, 153–4.

Opolon, P. (1984). Significance of middle molecules in the pathogenesis of hepatic encephalopathy. In *Advances in hepatic encephalopathy and urea cycle disease* (eds G. Kleinberger, B. Ferenci, P. Riederer, and H. Thaler), pp. 310–14 (Karger, Basel).

Patchell, R. A., White, C. L. III, Clark, A. W., Beschorner, W. E., and Santos, G. W. (1985). Neurologic complications of bone marrow transplantation. *Neurology*, 35, 300–6.

Peest, D., Schaper, B., Nashan, B., Wonigeit, K., Raude, E., Pichlmayr, R., *et al.* (1988). High incidence of monoclonal immunoglobulins in patients after liver or heart transplantation. *Transplantation*, 46, 389–93.

Penn, I. (1987). Cancers following cyclosporine therapy. *Transplantation Proceedings*, 19, 2211–13.

Petcher, T. J., Weber, H. P., and Ruegger, A. (1976). Crystal and molecular structure of an iododerivative of the cyclic undecapeptide cyclosporin A. *Helvetica Chimica Acta*, 59, 1480–9.

Peterson, L. R. and Ferguson, R. M. (1984). Fatal central nervous system infection with varicella-zoster virus in renal transplant recipients. *Transplantation*, 37, 366–8.

Peterson, J. W., Nishizawa, S., Hackett, J. D., Bun, T., Teramura, A., and Zervas, N. T. (1990). Cyclosporine A reduces cerebral vasospasm after subarachnoid hemorrhage in dogs. *Stroke*, 21, 133–7.

Powell-Jackson, P. R., Carmichael, F. J. L., Calne, R.Y., and Williams, R. (1984). Adult respiratory distress syndrome and convulsions associated with administration of cyclosporine in liver transplant recipients. *Transplantation*, 38, 341–3.

Powles, R. L., Clink, H. M., Spence, D., Morgenstern, G., Watson, J. G., Selby, P. J., *et al.* (1980). Cyclosporine A to prevent graft-versus-host disease in man after allogeneic bone marrow transplantation. *Lancet*, 1, 327–9.

Rabb, H. A., Niles, J. L., Cosimi, A. B., and Tolkoff-Rubin, N. E. (1989). Severe hyponatremia associated with combined pancreatic and renal transplantation. *Transplantation*, 48, 157–9.

Raby, N., Forbes, G., and Williams, R. (1990). Nocardia infection in patients with liver transplants or chronic liver disease: radiologic findings. *Radiology*, 174, 713–16.

Racusen, L. C., McCrindle, B. W., Christenson, M., Fivush, B., and Fisher, R. S. (1990). Cyclosporine lowers seizure threshold in an experimental model of electroshock-induced seizures in Munich–Wistar rats. *Life Sciences*, 46, 1021–6.

Randhawa, P. S., Markin, R. S., Starzl, T. E., and Demetris, A. J. (1990). Epstein–Barr virus-associated syndromes in immunosuppressed liver transplant recipients.

Clinical profile and recognition on routine allograft biopsy. *American Journal of Surgical Pathology*, 14, 538–47.

Reznik, M., Halleux, J., Urbain, E., Mouchette, R., Castermans, P., and Beaujean, M. (1981). Two cases of progressive multifocal leukoencephalopathy after renal transplantation. *Acta Neuropathologica—Supplement* (Berlin), 7, 189–91.

Richards, J. M., Vogelzang, N. J., and Bluestone, J. A. (1990). Neurotoxicity after treatment with muromonab-CD3 (letter). *New England Journal of Medicine*, 323, 487–8.

Rothenberg, R. J. (1985). Isolated angiitis of the brain. Case in a renal transplant recipient. *American Journal of Medicine*, 79, 629–32.

Rothfus, W. E., Hirsch, W. L., Latchaw, R. E., and Starzl, T. E. (1988). Neuroradiologic aspects of pediatric orthotopic liver transplantation. *American Journal of Neuroradiology*, 9, 303–6.

Rubin, A. M. and Kang, H. (1987). Cerebral blindness and encephalopathy with cyclosporin A toxicity. *Neurology*, 37, 1072–6.

Satya-Murti, S., Howard, L. K., Krohel, G., and Wolf, B. (1986). The spectrum of neurologic disorder from vitamin E deficiency. *Neurology*, 36, 917–21.

Saxton, C. R., Gailiunas, P. Jr., Helderman, J. H., Farkas, R. A., McCoy, R., Diehl, J., *et al.* (1984). Progressive multifocal leukoencephalopathy in a renal transplant recipient. Increased diagnostic sensitivity of computed tomographic scanning by double-dose contrast with delayed films. *American Journal of Medicine*, 77, 333–7.

Scheinman, S. J., Reinitz, E. R., Petro, G., Schwartz, R. A., and Szmalc, F. (1990). Cyclosporine central neurotoxicity following renal transplantation: Report of a case using magnetic resonance images. *Transplantation*, 49, 215–16.

Schober, R. and Herman, M. M. (1973). Neuropathology of cardiac transplantation. Survey of 31 cases. *Lancet*, 1, 962–7.

Settle, E. C. and Ayd, F. J. (1983). Haloperidol: a quarter century of experience. *Journal of Clinical Psychiatry*, 44, 440–8.

Shah, D., Rylance, P. B., Rogerson, M. E., Bewick, M., and Parsons, V. (1984). Generalized epileptic fits in renal transplant recipients given cyclosporin A. *British Medical Journal*, 289, 1347–8.

Sloane, J. P., Lwin, K. Y., Gore, M. E., Powles, R. L., and Smith, J. F. (1985). Disturbance of blood-brain barrier after bone-marrow transplantation (letter). *Lancet*, 2, 280–1.

Sokol, R. J., Guggenheim, M. A., Iannaccone, S. T., Barkhaus, P. E., Miller, C., Silverman, A., *et al.* (1985). Improved neurologic function after long-term correction of vitamin E deficiency in children with chronic cholestasis. *New England Journal of Medicine*, 313, 1580–6.

Starzl, T. E., Fung, J., Jordan, M., Shapiro, R., Tzakis, A., McCauley, J., *et al.* (1990). Kidney-transplantation under FK-506. *Journal of the American Medical Association*, 264, 63–7.

Stewart, R. S. and Stewart, R. M. (1979). Neuropsychiatric aspects of chronic renal disease. *Psychosomatics*, 20, 524–31.

Sullivan, K. M., Storb, R., Shulman, H. M., Shaw, C. M., Spence, A., Beckham, C., *et al.* (1982). Immediate and delayed neurotoxicity after mechlorethamine preparation for bone marrow transplantation. *Annals of Internal Medicine*, 97, 182–9.

Surman, O. S. (1989). Psychiatric aspects of organ transplantation. *American Journal of Psychiatry*, 146, 972–82.

Surman, O. S., Dienstag, J. L., Cosimi, A. B., Chauncey, S., and Russell, P. S. (1987). Liver transplantation: psychiatric considerations. *Psychosomatics*, 28, 615–21.

Takahashi, N., Hayano, T., and Suzuki, M. (1989). Peptidyl-prolyl *cis-trans* isomerase is the cyclosporin A-binding protein cyclophilin. *Nature*, 337, 473–5.

Tarter, R. E., Van Thiel, D. H., Hegedus, A. M., Schade, R. R., Gavaler, J. S., and Starzl, T. E. (1984). Neuropsychiatric status after liver transplantation. *Journal of Laboratory and Clinical Medicine*, 103, 776–82.

Tesar, G. E., Murray, G. B., and Cassem, N. H. (1985). Use of high-dose intravenous haloperidol in the treatment of agitated cardiac patients. *Journal of Clinical Psychopharmacology*, 5, 344–7.

van Thiel, D. H., Iqbal, M., Jain, A., Fung, J., Todo, S., and Starzl, T. E. (1990). Gastrointestinal and metabolic problems associated with immunosuppression with either CyA or FK 506 in liver transplantation. *Transplantation Proceedings*, 22, 37–40.

Thistlethwaite, J. R. Jr., Stuart, J. K., Mayes, J. T., Gaber, A. O., Woodle, S., Buckingham, M. R., *et al.* (1988). Complications and monitoring of OKT₃ therapy. *American Journal of Kidney Diseases*, 11, 112–19.

Thompson, C. B., June, C. H., Sullivan, K. M., and Thoman, E. D. (1984). Association between cyclosporin neurotoxicity and hypomagnesemia. *Lancet*, 2, 1116–20.

Tilney, N. L., Kohler, T. R., and Strom, T. B. (1982). Cerebromeningitis in immunosuppressed recipients of renal allografts. *Annals of Surgery*, 195, 104–9.

Tollemar, J., Ringden, O., Ericzon, B. G., and Tyden, G. (1988). Cyclosporine associated central nervous system toxicity. *New England Journal of Medicine*, 318, 788–9.

Trzepacz, P. T., Brenner, R. P., Coffman, G., and Van Thiel, D. H. (1988). Delirium in liver transplantation candidates: discriminant analysis of multiple test variables. *Biological Psychiatry*, 24, 3–14.

Tsanaclis, A. M. and de Morais, C. F. (1986). Cerebral toxoplasmosis after renal transplantation. A case report. *Pathology, Research and Practice*, 181, 339–43.

Tunkel, A. R. and Starr, K. (1990). Trimethoprim-sulfamethoxazole-associated aseptic meningitis (comment). *American Journal of Medicine*, 88, 696–7.

Tyden, G., Fehrman, I., Siden, A., and Persson, A. (1988). Hypophosphataemia and reversible neurological dysfunction in a patient subject to combined renal and pancreatic transplantation. *Nephrology, Dialysis and Transplantation*, 3, 823–5.

Urase, F., Shimotsuma, H., Hmazaki, H., Ashida, T., Satoh, M., Sueyoshi, A., *et al.* (1987). Two cases of allogeneic bone marrow transplantation with psycho-neurological symptoms possibly due to hypomagnesemia caused by cyclosporin A. *Rinsho Ketsueki*, 28, 2198–203.

Vazquez, L., Ellis, A., Saint Genez, D., Patino, J., and Nogues, M. (1988). Epidural lipomatosis after renal transplantation—complete recovery without surgery. *Transplantation*, 46, 773–4.

Vellodi, A., Jayatunga, R., and Hugh-Jones, K. (1987). Hemiplegia and focal convulsions as a manifestation of cyclosporine A toxicity. *Journal of Clinical Pharmacology*, 27, 914–15.

Vogt, D. P., Lederman, R. J., Carey, W. D., and Broughan, T. A. (1988). Neurologic complications of liver transplantation. *Transplantation*, 45, 1057–61.

Wade, J. C. and Meyers, J. D. (1983). Neurologic symptoms associated with parenteral acyclovir treatment after marrow transplantation. *Annals of Internal Medicine*, 98, 921–5.

Wamboldt, F. W., Weiler, S.J., and Kalin, N. H. (1984). Cyclosporin-associated mania (letter). *Biological Psychiatry*, 19, 1161–2.

Waniek, W., Pach, J., Hartmann, H. G., and Beersiek, F. (1977). Disorders of the cerebral function in patients in a dialysis-transplantation program. *Schweizerische Medizinische Wochenschrift (Journal Suisse De Medicine)*, 107, 832–40.

Wilczek, H., Ringden, O., and Tyden, G. (1985). Cyclosporine-associated central nervous system toxicity after renal transplantation. *Transplantation*, 39, 110.

Wilkinson, A. H., Smith, J. L., Hunsicker, L. G., Tobacman, J., Kapelanski, D. P., Johnson, M., *et al.* (1989). Increased frequency of posttransplant lymphomas in patients treated with cyclosporine, azathioprine, and prednisone. *Transplantation*, 47, 293–6.

Williams, L. C. and Doak, P. B. (1977). Fits in association with methylprednisolone treatment of transplant rejection (abstract). *Australian and New Zealand Journal of Medicine*, 7, 218.

Wilson, S. E., de Groen, P. C., Aksamit, A. J., Wiesner, R. H., Garrity, J. A., and Krom, R. A. F. (1988). Cyclosporin A-induced reversible cortical blindness. *Journal of Clinical Neuro-Ophthalmology*, 8, 215–20.

Wiznitzer, M., Packer, R. J., August, C. S., and Burkey, E. D. (1984). Neurological complications of bone marrow transplantation in childhood. *Annals of Neurology*, 16, 569–76.

Wszolek, Z. K., McComb, R. D., Pfeiffer, R. F., Steg, R. E., Wood, R. P., Shaw, B. W. Jr., *et al.* (1989). Pontine and extrapontine myelinolysis following liver transplantation. Relationship to serum sodium. *Transplantation*, 48, 1006–12.

Zaal, M. J. W., de Vries, J., and Boen-Tan, Y. T. N. (1988). Is cyclosporin toxic to endothelial cells? (letter) *Lancet*, 2, 956–7.

Zampella, E. J., Duvall, E. R., Sekar, B. C., Langford, K. H., Epstein, A. E., Kirklin, J. K., *et al.* (1987). Symptomatic spinal epidural lipomatosis as a complication of steroid immunosuppression in cardiac transplant patients. Report of two cases. *Journal of Neurosurgery*, 67, 760–4.

Zazgornik, J., Shaheen, F. A., Kopsa, H., Biesenbach, G., Kaiser, W., and Waldhaus, W. (1988). Severe hyperkalaemia, hyperchloraemia, hyporeninaemia and hyperaldosteronism in a cyclosporine-treated renal-transplant patient. *Nephrology, Dialysis and Transplantation*, 3, 826–9.

7 Psychotherapy and counselling with transplant patients

J. Soos

Patients undergoing transplantation do not require a new type of psychotherapy. A huge variety of treatment approaches already exist (Herink 1980). Rather, the fundamental principles of psychotherapy need to be applied to the transplant situation. Adaptation of existing therapies for these clients involves the alteration of some technical aspects of the psychotherapy process and requires an awareness on the part of the therapist of the intrapsychic and interpersonal issues which arise in this context.

As this volume attests, understanding of the psychological aspects of transplantation has grown rapidly over the past decade. However, empirical information regarding the psychotherapeutic treatment of these patients has lagged behind other areas. A computerized literature search spanning back to January 1967 found less than a dozen articles which specifically address the provision of psychological treatments to transplant patients. This chapter will briefly outline the indications for psychotherapy in the transplant situation and draw upon published literature and clinical experience to discuss the treatment of these patients and their families. Interested readers are referred also to general reviews of psychotherapy in the medically ill (Stein *et al.* 1969; Freyberger 1975; Karasu 1980; Rodin 1990).

Indications for psychotherapy

Supportive psychotherapeutic interaction may be indicated for patients with any chronic medical illness and who are experiencing psychological distress (Rodin 1990). This distress is typically the result of a discordant interaction between the medical circumstances and the expectations or personality of the patient. Although this indication encompasses a large group of persons, the likelihood of a patient engaging in psychotherapy is mediated by several other factors, including the patient's interest and attitudes towards such discussions and the availability of alternate sources of support. In practice, it is usual for the largest group of patients to show interest in group processes, for fewer to attend individual counselling and for a very small subgroup to be motivated for an insight-oriented approach. Regardless of the approach undertaken, the time course of therapy will be dictated in part, by illness related events. A worsening of medical state may initiate the search for help, breaks in therapy may occur during hospitalization, and therapy may at times terminate following the resolution of a health crisis or worse, with the death of the patient.

In the context of organ transplantation, the emotional intensity of the events encountered may stimulate personal reflection on fundamental issues of personhood and dispose certain patients to insight-oriented therapy. However, the majority of patients will be best suited to a brief and supportive type of interaction which facilitates their goals of obtaining and coping with an organ transplant. Basic education about coping skills and an explanation that pronounced and conflicting emotions are normal in this situation are of benefit to many patients. Some examples of transplant-related events which may stimulate emotional distress are briefly discussed.

Pre-transplant

Although some patients may experience the decision to undergo evaluation for transplantation as an expected progression of their illness, this event may disrupt the psychological equilibrium of many others (Kuhn *et al.* 1990). A physician's recommendation of a transplant is a potent validation of illness severity and may interfere with common defences, such as minimization and denial. The applicant may become acutely aware of previously unacknowledged fears concerning invalidism or death. Death anxiety may underlie worries about being found unsuitable for a transplant and be manifest clincially as performance anxiety during assessment procedures.

Once a transplant is recommended, many patients will make an immediate decision to proceed. This may reflect adequate adjustment and preparation on the part of the applicant prior to the time of the recommendation. Alternatively, a rapid decision may function defensively to minimize the patient's reflection on an emotionally charged predicament. Other patients will agonize thoughtfully over the decision, and must weigh the certainty of further disability or death without a transplant against the many uncertainties and demands which are involved with a decision in favour of surgery. For patients to proceed in an informed manner, some appreciation of possible outcomes following the transplant is required. While up to 89 per cent of surviving transplant recipients rate their overall quality of life as good to excellent (Brennan *et al.* 1987), the likelihood of complications is great (House and Thompson 1988). However, patients and their families may deny the possibility of untoward events and assume that the postoperative course will be trouble-free. This may predispose the patient to demoralization or depression if major complications occur following the procedure (Dubovsky and Penn 1980). Brief counselling may be in order for applicants who experience the most difficulty with the decision for a transplant, or when the decision-making processes indicate problematic adjustment. As the following case illustrates, patients' unrealistic expectations may be challenged most by the progression of disease in themselves or in others.

Case history Mr A., a 37 year old man with endstage cardiomyopathy was referred for heart transplant evaluation. He had experienced a rapid progression of disability over the previous year. However, he had remained employed at home as a computer programmer for small businesses. At the time of assessment, he presented as highly motivated for surgery, stating that he would like to get it over with soon so as to get on with his career. Staff were concerned about his apparent lack of interest in learning about the postoperative course. He stated that he did not believe in worrying about events before they occurred and further, that there was no point in becoming depressed over things that may not happen anyway. Mr A. declined an offer to talk with the psychologist affiliated with the team.

During his assessment for transplant, Mr A. interacted amicably with other patients and made acquaintance with several of the candidates. The transplant team questioned his preparedness for complications should they occur following surgery. Nevertheless, they accepted Mr A. to the waiting list, expecting him to learn more about the transplant process by attending a weekly support group.

After waiting ten weeks for surgery, the patient announced that he would not continue to attend the support group. He stated that he had made good friends with another candidate who 'saw things his way' and did not need to 'listen to other people's problems'. Several weeks later, a heart transplant recipient died following a prolonged intensive care stay and Mr A.'s friend, who was also still waiting for surgery, died abruptly from pneumonia. Initially, Mr A. voiced concerns about the competence of the transplant team. Later, he came to accept that the deaths were beyond the control of the staff and he became demoralized and pessimistic about his own future.

Mr A. recognized that he was becoming depressed and now agreed to meeting the psychologist. For the first time, he expressed a great sense of personal vulnerability and his fears of succumbing to his disease. Further, he expected and feared overwhelming depression and anxiety should he allow himself to 'dwell' on these thoughts. It became apparent that the patient equated the experience of fear with either 'giving up' or as a manifestation of a 'negative' attitude. Although normal given his situation, fears were perceived as a sign of personal weakness. His sense of mastery and strength was challenged by his increasing difficulty in extruding fears from awareness. Mr A.'s attitudes towards these emotional experiences appeared related to early family life in which there was little acceptance of expressed emotions.

Mr A. responded with relief to the explanation that fear was a normal and expected reaction to severe illness and transplant. He was helped to see how he had been expending enormous energies by his attempts to suppress experiences which reflect the reality of the transplant situation. These preliminary discussions facilitated a thera-peutic alliance which persisted throughout the transplant process. For this patient, periodic psychotherapeutic interaction not only increased his ability to cope adequately with the situation, but also helped him to reconceptualize the transplant experience as a stimulus for increased personal awareness and psychological development.

Denial is a common and adaptive defence which may help to protect patients from feeling overwhelmed by fears or ruminative worry (Lazarus and Folkman 1984). This may include denial of prognosis, denial of the emotional impact of certain facts, or commonly denial of the personal relevance of facts or events. Mai (1986) has described the protective role which denial may play in the transplant patient who is confronted with multiple and uncontrollable dangers. However, as the above case illustrates, the medical severity of the transplant situation persistently confronts denial and leaves some patients feeling overwhelmed. Others may demonstrate problematic medical (e.g. noncompliance) or social (e.g. refusal to complete a will) complications of denial. Psychotherapeutic interaction may benefit interested patients, but will best proceed when the patient recognizes a need for assistance. Previously unacknowledged fears may be discussed in the protective environment of the therapeutic relationship.

Psychotherapeutic treatment of a patient with massive denial is a complex task. Patients may be referred by staff who are concerned about manifestations of denial, but therapeutic challenge to denial may not necessarily be indicated. Alternatively, the patient may not be agreeable or ready to tolerate the expression of disavowed beliefs or emotions. Many patients do not wish to acknowledge that in addition to suffering with physical illness, they are also experiencing psychological difficulty. Some fear that discussion of certain topics will lead to depression and compromise their chance for a successful transplant. When necessary, the therapist may wish to encourage the attitude that it is best to hope for the best, but prepare for the worst. However, he or she risks becoming the object of displaced hostility, particularly if placed in the position of confronting the patient with harsh medical realities. It is ideal in this situation for the therapist to ensure that the medical staff clearly and repeatedly inform the patient and family of necessary information. This leaves the therapist in a more neutral and supportive position, free to work with the patient's response and to facilitate adjustment to the information provided. A permissive and flexible approach to therapy is required with these patients.

Additional emotional challenges to both the potential organ recipient and the donor may occur when a live donor is being considered. Most researchers have found that the psychological benefits of donating a kidney to a family member far outweigh any negative psychosocial sequelae (Simmons 1981). Nonetheless, the symbolic implications of sustaining a family member by sacrificing one's own healthy organ may have both intrapsychic and interpersonal sequelae for both parties. Problems may arise, for example, if a family member feels pressured to donate (Gulledge *et al*. 1983). How does one negotiate interpersonal closeness and distance, if one feels dependent on the donor's kidney? Might a donor not use the 'gift of life' manipulatively to influence the recipient? (Steinberg *et al*. 1981). Individual and/or family therapy may be of benefit to explore such questions before the parties can both feel comfortable proceeding with the renal transplant.

In families with more severe psychopathology, the implications for both the potential donor and recipient are especially complex. For example, the donation of an organ from an overly controlling parent may further impair a child recipient's attempts at separation-individuation. Remarks made by a young woman during evaluation for a living-related kidney transplant from her mother illustrates this phenomenon. 'I don't want my mother to have that control over me. It's like I'll owe her something for the rest of my life. It hurts me when she uses the kidney as a leverage.' Later in the same interview, the potential recipient voiced the reverse side of her conflicted and ambivalent relationship with her mother. 'It feels like I would finally be really bonding with my mother. I can't get closer to her than by having part of her in me.'

The intrapsychic ambivalence related to oscillations between the felt need for psychic merger and the concurrent fear of engulfment are readily apparent. This mother and daughter were seen in both individual and family sessions by the psychologist affiliated with the transplant team. The aims of treatment were not to attempt correction of persistent characterological difficulties. Instead, a more modest goal of helping each family member to identify and in turn communicate their respective feelings and needs was attempted.

The type of transplant may also stimulate particular concerns to emerge. For example, it may be complicated psychologically for patients with terminal lung disease who receive a combined heart/lung transplant. Their own heart may have been healthy, and these patients will simultaneously become both a transplant recipient and an organ donor. The person will need to grieve the loss of a fully functioning vital organ, before he or she can adjust to the eventual psychological internalization of the new organs (Basch 1973). Each of the intrapsychic and interpersonal phenomena which arise with live donor transplants apply in this situation (Simmons 1981).

Case history   Ms R. is a 29 year old female with cystic fibrosis who was awaiting transplantation for six months. She was largely asymptomatic until two years prior to the evaluation. She was referred because of depression and an increasing sense of frustration and helplessness. In therapy she began to voice concerns about giving up her healthy heart. While she understood the rationale for the surgery, she felt disturbed by the thought of losing her own disease-free heart. Ms R. experienced her heart as having a life of its own. She displaced many of her own feelings of loss and her need for support on to her heart which was perceived as if it were a separate individual with whom she had a close, confiding relationship. She said 'I can't imagine my heart in someone else's body. I mean it's not like I'm going to die; I'll be alive. Knowing that a healthy part of me is alive in someone else's body is very weird. We [referring to her and her heart] have been together a lot through the years. It'll be like losing a close friend'. She added 'I look at my heart like a very close friend, somebody I can trust to tell my deepest, dark secrets to. My heart knows everything that I have ever felt since the first day of my life. It has held out for me when times were very bad, such as in the intensive care unit. It has never let me down. It has felt every pain and every joy throughout my life. My heart, when it leaves me, will be like giving up a part of my soul. I hope that whoever receives my precious little heart appreciates it and takes care of it and treats it like gold. I feel sad that my heart has to leave me, it is a feeling like my best friend or parents are going away, and I can never see them again'. In a similar vein, she described the loss of her heart as akin to 'putting one's little baby up for adoption'. This language poignantly symbolizes the very private and fundamental nature of her grief. Undoubtedly, her own history of failed attempts to adopt influenced her choice of this imagery.

Ms R.'s psychotherapy addressed issues of anticipatory grief. Her nagging 'weird feelings' were reconceptualized as normal feelings of loss associated with losing her own body part. Her own metaphors of putting up a baby for adoption, and losing a friend were used to understand her current distress. Expressing the feelings also rendered them less bewildering and promoted the working through of the confusion and dysphoria.

The two-chair technique associated with Gestalt Therapy was used in this case to help resolve her conflict (Greenberg and Higgins 1980). Ms R. 'placed' her heart in the empty chair in front of her and began a dialogue, shifting back and forth between the two chairs, as she oscillated between the role of her heart and herself. Ms R. stated 'I feel empty, thinking that you won't be inside of me; you're a part of me, and you'll be gone. I will miss you. Also, will I feeling differently about others with someone else's heart inside me? Will my feelings towards those I love change? For example, will I still feel attracted towards the same kind of guy?'. Heart: 'I too will miss you, but think of how much better you will feel with your new heart and lungs. We'll all be better off. You'll be able to enjoy the things you like doing, and I'll be able to keep a person alive. That will make us both feel good'.

Focusing on the life-sustaining aspect of giving up her heart was tremendously useful in coming to terms with her anguish. However, the overall focus of therapy was much broader in scope. The Gestalt-oriented grief work is presented to highlight how diverse treatment techniques can be brought to bear on transplant-related psychological issues. Ms R.'s concerns about internalizing qualities associated with the donor heart were not psychotic distortions. That she was deeply troubled by the prospect of giving up her heart is not surprising given the central role the heart plays in religious thought, poetic expression, and the culture's ongoing references to the intimately personal and symbolic qualities of this organ (Meserve 1984; Siebert 1990). In addition, this woman had developed a special appreciation for the organ which had helped her survive episodes of serious illness.

Although acceptance to a transplant programme may be an important source of hope, the period following acceptance to a waiting list is one of the most stressful periods of the transplantation process (Levenson and Olbrisch 1987). The uncertainty about whether and when an appropriate organ will be made available is anxiety-provoking, particularly if the patient's condition deteriorates (Allender *et al.* 1983). Such patients may fear death before the new organ is made available. It is not uncommon for patients to make funeral preparations prior to their transplantation. This may not be unreasonable given the fact that as many as one-third of patients may die on the waiting list for heart or lung transplants (McGregor 1987; Bright *et al.* 1990). A prolonged wait for transplant stimulates a wide variety of additional concerns (Levenson and Olbrisch 1987) which may benefit from discussion. For this reason, group counselling has been recommended routinely for candidates (Suszycki 1986; Bright *et al.* 1990). During this time, when a sense of helplessness may pervade, supportive interaction amongst patients is to be encouraged.

Interpersonal disruptions are also common during the waiting period. The patient's original source of social support may become less available. Previously close friends may gradually drift out of their lives due to prolonged hospitalizations, immobility, or lack of interest by the patient in social inter-actions. Long periods of fear and uncertainty may also undermine marital cohesion (Krausz 1988). In many families, traditional marital roles are reversed due to demands created by the patient's forced helplessness (Mishel and Murdaugh 1987). The spouse may need to take on duties that previously were handled by the patient, now largely incapacitated by endstage organ disease. Such unanticipated realignments of role behaviours can seriously undermine the sense of stability at a time when comfort and predictability are most needed (Mishel and Murdaugh 1987). Indeed, rates of divorce are higher than usual among transplantees (Rodgers 1984; Wolcott 1990). Individual psychotherapy may be indicated for some candidates to ensure that maladaptive behaviours will not erode their much needed social support. Couple or family counselling may be indicated solely, or interspersed with individual counselling.

Post-transplant

Strain and Grossman (1975) have described the multiple psychological stresses that confront the surgical patient. Hospitalization and its attendant fear of death undermines the patient's belief that he or she is self-sufficient and independent. The hospitalized patient may also experience fear of strangers, feelings of isolation, anxiety about separation from significant others, fear of the loss of love and approval, fear of the loss of control of developmentally achieved functions (e.g. bladder control, speech), fear of loss or injury of bodily parts, and fear of pain. Feelings of guilt and shame may also be revived by physical symptoms.

Postoperative patients may need assistance with pain management. While many patients experience distressing levels of pain, it is often overlooked in face of the more dramatic surgical outcome (Strain 1986). In addition to analgesics, psychological methods of pain management can be taught to patients while they are still in hospital. These include relaxation techniques, systematic desensitization, the provision of sensory and procedural informa-tion (Suls and Wan 1989), or instruction in self-hypnosis. These self-control techniques may help the patient to tolerate stressful medical procedures such as transbronchial lung biopsies, jugular intravenous insertions for drug access or nasogastric feedings. Others may require assistance with needle phobias, or anxiety about confining procedures (e.g. magnetic resonance imaging) (Quirk *et al.* 1989). Certain patients may refuse to adhere to the medical regime because of fear, confusion, anger, or unresolved conflicts over authority (Meichenbaum and Turk 1987; Kaplan and Simon 1990). An enhanced sense of control and mastery may result from the use of psycho-behavioural techniques and help compensate for patient's sense of helpless-ness and vulnerability. Taylor (1986) contends that a central element in the management of the stressful medical procedures is the notion of psychological control. If patients can be allowed to exert control over the procedure, or else learn means of controlling their subjective reaction to the procedure, they will probably be able to cope more adequately with the distress, and hence be more likely to comply.

For the transplant recipient, hypnosis may be indicated in treating post-surgical pain, assisting with the management of stressful medical procedures, and in helping counter hopelessness and demoralization (Golden *et al.* 1987; Hammond 1990). Both during an extended waiting period, and amidst a protracted, difficult postoperative course, being able to visualize one's self in a state of health, enjoying a favoured, sought-after goal, may help to counter hopeless, depressive thoughts, and to instill a renewed sense of positive expectancy and elevated mood.

Cue-controlled relaxation (Philips 1988), is commonly taught to the patient as part of the self-hypnosis training. 'Each time you exhale, say to yourself the word "calm". With time the association with the outbreath and the word will serve as a cue to bring forth these deep states of calm and well-being whenever you require it.' The patient thereby learns an additional strategy to allay discomfort and to foster a feeling of self-control to counter demoralization and excess dependency. Frequently a hypnosis tape is made for the patient, employing personally meaningful and relaxing imagery coupled with mutually-derived therapeutic suggestions. Hospitalized patients can readily listen to such cassette tapes on their personal tape players with headsets, thereby not disturbing other patients.

Transplant recipients are faced with substantial adjustment challenges following discharge from hospital. These are discussed in other chapters and include: readjustment to family and vocational roles; body image changes; coping with the persistent threat of rejection; multiple expectations of medical staff and the intrusion of follow-up protocols; dealing with the side-effects of immunosuppressants; and potential loss of long-term disability incomes. Patients may benefit from brief psychotherapy to help assuage anxieties engendered by the first allograft rejection (Beidel 1987). Depression and suicidal ideation may result from unfulfilled expectations (Surman 1989). One recipient reported the following to the author. 'Sometimes I long for the peace that would come from death. If I would have really known the hardships that follow, I don't know if I would have wanted the transplant. This is not like a regular sickness where you are ill and then you get cured. You can never ever stop worrying.'

Thoughts about the new organ may be troubling for some patients. Some writers describe the need for an intrapsychic integration of the new organ, a task that demands that the patient psychologically accept and internalize the new body image (Basch 1973). One patient who was assessed by the author wondered whether her new heart would be strong enough to allow her to return to her pre-morbid love of swimming. In addition, she hated the idea that the donor may have been a 'meat eater'. Survival guilt may also impair the patient's postoperative quality of life.

Case history   Mr M. was a heart transplant recipient who requested assistance with lingering concerns about his otherwise uncomplicated procedure. He readily reported that he was troubled by the fact that his father had died an early death due to heart failure, while he had been spared this fatal outcome. He had previously considered this risk as part of his genetic heritage.

The patient initially spoke of a vague, troubling sense of family betrayal. With further discussion, additional symbolic meanings became apparent. His own survival had awakened feelings of unresolved grief over the loss of his father. Further, Mr M. acknowledged having assumed for much of his youth that he would not live past the age of his father. He had accomplished much at an early stage of his career, in part motivated by a deeply felt belief that he should meet his goals and be ready for an early demise. In fact, it was likely that as a youth, he had coped with the loss of his father by identifying with both the time and cause of death, and with fantasies of rejoining his father after his own, similar death at a later date. Acceptance of this interpretation facilitated Mr M.'s reconceptualization of his own life in relation to that of his father. He realized that his father would have wished him to enjoy the opportunities for further life which the heart transplant had provided. Therapy completed itself with a preliminary discussion of his ideas about how to use his life fruitfully.

Survival of the post-operative phase can force the patient to confront existential issues and renewed uncertainty as to the meaning and purpose of their life. The therapist can assist these patients with the enormous psychological shift that accompanies the transition from near death to renewed life. For example, one heart–lung transplant recipient who was referred to the author for depression and suspected non-compliance wondered if it was not fundamentally wrong to be given a new life when she otherwise would have faced certain death. This deeply religious patient felt that such 'human tampering' was perhaps in some way morally incorrect. During brief individual therapy, this recipient's disquieting feelings and troubling thoughts were interpreted as a result of trying to come to terms with a sense of having 'violated the dictates of nature' by being 'brought back from the dead', but without a recognizable meaning or purpose in her life. From this point on, the therapist attempted to provide a facilitative interpersonal environment for the patient to search within her self for new meaning to her life.

Treatment of the transplant patient

Basic principles of brief therapy (Garfield 1989) are applicable in treatment of the transplant. During the initial meetings, facilitation of the therapeutic alliance is a major goal. This is accomplished in a number of ways, including the adoption of a supportive, but not intrusive, attitude; the use of language and imagery which is congruent with the patient's mode of functioning; helping clients to identify and prioritize problems for discussion; the explanation of an understandable formulation of the patient's distress; and providing a rationale for treatment. The interpretation of many transplant patients' distress as normal, albeit uncomfortable or problematic, may rapidly ameliorate their concerns about being abnormal or out of control. As many medical referrals fear psychiatric labelling by the therapist, this conceptualization will also assist with the development of a working alliance. It is useful to explore at an early stage the patient's subjective perception of the illness (Rodin 1984; Viederman 1986) and the impact of these perceptions on coping. Each of the techniques will help initiate an alliance and may reduce distress.

Therapy with a transplant candidate will usually require an active approach on behalf of the therapist. Typically, a wide variety of real and fantasized issues are brought for discussion. The therapist must help to counter feelings of demoralization and aimlessness while facilitating adjustment to the patient's realistic circumstance. Defensive postures must be respected during this time, unless severely compromising medical care. The ability to maintain a viable sense of purpose in life, amidst the apparent meaninglessness of endstage organ disease, is an essential component of an effective coping strategy. In her paper, aptly titled 'Cardiac transplant: preparation for dying or for living', Christopherson (1976) has discussed the difficulties encountered in psychotherapy with patients facing such an ambiguous and dichotomized outcome.

Each of psychodynamic, cognitive, and behavioural perspectives has applicability for counselling and therapy with transplant patients. In fact, the spectrum of problems which transplant patients will bring to therapy lends itself well to a integrative model (Reid 1990) which borrows from varied perspectives. Although an approach which emphasizes genetic interpretations is unlikely to be suitable for more than a few selected patients, an appreciation of the patient's intrapsychic structure and its influence on his or her perception of the current circumstances is invaluable. Appropriate instruction in cognitive and behavioural stress management techiques will encourage a sense of mastery over symptomatic distress. Cognitive techniques have been described to help calm health-related anxiety (Warwick 1989). Regardless of the predominate approach, the therapist should engender a permissive attitude towards emotional expression. By the time a transplant patient attends therapy, he or she has typically been struggling with major life disruption. The ventilation of concerns is itself therapeutic and allows for further clarification of the personal meaning of the changes which illness has forced on the patient.

The nature of the developing relationship between therapist and transplant patient requires monitoring in any approach to therapy. Chronic and endstage organ disease is typically associated with alteration of a person's sense of autonomy. This may involve a tendency for regression and heightened dependency wishes (Viederman 1986) or, alternatively, pseudo-independence, with denial of vulnerability, may be demonstrated. For these patients, the naive offerings of a supportive relationship without adequate understanding of their personality style may respectively foster regression or stimulate unconscious dependency fears. The latter may lead to discontinuation of therapy or flight into health.

The therapist's reaction to seriously ill transplant patients has great potential for influence on therapy. The finality of life-threatening physical illness forces the therapist to confront not only the limitations of therapeutic efficacy but ultimately the therapist's own mortality (Rodin and Garfinkel 1984). Feelings of helplessness and powerlessness on the part of the therapist may, if not recognized, contribute to counter-transference acting out. This may take the form of overprotectiveness (e.g. meeting too frequently), rescue fantasies with inappropriate therapeutic endeavours, or, alternatively, avoidance of interaction by prematurely discontinuing therapy. Guilt may develop in the therapist who experiences fantasies of a patient's transplant or death. In these instances, therapy may be prematurely terminated to relieve the therapist's discomfort. In addition, therapists may wrongly collude with a patient's fantasies that psychological work may cure them from serious physical illness (Adler 1984). While confrontation of a patient's magical hopes for recovery is not necessarily indicated, it is potentially harmful to both the therapeutic process, and to the patient, to accept an implicit contract that psychotherapy may directly contribute to the resolution of disease. Finally, counter-transference hate may arise in psychotherapy with medical patients (Adler 1984). This may result from the sense of powerlessness which severe illness may stimulate in both the patient and therapist. Alternatively, therapists who allow or encourage unrealistic expectations on the part of the medical or surgical staff may be infuriated by a referred patient who is unresponsive to their interventions. Psychotherapeutic involvement with these patients will inevitably demand of the therapist reflection upon personal attitudes towards therapy and one's own vulnerability and mortality.

Case history   Mr W. is a 31 year old male who received a double lung transplant two years prior to being referred for suicidal ideation. He was diagnosed at age 11 with cystic fibrosis and the patient recalled how he was repeatedly informed throughout his life that he would not reach adulthood. During his adolescence, he tried to deny the grave implications of his life-threatening illness by adopting a defiant attitude. He said 'I would argue with the teachers all the time, and smoke constantly in spite of everyone's concern'.

One year following transplant, the patient's mother died. This unexpected tragedy led to profound levels of hopelessness and despair. Nightmares involving vivid scenes of animals' chests being cut open, which were present before surgery, now returned. He felt guilty about his mother's death, repeatedly asking himself why it was his mother and not he who died. The death of his mother and the new opportunity for his own survival forced this patient to raise such fundamental questions as 'What is the reason for my life? Why is God letting me live, while my mother suddenly dies? Who do I really have left now, and why bother going on?'. While answers to these questions evaded him, his state of demoralization intensified. While he was afraid to 'directly kill' himself, he began to think increasingly about stopping his immunosuppressant drugs as that would be a 'very easy way to go'. Finally, he became frightened by despair and he referred himself. His grief and the lack of purpose in life became the goals of therapy.

A post-transplant existential crises may commonly occur. Helping patients to develop personally meaningful life goals may not only contribute to an improved quality of life, but may be life-sustaining. The importance of fostering, through the psycho-therapeutic process, a viable purpose of life and a will to live throughout the transplantation process appears to be an important focus of treatment.

In addition, the cognitive–behavioural approach (Persons 1989) was used in therapy with Mr W. The patient was taught how to identify automatic negative thoughts accompanying feelings of depression. For him, the underlying themes often related to self deprecation. Once he pinpointed these maladaptive thoughts, Mr W. was taught to replace them with encouraging coping self-statements where he would either remind himself of positive personal attributes and accomplishments or else refute negative appraisals of situations and generate alternative explanations. Between sessions, he kept a record of dysfunctional thoughts that accompanied negative emotions and un-satisfactory behaviours. In time, he was able to dismiss the written exercises and did not need any assistance with the challenging of irrational thinking. The patient thus developed a coping strategy to monitor and positively influence his experience and behaviour.

Psychotherapy ended after several months. Mr W. no longer felt suicidal. He began a career as manager of a rural restaurant. In addition, he spends considerable time speaking to other patients with cystic fibrosis about the benefits of transplantation. He met his first girlfriend in over a decade, and states that he feels more confident than ever before. As can be seen from the clinical material, an eclectic and problem-focused approach to individual therapy was used. The healing properties of the therapeutic relationship are enhanced by the judicious use of well established therapeutic techniques.

Group therapy

Group therapy has an established place in the psychosocial treatment of transplant patients and their families (Buchanan 1975; Gold *et al.* 1986; Suszycki 1986; Bright *et al.* 1990). Many programmes have an open-ended, unstructured support group which is available to patients during all stages of the transplant process. The support group creates a context where curative factors come into play (Yalom 1985). These include the instillation of hope and a sense of universality, the imparting of information and altruism. Helping and observing others cope may contribute to an increased sense of personal mastery. Group feedback may facilitate adaptative ways of interacting. Catharsis, and discussion of fears of death and of the future, may also be addressed by the group format.

In addition to providing accurate information, a group offers a predictable opportunity to experience social support. The role of social support in ameliorating illness related stressors is well established (LaRocco *et al.* 1980). An ongoing support group also allows the therapist associated with the transplant group to remain attuned to the fluctuating needs of the patients, to address rumours and inaccuracies which are commonly passed amongst candidates and recipients and to identify patients who are having significant emotional problems. Bright *et al.* (1990) have reported that limits needed to be affirmed when lung transplant patients in an unstructured group expected to be informed in detail about the medical progress of other patients. These requests can be managed with explanations regarding confidentiality and families' right to decide with whom they wish to communicate medical information.

In addition to an open-ended support group, the Vancouver transplant group offer a series of coping skills training modules that are made available to the patients and their families on a periodic basis. These consist of four $1\frac{1}{2}$ hour group sessions organized around specific transplant-related issues. Bereavement, family adaptation, stress and anger management, communication and conflict resolution, and modifying coronary-prone behaviour (Roskies 1987) are modules currently in place. Didactic information is presented for the first 15–30 minutes of each session. The remaining time is spent in informal discussion where group members share their experiences and practice the new coping behaviours presented.

Marital therapy

There may be eroding effects on marital relationships during all phases of the transplant process (Mishel and Murdaugh 1987). One of the important post-hospitalization psychosocial tasks the individual needs to accomplish is the gradual relinquishing of the sick role and the eventual return to non-patient status (Christopherson 1987). Chronic illness and repeated hospitalizations are likely to have fostered a sense of relative helplessness within the patient. Family adjustments are made, where often a previously high-functioning, capable individual is placed into a state of illness-induced dependency. Meanwhile, a previously non-assertive spouse may have had to accept greater family responsibilities. Following transplant, the recipient may be reluctant to give up the security of the patient role, although the spouse may resent this continued, now inappropriate, passivity. Alternatively, the patient may be eager to resume the pre-illness position of authority within the family, but the spouse might be disinclined to forfeit the newfound leadership role during the patient's illness (Rauch and Kneen 1989).

These and other couples' issues can readily be treated from within the framework of brief behavioural marital therapy (Wishman and Jacobson 1990). Conflict resolution skills may, for example, need to be taught before they can negotiate interpersonal problems precipitated by transplant-induced role strain.

Case history Shortly after a middle-aged male patient, Mr G., was accepted for cardiac transplantation, his wife announced that she was considering separation. This pronouncement surprised the transplant team, as less than a week earlier they presented as a caring, mutually supportive, and knowledgeable couple. However, she angrily stated that she felt alone and shut out as the patient's physical condition gradually deteriorated. She complained that his increasing self-preoccupation led him to neglect her emotional needs completely. Moreover, she noted that Mr G. had begun to sleep an inordinate amount during the day and she wondered if he was depressed. When the patient heard that his spouse informed the transplant coordinator of his apparent depression, he feared that he would consequently be removed from the waiting list. He told his wife that she would be responsible for his death should he no longer be found to be a suitable transplant candidate.

The two were referred for couple therapy. They were helped to see that their current distress was largely situationally mediated. Prior to the patient being accepted for transplantation, they had a relatively sound, working relationship. Moreover, it was pointed out that, if at all possible, major life decisions ought not be implemented amidst a crisis (Krausz 1988). They were helped to pinpoint interpersonal problems that were felt to be vital, and to relinquish irritants that were of relatively less concern.

A dysfunctional pattern of communication was identified as contributory to the conflict. Mr G. had withdrawn socially and wished to be left alone for longer periods of time than was previously characteristic for him. He was physically too weak to participate in extended social activities with his wife. His wife experienced his increased need to be alone as a rejection of her supportive efforts. The more she attempted to engage him, the more angry and withdrawn he became. He viewed her supportive overtures as irritating intrusions. Mrs G. had come to feel increasingly helpless and angry at him for behaviour which she believed was maladaptive.

The therapist helped each spouse to identify and in turn voice their respective needs in a non-judgemental manner. Communication and negotiation skills were taught. A compromise solution was arrived at where Mrs G. agreed to recognize his need for increased private time. He, in turn, agreed to go out to lunch with her at least three times per week. Most importantly, they agreed that this was not the time to think of divorce, and that they would reassess their marriage further at some time after the transplant.

Marital distress, of course, is not always resolved so readily. After a successful transplant, long-suppressed unresolved and contentious issues may gradually re-surface (Mishel and Murdaugh 1987). Therapy may not be able to redress long-standing marital dysfunction. In such a case, individual and/or couple therapy may help the couple disengage with as little acrimony as possible.

Rationale for psychotherapy with transplant patients

A basic thesis of this chapter is that current approaches to psychotherapy can be readily adapted to the emotional needs of this population. The reduction of psychological distress can improve the patient's quality of life throughout the various phases of the transplantation process. This is an important and valuable goal in its own right; in spirit with Engel's (1977) biopsychosocial approach to understanding and treating disease.

It is possible, but not proven, that psychological interventions may contribute to increased post-transplant recovery and survival (Schultheiss *et al*. 1987). Pre-surgical stress management and patient preparation is associated with improved surgical outcome (Anderson 1987). Behavioural interventions designed to enhance compliance with immunosuppressive medication may save the non-compliant, depressed patient's life (Lesko and Hawkins 1983). Psychotherapy to ameliorate postoperative depression can prevent the patient from committing suicide. Smoking and alcohol abuse are potentially lethal means of maladaptively managing post-transplant induced stressors. Stress mangagement techniques can readily teach patients adaptive coping strategies that do not jeopardize their physical well-being.

Recent work in psychoneuro-immunology has shown that the central nervous system is capable of influencing both humoral and cell-mediated immune processes via the hypothalamic–pituitary–adrenal cortical axis, and by numerous other pathways (Stein *et al*. 1986; Geiser 1989; Vollhardt 1991). Might an acute episode of psychosocial stress potentiate helper T-cell activity, and thus increase the likelihood of allograft rejection? The corollary is that perhaps improved coping ability may, via neuroendocrine pathways, contribute to an internal environment more conducive to graft acceptance. The data are not yet available to answer the question of whether or not effective coping can enhance immunological factors controlling rejection (Lesko and Hawkins 1983; Pennebaker *et al*. 1988). Multi-centre longitudinal outcome studies are needed to clarify this intriguing possibility.

Conclusions

This chapter has outlined some of the psychosocial stressors that may become indications for psychotherapy or counselling with some transplant patients. Psychological interventions can be of assistance throughout the process. Individual and group psychotherapy can teach the patient coping skills necessary to help assuage anxieties associated with both the waiting period and the post-transplant course. Cognitive–behavioural techniques may assist with post-surgical pain and with stressful medical procedures while recovering in the hospital. Marital therapy can address role adjustment problems during the various phases of transplantation. Anxiety and depression secondary to interpersonal struggles can thus be ameliorated.

Ongoing advances in surgical technique and immunosuppression will probably continue to improve the results of transplantation. By addressing our patients' fundamental human concerns, the psychotherapist is in the position to contribute to enhanced quality of life. Moreover, psychological assistance before surgery may contribute to enhanced postoperative recovery.

References

Adler, G. (1984). Special problems for the therapist. *International Journal of Psychiatry in Medicine*, 14, 91–8.

Allender, J., Shisslak, C., Kasniak, A., and Copeland, J. (1983). Stages of psychological adjustment associated with heart transplantation. *Heart Transplantation*, 2, 228–31.

Anderson, E. A. (1987). Preoperative preparation for cardiac surgery facilitates recovery, reduces psychological distress, and reduces the incidence of acute postoperative hypertension. *Journal of Consulting and Clinical Psychology*, 55, 513–20.

Basch, S. H. (1973). The intrapsychic integration of a new organ: A clinical study of kidney transplantation. *Psychoanalytic Quarterly*, 42, 364–84.

Beidel, D. C. (1987). Psychological factors in organ transplantation. *Clinical Psychology Review*, 7, 677–94.

Brennan, A. F., Davis, M. M., Buchholz, D. J., Kuhn, W. F., and Gray, L. A. (1987). Predictors of quality of life following cardiac transplantation: Importance of compliance with medical regimen, especially immunosuppressant therapy. *Psychosomatics*, 28, 566–71.

Bright, J., Craven, J., Kelly, P., and the Toronto Lung Transplant Group (1990). Psychosocial stress in lung transplant candidates. *Health and Social Work*, 15, 125–32.

Buchanan, D. C. (1975). Group therapy for kidney transplant patients. *International Journal of Psychiatry in Medicine*, 6, 523–31.

Christopherson, L. K. (1976). Cardiac transplant: preparation for dying or for living. *Health and Social Work*, 1, 58–72.

Christopherson, L. K. (1987). Cardiac transplantation: A psychological perspective. *Circulation*, 75, 57–62.

Dubovsky, S. L. and Penn, I. (1980). Psychiatric considerations in renal transplant surgery. *Psychosomatics*, 21, 481–91.

Engel, G. L. (1977). The need for a new medical model: a challenge for biomedicine. *Science*, 196, 129–36.

Freyberger, H. (1975). Psychotherapeutic possibilities in medically extreme situations. *Psychotherapy and Psychosomatics*, 26, 337–43.

Garfield, S. L. (1989). *The practice of brief psychotherapy* (Pergamon, New York).

Geiser, D. S. (1989). Psychosocial influences on human immunity. *Clinical Psychology Review*, 9, 689–715.

Gold, L. M., Kirkpatrick, B. S., Fricker, F. J., and Zitelli, B. J. (1986). Psychosocial issues in pediatric organ transplantation: the parents' perspective. *Pediatrics*, 77, 738–44.

Golden, W. L., Dowd, E. T., and Friedberg, F. (1987). *Hypnotherapy: a modern approach* (Pergamon, New York).

Greenberg, L. S. and Higgins, H. M. (1980). Effects of two-chair dialogues and focusing on conflict resolution. *Journal of Counselling Psychology*, 27, 221–4.

Gulledge, A. D., Buszta, C., and Montague, D. K. (1983). Psychosocial aspects of renal transplantation. *Urologic Clinics of North America*, 10, 327–35.

Hammond, D. C. (ed.) (1990). *Handbook of hypnotic suggestions and metaphors* (Norton, New York).

Herink, R. (ed.) (1980). *The psychotherapy handbook* (New American Library, New York).

House, R. M. and Thompson, T. L. II (1988). Psychiatric aspects of organ transplantation. *Journal of the American Medical Association*, 260, 535–9.

Kaplan, R. M. and Simon, H. J. (1990). Compliance in medical care: reconsideration of self-predictions. *Annals of Behavioral Medicine*, 12, 66–71.

Karasu, T. B. (1980). Psychotherapy with physically ill patients. In *'Specialized techniques in individual psychotherapy'* (eds T. B. Karasu and L. Bellak), pp. 258–76 (Brunner/Mazel, New York).

Krausz, S. (1988). Illness and loss: helping couples cope. *Clinical Social Work Journal*, 16, 52–65.

Kuhn, W. F., Brennan, A. F., Lacefield, P. K., Brohm, J., Skelton, V. D., and Gray, L. A. (1990). Psychiatric distress during stages of the heart transplant protocol. *Journal of Heart Transplantation*, 9, 25–9.

LaRocco, J. M., House, J. S., and Freud, R. P. (1980). Social support occupational stress and health. *Journal of Health and Social Behaviour*, 21, 202–18.

Lazarus, R. and Folkman, S. (1984). Coping and adaptation. In *Handbook of behavioural medicine* (ed. W. D. Gentry), pp. 282–325 (Guilford, New York).

Lesko, L. M. and Hawkins, D. R. (1983). Psychological aspects of transplantation medicine. In *New psychiatric symptoms: DSM-III and beyond* (ed. S. Akhtar), pp. 265–309 (Jason Aronson, New York).

Levenson, J. L. and Olbrisch, M. E. (1987). Shortage of donor organs and long waits: New sources of stress for transplant patients. *Psychosomatics*, 28, 399–403.

McGregor, C. G. A. (1987). Cardiac and cardiopulmonary transplantation. In *Clinical transplantation: current practice and future prospects* (ed. G. R. D. Catto), pp. 211–31 (MTP Press, Lancaster).

Mai, F. M. (1986). Graft and donor denial in heart transplant recipients. *American Journal of Psychiatry*, 143, 1159–61.

Meichenbaum, D. and Turk, D. C. (1987). *Facilitating treatment adherence* (Plenum, New York).

Meserve, M. C. (1984). The matter of the heart. *Journal of Religion and Health*, 23, 263–7.

Mishel, M. H. and Murdaugh, C. L. (1987). Family adjustment to heart transplantation: redesigning the dream. *Nursing Research*, 36, 332–8.

Pennebaker, J. W., Kiecolt-Glaser, J. K., and Glaser, R. (1988). Disclosure of traumas and immune function: health implications for psychotherapy. *Journal of Consulting and Clinical Psychology*, 56, 239–45.

Persons, J. B. (1989). *Cognitive therapy in practice: a case formulation approach* (Norton, New York).

Philips, H. C. (1988). *The psychological management of chronic pain: a treatment manual* (Springer, New York).

Quirk, M. E., Letendre, A. M., Ciottone, R. A., and Lingley, J. F. (1989). Anxiety in patients undergoing MR imaging. *Radiology*, 170, 463–6.

Rauch, J. B. and Kneen, K. K. (1989). Accepting the gift of life: heart transplant recipients' post-operative adaptive tasks. *Social Work in Health Care*, 1, 47–59.

Reid, W. J. (1990). An integrative model for short-term treatment. In *Handbook of the Brief Psychotherapies* (eds. R. A. Wells and V. J. Giannetti), pp. 55–77 (Plenum, New York).

Rodgers, J. (1984). Life on the cutting edge. *Psychology Today*, October, 58–67.

Rodin, G. M. (1984). Expressive psychotherapy in the medically ill: resistance and possibilities. *International Journal of Psychiatry in Medicine*, 14, 99–108.

Rodin, G. M. (1990). Psychotherapy of patients with chronic medical disorders. In *Review of General Psychiatry* (ed. H. H. Goldman), pp. 567–73 (Appleton & Lange, Norwalk).

Rodin, G. M. and Garfinkel, P.E. (1984). Psychotherapy of the medically ill: introduction and overview. *International Journal of Psychiatry in Medicine*, 14, 87–8.

Roskies, E. (1987). *Stress management for the healthy type A* (Guilford, New York).

Schultheiss, K., Peterson, L., and Selby, V. (1987). Preparation for stressful medical procedures and person by treatment interactions. *Clinical Psychology Review*, 7, 329–52.

Siebert, Z. C. (1990). The rehumanization of the heart. *Harper's Magazine*, February, 53–60.

Simmons, R. G. (1981). Psychological reactions to giving a kidney. In *Psychonephrology 1: psychological factors in hemodialysis and transplantation* (ed. N. B. Levy), pp. 227–45 (Plenum, New York).

Stein, E. H., Murdaugh, J., and MacLeod, J. A. (1969). Brief psychotherapy of psychiatric reactions to physical illness. *American Journal of Psychiatry*, 125, 76–83.

Stein, M., Schleifer, S. J., and Keller, S. E. (1986). Brain behavior and immune processes. In *Consultation—liaison psychiatry and behavioural medicine* (eds J. L. Houpt and H. K. H. Brodie), pp. 401–19 (Basic Books, New York).

Steinberg, J., Levy, N. B., and Radvila, A. (1981). Psychological factors affecting acceptance or rejection of kidney transplants. In *Psychonephrology I: psychological factors in hemodialysis and transplantation* (ed. N. B. Levy), pp. 185–93 (Plenum, New York).

Strain, J. J. (1986). The surgical patient. In *Consultation—liaison psychiatry and behavioural medicine* (eds J. L. Houpt and H. K. M. Brodie), pp. 379–89 (Basic Books, New York).

Strain, J. J. and Grossman, S. (1975). *Psychological care of the medically ill: A primer in liaison psychiatry* (Appleton-Century-Crofts, New York).

Suls, J. and Wan, C. K. (1989). Effects of sensory and procedural information on coping with stressful medical procedures and pain: A meta-analysis. *Journal of Consulting and Clinical Psychology,* 57, 372–9.

Surman, O. S. (1989). Psychiatric aspects of organ transplantation. *American Journal of Psychiatry*, 146, 972–82.

Suszycki, L. H. (1986). Social work groups in a heart transplant program. *Journal of Heart Transplantation*, 5, 166–70.

Taylor, S. E. (1986). *Health psychology* (Random House, New York).

Viederman, M. (1986). Psychotherapeutic approaches in the medically ill. In *Consultation—liaison psychiatry and behavioural medicine* (eds J. L. Houpt and H. K. H. Brodie), pp. 261–72 (Basic Books, New York).

Vollhardt, L. T. (1991). Psychoneuroimmunology: A literature review. *American Journal of Orthopsychiatry*, 61, 35–47.

Warwick, H. M. C. (1989). A cognitive–behavioural approach to hypochondriasis and health anxiety. *Journal of Psychosomatic Research*, 33, 705–11.

Wishman, M. A. and Jacobson, N. S. (1990). Brief behavioural marital therapy. In

Handbook of the brief psychotherapies (eds R. A. Wells and V. J. Giannetti), pp. 325–49 (Plenum, New York).

Wolcott, D. L. (1990). Organ transplant psychiatry: psychiatry's role in the second gift of life. *Psychosomatics*, 31, 91–7.

Yalom, I. D. (1985). *The theory of practice of group psychotherapy*, 3rd edn (Basic Books, New York).

8   Ethical considerations in transplantation

F. Lowy and D. Martin

The successful application of basic science and technological discoveries is the most striking feature of medical care during the past three decades. Yet this triumph over natural disease and suffering, which has greatly improved the human condition, has not been an unqualified blessing. A number of secondary medical, psychological, economic, and ethical problems have resulted.

Organ transplantation is paradigmatic. Thousands of persons with endstage renal, hepatic, cardiac, and pulmonary disease have benefited from an extension of life, sometimes for many years. However, the ever-expanding scope of organ transplant and its widespread utilization have also raised serious ethical questions. Jonsen (1989) has stated that the Age of Transplantation has ushered in the Age of Bioethics. Ethical questions revolve around practical issues about the benefit:harm ratio (for example, the added social and psychological burdens for transplant recipients and their families); the benefit:cost ratio (economic burdens for recipients, families, and society); and issues of justice (problems of micro- and macro-allocation of resources). But they also touch on fundamental ethical issues that concern the obligations of human beings to each other. Except for the sacrifice of life itself, there is no more personal gift than the gift of part of one's body.

Both secular and religious ethicists throughout the western world have approved life-extending organ transplantation after some initial misgivings among some of the latter. Both Judaism and Roman Catholicism have long-standing prohibitions against self-mutilation. As the benefits of organ transplantation were persuasively demonstrated, theologians in both faiths have re-examined the issue and have concluded that, so long as the donor does not suffer serious harm, organ donation is not only permissible, but a morally praiseworthy act of charity. However, religious as well as secular ethicists condemn the removal of organs before death, even if natural death is imminent and the earlier removal of the organ would improve the chance of a successful transplantation.

A detailed discussion of each of all relevant questions is beyond the scope of this chapter. Several are alluded to in other chapters. Youngner (Chapter 9) has included ethical dimensions in his discussion of organ retrieval for transplantation. Dixon (Chapter 10) has discussed in detail the religious perspectives on these procedures. Here we offer a general survey of ethical issues related to organ transplantation and a more detailed consideration of ethical problems in situations where the psychiatrist is most likely to be involved as a consultant.

Recipient considerations

Transplantation is subject to two ethical requirements that apply to all medical interventions. The first demands a favourable benefit to risk ratio, i.e. minimal risk to the organ donor and an acceptable, though obviously greater, risk to the recipient, which is offset by a substantial likelihood of benefit. The second requirement is consent to donate, which must be competent, fully informed, comprehending, and voluntary on the part of the living organ donor, or expressed by either a valid advance directive or familial consent for cadaveric organ donation. But the recipient also must provide informed consent. Here there are ethical considerations that sometimes involve psychiatric consultants. The prospective organ recipient is inevitably seriously ill and, at times, mentally impaired to the point where competence to give or refuse consent for the treatment is in question. The physicians involved, including the transplant team, are understandably eager to proceed if transplantation is the only, or the best, way of extending the patient's life. It is their duty to explain the consequences of accepting or rejecting transplantation and persuading (though not coercing) the patient to accept what seems best. When the patient refuses a recommendation advocated by physicians and the family, the consultant psychiatrist may well be called in to assess competence. It is important for this consultant not to be swayed by familial or medical peer pressure to declare incompetence prematurely in order to permit substitute decision makers to agree to treatment, but, in the process, deprive the patient of self-determination. As Tancredi (1985) has pointed out, physicians 'tend to believe that psychiatrists can persuade patients of the benefits of treatment, and if for some reason they cannot, then it is at least expected that psychiatrists will find such patients incompetent'.

The importance of giving patients a genuine opportunity to accept or reject the offer of a transplant is underscored by the outcome literature, considering quality of life as well as survival rates. That transplantation involves painful surgery and an operative death risk is well known to potential recipients. However, they may not realize that post-transplant follow-up regimens are arduous and that return to ambulatory activity, and especially to employment, is by no means assured.

A recent task force, reviewing the success of organ transplantation, has repeated the well documented survival statistics: 92–95 per cent of kidney recipients, 75–85 per cent of heart recipients, and 60–70 per cent of liver recipients are still alive at one year (New York State Task Force on Life and the Law 1988). But they also note that 80 per cent of kidney recipients develop infections, and 25 per cent of these lead to death. Kidney recipients are also at higher risk for hypertension, hepatitis, and cancer. This report is typical of the outcome literature. What is needed as well is an examination of the quality of life of organ recipients, measured both subjectively and objectively, as compared with the quality of life they would be likely to have had had transplant not been carried out.

Unfortunately, few relevant studies are satisfactory and this limits disclosure of benefits and risks to patients considering giving consent to transplant. Most reported outcome studies, such as that of Shaw *et al.* (1985), are optimistic in tone, but do not provide readers with the evidence upon which the conclusion of good quality of life is based. In careful cost–benefit analyses, Evans (1986) examined not only heart and kidney post-transplant survival rates, but also objective and subjective quality of life scores for patients and a control group. On subjective quality of life measures (sense of well-being, life satisfaction) recipients compared favourably with the general population sample. However, they did rather less well on objective quality of life measures which included functional ability, ability to work, and health status.

Scharschmidt (1984) reported several quality of life indices for liver transplant recipients. However, on the first, 'number of weeks spent in hospital', the data are reported on only 45 out of the total patient population of 540; the analysis of 'functional status' (defined as (1) fully rehabilitated; (2) able to care for self; (3) needs care), is based on data from 184 patients. Also reported is that 80 per cent of patients in one of the four centres surveyed 'resumed their former occupation or activities'. The conclusion drawn from these rather sparse data is that 'the quality of life for transplant recipients surviving at least four or more months appears to be good'.

Reports of post-transplant side-effects lead to further worry about the quality of life of some recipients. One review concluded that, within five years, 40–50 per cent of heart recipients develop accelerated coronary artery disease in their donor hearts (*Medical World News* 1988). Concern has also been expressed regarding the myriad of medications required by organ recipients, and the effects that these and chronic patienthood have on quality of life. 'Lack of social activities and exposure deprive the young individual of the interaction and experience necessary for emotional growth and development. When the treatment itself becomes central, as in hemodialysis or transplantation, it can replace other dimensions of life and virtually become life itself' (Scharschmidt 1984). Some patients grow tired of the frequent visits to the hospital for tests, come to resent the drug regimen, and want to break free from the strict lifestyle (Caplan *et al.* 1989). These patients are then often labelled noncompliant, and sometimes disparaged.

As with any treatment that carries risk, the decision to recommend an organ transplant requires a careful balancing of benefits and harms. It is a matter of net health risk reduction; short- and long-term risks of transplantation are weighed against the risks of not offering a transplant to a patient with progressive, usually endstage, disease. Where the extension of life is the major objective of organ transplantation, it is the best possible treatment for carefully selected patients. However, it is a mistake to conclude automatically that every person whose life would be extended prefers this to a quicker death whereby he or she would be spared further pain, disability, dependency, and, at times, concern over heavy financial and psychosocial burdens for loved ones.

The problem for physicians attending potential organ recipients (including consultation psychiatrists) is to be clear that they must act in the best interests of the patient as the patient sees them, not as family members or the medical team defines them. Whether because of love or guilt, some families attempt to coerce patients to accept transplantation when this is unwelcome. Physicians must bear in mind that patients alone, when competent, have the final say (Annas 1983).

Selection of recipients

Throughout the world, tragically, many people die while awaiting a donor organ for a needed transplant. In the United States, some 15 000 more donor hearts (Evans *et al.* 1986) and more than 20 000 kidneys (Kolata 1983) are thought to be needed annually. As will be noted below, it is likely that organs will remain in short supply for the foreseeable future. How, then, should this scarce resource be allocated? As Childress (1970) asked more than 20 years ago 'Who shall live when all cannot live?'. This question, which arises whenever a scarce new drug or procedure first becomes available, is as much moral as it is technical. On which principles can life-preserving resources be provided to some while being denied to others? The first successful kidney transplants focused public and scholarly attention on this age-old problem. Philosophers and theologians in profusion joined health care professionals and the lay media in debating this issue. Jonsen (1989) has lucidly summarized the voluminous arguments concerning organ allocation by pointing out that the basic question is whether social utility or egalitarianism should be the guiding principle. Proponents of social utility (e.g. Basson 1979; Rescher 1969) point out that some persons are in a position to return more to society for the investment that society makes in all its members, and they argue that social worth should be a major explicit consideration in allocation. Others note that, whatever the publicly declared criteria might be for receiving a scarce organ, social worth or even frank personal favouritism in any event motivates transplant teams to allow certain potential recipients to 'jump the queue' (Willard 1980). Opponents of this utilitarian approach, for example, Childress (1970), Katz and Capron (1975), and Winslow (1982), point out that it is not possible to design standards of social contribution that take into account the multiplicity of human characteristics that are socially useful, and even if it were possible they could not be applied fairly. More fundamentally, assessments of social worth ignore the dignity and value of all human lives. In all major religions, human beings are regarded as equal in the sight of God.

During the past three decades, hospital transplant teams have developed procedures for justly allocating organs. As Rawls (1971) pointed out, while it is not possible to guarantee a just outcome for all persons, we can attempt to create just procedures. Generally, technical medical criteria are employed to determine the relevant pool of potential recipients for transplants, using conventional standards which are more or less objective. They include constituency factors (e.g. geographic boundaries), progress-of-science factors (e.g. during the experimental phase good prognosis candidates may be favoured to establish the procedure) and prospect-of-success factors (Rescher 1969). To the extent that these factors are not strictly objective and call for judgements, it is important to ensure that these are made on relevant factors. For example, since both benefit and burdens of medical research should be justly distributed, it would be unfair for the poor and the unsophisticated to be subjects for transplantation in the experimental phase while the well-off and well-educated are over-represented among recipients once the procedure has become routine (Christopherson 1982).

Psychiatrists and psychologists are often called upon to predict the potential impact of psychiatric disorders or personality features on the prospect of success following a transplant. The considerations involved in this assessment are discussed in Chapters 2 and 3 and elsewhere in this book. As described in these chapters, much controversy has been generated with regard to the role of psychiatric factors in selecting patients for transplants. To deny patients a medical procedure purely on the basis of a psychiatric disorder is unwarranted, and a careful assessment of the individual case is necessary. Further, by means of death by suicide, serious psychiatric disorders are well represented in persons providing cadaveric organs for donation. To deny this same resource to emotionally disturbed patients risks a substantial disruption in the fair distribution of health care resources. Others have argued previously that the resources allocated to transplantation could be used in other ways to improve the condition of many more persons (The National Task Force on Organ Transplantation 1986; Welch and Larson 1988; Leaf 1980).

Psychiatrists who provide consultations on applicants to transplant pro- grammes are in a position of divided loyalties (Gellman 1986; Murray 1986) between their obligations to the patient, the transplant team, and to society. Psychiatrists and others are trained to elicit personal information from patients. Typically, this skill is used to facilitate a therapeutic alliance with the patient and to assist with the resolution of their emotional distress. However, in the context of a transplant assessment, the information elicited may be used to deny the person a life-sustaining surgical treatment. Due to this discrepancy between how patients may expect psychiatrists to conduct themselves, and the reality of the consulting relationship with the transplant team, patients need to be informed beforehand that information which they provide to psychosocial assessment personnel may be considered in making a decision about whether to offer transplantation.

Organ procurement

As has already been noted, there is a shortage of organs for transplantation, relative to need. As improvements in surgical techniques and immuno-suppressive therapy make organ transplantation the treatment of choice for more and more seriously ill people, the demand for donated organs has increased more rapidly than the supply. Making more organs available has become a health policy imperative. However, there are ethical as well as technical problems associated with the procurement of both cadaveric and living donor organs.

Cadaveric organ donation is, of course, more desirable in that the recipient is likely to benefit and the donor, having been declared dead due to the cessation of cardiac or respiratory function or having undergone brain death, cannot suffer physical harm. Unfortunately, no method of ensuring sufficient donation of cadaveric organs that is both effective and ethically acceptable has been found to date.

Familial consent for removal of organs in anticipation of the imminent death of an injured family member is the most common method. However, health care professionals in intensive care units and emergency rooms find it difficult to approach distraught grieving families and, busy with the care of other seriously ill patients, often do not take the time required to help them to feel comfortable about the organ donation. Staff must be sensitive enough to encourage organ donation without pressuring or coercing families (Caplan 1983). A further problem is that family members do not necessarily know what the dying patient would have wanted and, therefore, may not be morally valid substitute decision makers. Indeed, at times families will refuse permission for organ retrieval even when the patient has previously indicated preparedness to donate organs. It is not surprising, in view of these problems and the reluctance on the part of health care professionals to undertake a requesting procedure for which they may not be trained or inclined, that familial consent yields insufficient organs.

Required request is an attempt to overcome this difficulty. Laws obliging physicians and/or hospitals to ensure that the family is asked to donate the organs of the deceased have been enacted in over 40 US states (Caplan 1988) and the Canadian provinces of Ontario and Manitoba. The practical difficulty with legally mandated required request is that the compliance can be perfunctory and ineffective when health professionals resent the imposed obligation (Houlihan 1987). The ethical problems of encouraging organ donation without coercion, and families not knowing or not respecting the wishes of the deceased, remain.

Routine referral is a variant of required request proposed by Prottas (1988) to bypass the reluctance of intensive care unit staff. Hospitals would be required to inform trained organ procurement teams of all admissions which could result in death compatible with transplantable cadaveric organs. These teams, rather than the professionals treating the patient, would be responsible for obtaining consent for organ retrieval at the point of death. However, their involvement might well be experienced as an intrusion by the treating team. Patients and their families could become concerned that all necessary treatment might not be given in the interests of securing organs for transplantation. Further, this approach would necessitate some loss of confidentiality about the diagnoses and prognoses of these patients.

Voluntary donations by advance directive, for example through donor cards or signed authorization on drivers' licences, is an ethically desirable approach. The donor, presumed to be competent and informed, altruistically donates body parts to be retrieved posthumously. Altruism and autonomy, both cherished values in our society, are thereby expressed. Unfortunately, there seems to be considerable resistance to carrying donor cards: in one survey only 14 per cent of people reported carrying these (Manninen and Evans 1985) and, in another, only 23 per cent of people who become donors did so as a result of carrying a donor card (Miller 1987). As psychiatrists well know, many people have difficulty considering the inevitability of their death and others have disturbing fantasies about posthumous dismemberment. For some persons, signing an advance directive permitting organ retrieval seems to be emotionally equivalent to having their deaths declared prematurely or even hastened. Furthermore, when familial consent is sought and denied, even in the presence of a signed organ donor card, the family's wishes are usually given precedence, despite the infringement on the self-determination of the deceased.

Presumed consent is a policy adopted in some countries (Stuart *et al.* 1981). Individuals are presumed to have consented to the removal of their organs upon death unless they have indicated otherwise during their lifetime. A more paternalistic version of this policy, adopted by several countries, grants physicians complete authority to remove organs for transplant irrespective of the previously-expressed wishes of the deceased or the family. Nevertheless, in most countries with presumed consent legislation, physicians are not prepared to retrieve organs without the family's agreement because of the obvious risk of infringing on the family's sensibilities or religious beliefs. In societies where personal autonomy is highly valued, a presumed consent policy will clearly be unacceptable; indeed in one United States poll, only 7 per cent of respondents stated that doctors should have the authority to remove organs without the consent of the deceased and the next of kin (Manninen and Evans 1985). Although it is not yet entirely clear to what extent a person continues to have legal rights to tissues or organs once these are removed from the body, or after death, in our society there is consensus that in both life and death the integrity of the body should be respected and not violated without consent.

An incentive-based advance directive organ registry has been proposed in which all adults are encouraged to register their directives regarding organ donation (Kleinman and Lowy 1989). Those persons who, voluntarily, agree to permit all usable organs to be retrieved for transplantation at the time of death would receive priority should they themselves require a transplant at a time when there is a shortage of organs. This proposal would shift the focus of decision making from the families of the deceased to all individuals who are both potential organ donors and recipients. The attempt is to strike an acceptable balance by creating an incentive to donate organs while respecting the autonomy of potential donors.

The need to develop imaginative ways of increasing the supply of cadaveric organs is emphasized by the recent resurgence of enthusiasm for living organ donations. In the early days of solid organ transplantation, living donor kidney transplants were decidedly more successful than cadaveric transplants. With the great improvement in immunosuppressant and surgical techniques, the advantage of living donor transplants has been greatly reduced. Although there remain situations where only living organ transplants are possible, many of these are performed nowadays when there is a shortage of cadaveric organs.

There are a number of ethical problems associated with living organ donations. Foremost, of course, is the risk to the donors. Nowhere else in medicine is a healthy organ removed from a healthy person without the procedure intended to be of benefit to that individual. When an organ is transplanted from a volunteer living donor the major benefit is to the recipient, the donor receiving only the satisfaction of having helped a fellow human being, often a close relative. It is assumed that the risk to the donor, presumed to be low, is outweighed by the prolongation of or improvement to the life of the recipient. However, while every effort is made to minimize the risk to the donor, the perioperative and long-term complications are not negligible (Dunn *et al.* 1986). Living donors of a kidney are subject to infection, pulmonary emboli, injury to liver, spleen and adrenal glands, pancreatitis, and the long-term risk of hypertension. Transplantation of parts of single organs such as lung, liver, or pancreas are even more risky for donors. It is essential for donors to be fully informed of these risks before they consent.

That ethical concerns in such situations can be identified, studied and addressed adequately has been shown by Singer *et al.* (1989). Nevertheless there are some problem areas that, together with the risks to healthy donors, make living organ donation at best an ethical compromise. Truly voluntary informed consent is the ethical bedrock of all medical procedures, including of course, the removal of organs for transplantation. But when a close relative's life is in the balance can consent be truly voluntary? The prospective donor must contend with feelings of guilt about any reluctance to donate an organ and the fear of criticism or rejection by other family members. Subtle or overt pressure by the family can occur. The medical team, including the psychiatric consultant who is very often involved, must delicately balance encouragement of life-extending organ donation and protection of the right of the potential donor to refuse without guilt. To facilitate this, careful psychiatric and psychological evaluation is indicated and, often, psychiatric intervention as well.

While living organ donation is an altruistic, praiseworthy act of self-sacrifice, physicians must reconcile it with the need to override a fundamental principle of medical ethics, to do no harm, and with the traditional reluctance to use one human being, the donor, as a means to benefit a second person rather than as an end in itself. Needless to say, where these problems are properly taken into account and the decision is made to proceed with a living organ transplant, the result can be most gratifying for recipient, donor, and treatment team.

Trade and commerce in organs

Like any commodity that is both desirable for some people and in short supply, transplantable organs have economic value. It is not surprising that a commerce in organs has developed surreptitiously in countries where this is considered unethical, and more openly elsewhere (Sells 1989). American cadaver organs have been transplanted into wealthy patients from other countries while thousands of Americans who cannot match the fee requested for the surgery remain on waiting lists. Living organs (mostly kidneys) have been sold by poor people in Latin America for transplantation in the United States and by poor people in India, Pakistan, and Bangladesh for transplantation in Britain and Saudi Arabia. Prisoners in the Philippines have been reported to donate organs in the hope of gaining an early parole. These are only examples of what appears to be a widespread phenomenon.

The reactions of both ethicists and the public in North America and Western Europe has largely been negative on several grounds. First, commerce in organs obviously favours rich recipients who often come from countries where cadaveric organs or surgery are in especially short supply due to religious, cultural, or budgetary restrictions (Sells 1989). Therefore, it is considered unjust, especially in countries such as Britain, Canada, and the Scandinavian countries, where a right to all necessary health care irrespective of ability to pay has been publicly accepted. Second, in the Judaeo-Christian tradition the human body is regarded as a sacred God-given gift which, in the most fundamental view, does not belong to the person and is not his or hers to dispose of. To sacrifice an organ to save another's life is considered virtuous, but if the object is financial profit it is considered demeaning to personhood. A similar objection stems from the idea that we do not possess our bodies; we *are* our bodies. Third, some argue that altruism in giving and gratitude in receiving are fundamental foundations of human relations (Murray 1987). Organ donation is an expression of altruism and to replace this with free market trade in organs would alter the very nature of our being in an undesirable fashion (Dickens 1987). Finally, were trade in organs to become socially accepted, a number of undesirable scenarios can be envisioned: would poor persons without health insurance be pressured into providing a kidney to cover hospital costs (Ad Hoc Committee of the Harvard Medical School 1968)? Just as a US citizen with $50 000 in the bank would be considered ineligible for welfare, would a person with two healthy kidneys valued at $50 000 each be regarded as ineligible? Would a potential organ seller be less truthful about medical history or lifestyle in order to protect the market value of the organ? Would patients and their families lean against long-term or palliative care if profit can be made from a more immediate death and organ sale?

While these arguments against commerce in organs seem persuasive, important points are made in rebuttal. If free market enterprise, in which one's assets are exploited creatively, is valued in our culture, then why is trade in organs, which can be mutually beneficial to seller and buyer, so repugnant? The idea will certainly not be repugnant to the patient about to die or tied to burdensome haemodialysis because no donated kidneys are available. Further, depriving the poor of what may be their only means of improving their families' circumstances in countries of low opportunity can be seen as unjust. Dickens (1987) has pointed out that the English Common Law tradition does not necessarily oppose commerce in organs: 'when a person at imminent risk of death purchases a potential means of survival in apparent contradiction of legislation, the defence of necessity might be accepted'.

Nevertheless, the weight of opinion in North America and Europe is clearly against trade in organs and either legislation or guidelines prohibiting payment for organs have been enacted. Organs are to be transplanted into the most appropriate recipients on the basis of medical, not financial criteria. However, in India and some other countries, it has been impossible to pass such laws and many physicians are satisfied that the sum of benefits to both organ donor and recipient justify the practice (Sells 1989).

Other ethical issues

Because of space limitations, this chapter will not include discussions of other transplant-related issues. Some of these will simply be mentioned briefly and a few key references provided.

Brain death criteria

Brain death criteria have become accepted largely because of the need to preserve organs between the point of cessation of brain function (including brain stem) and the time when a transplant can be carried out (Ad Hoc Committee of the Harvard Medical School 1968). Criteria applying in the USA are specified in the Uniform Determination of Death Act and the report of the President's Commission for the Study of Ethical Problems in Medicine and Biomedical and Behavioral Research (1981). Some physicians are prepared to alter the definition even further, believing that cerebral death alone, even with some brain stem activity, should be sufficient to determine death (Grenvik 1988). This would enable anencephalic infants to be certified dead so that their organs can be legally transplanted. Needless to say, ethical concerns arise immediately.

Anencephalic infants as organ donors

Because there is an even greater shortage of children's organs for transplantation than adult organs, there has been, in some quarters, enthusiasm for the use of organs from anencephalics, infants born without most of the brain. Organs cannot legally be removed until at least brain death criteria are met. However, since anoxia may by that time render potential donor organs unfit for transplantation, anencephalic infants have been placed on life support systems until transplantation can be performed. While some justify this on utilitarian grounds, others are concerned about a procedure that is not for the benefit of the infant and treats him or her as a means to an end. A lively debate among ethicists has resulted (Harrison 1986; Annas 1987; Botkin 1988).

Xenografts

Transplants of a non-human organ to a human being have captured public attention particularly since the Baby Fae case (Kushner and Belliotti 1985). The ethical as well as the technical problems remain to be solved (American Medical Association Council on Scientific Affairs 1985; Drugan *et al.* 1989).

Conclusions

Organ transplantation is a modern medical marvel, dreamed of for centuries, but technically impossible until the present time. However, ethical implications of transplantation abound and have led to a large body of literature. Issues including informed consent, the distribution of resources, and commerce in donor organs have been reviewed in the present chapter. Each major development in the field (e.g. living–related donor transplant) entails complex ethical dilemmas which challenge our ability to synthesize moral opinions. The dialectic between organ transplant and bioethics will undoubtedly broaden in the future.

References

Ad Hoc Committee of the Harvard Medical School to Examine the Definition of Brain Death (1968). A definition of irreversible coma. *Journal of the American Medical Association*, 205, 337–40.
American Medical Association Council on Scientific Affairs (1985). Xenografts—

review of the literature and current status. *Journal of the American Medical Association*, 254, 3353–7.

Annas, G. J. (1983). Consent to the artificial heart: the lion and the crocodiles. *Hastings Center Report*, 13, 20–2.

Annas, G. J. (1987). From Canada with love: anencephalic newborns as organ donors? *Hastings Center Report*, 17, 36–8.

Basson, M. D. (1979). Choosing among candidates for scarce medical resources. *Journal of Medical Philosophy*, 4, 313–33.

Botkin, J. R. (1988). Anencephalic infants as organ donors. *Pediatrics*, 82, 250–6.

Caplan, A. L. (1983). Organ transplants: the costs of success. *Hastings Center Report*, 13, 23–32.

Caplan, A. L. (1988). Professional arrogance and public misunderstanding. *Hastings Center Report*, 18, 34–7.

Caplan, A. L., Annas, G., Bazell, R., Burrows, L., Miller, C., and Swazey, J. (1989). The gift of life: dilemmas in organ transplantation. *Mount Sinai Journal of Medicine*, 56, 395–405.

Childress, J. (1970). 'Who shall live when all cannot live'. *Soundings*, 53, 339–55.

Christopherson, L. K. (1982). 'To mend the heart': ethics and high technology. 2: heart transplants. *Hastings Center Report*, 12, 18–21.

Dickens, B. M. (1987). Legal and ethical issues in buying and selling organs. *Transplantation/Implantation Today*, 4, 15–21.

Drugan, A., Evans, W. J., and Evans, M. I. (1989). Fetal organ and xenograft transplantation. *American Journal of Obstetrics & Gynecology*, 160, 289–93.

Dunn, J. F., Nylander, W. A. Jr, Richie, R. E., Johnson, H. K., MacDonell, R. C. Jr, and Sawyers, J. L. (1986). Living related kidney donors: a 14-year experience. *Annals of Surgery*, 203, 637–43.

Evans, R. W. (1986). Cost-effectiveness analysis of transplantation. *Surgical Clinics of North America*, 66, 603–16.

Evans, R. W., Manninen, D. L., Garrison, L. P. Jr, and Maier, A. M. (1986). Donor availability as the primary determinant of the future of heart transplantation. *Journal of the American Medical Association*, 255, 1892–8.

Gellman, R. M. (1986). Divided loyalties: a physician's responsibilities in an information age. *Social Science and Medicine*, 23, 817–26.

Grenvik, A. (1988). Ethical dilemmas in organ donation and transplantation. *Critical Care Medicine*, 16, 1012–18.

Harrison, M. R. (1986). The anencephalic newborn as organ donor. *Hastings Center Report*, 16, 21–3.

Houlihan, P. (1987). Requesting organ donations: the hardest question to ask. *Canadian Medical Association Journal*, 137, 537–9.

Jonsen, A. R. (1989). Ethical issues in organ transplantation. In *Medical Ethics* (ed. R. M. Veatch). (Jones and Bartlett, Boston.)

Katz, J. and Capron, A. M. (1975). *Catastrophic diseases: who decides what?* (Russell Sage Foundation, New York).

Kleinman, I. and Lowy, F. H. (1989). Cadaveric organ donation: ethical considerations for a new approach. *Canadian Medical Association Journal*, 141, 107–10.

Kolata, G. (1983). Organ shortage clouds new transplant era. *Science*, 221, 32–3.

Kushner, T. and Belliotti, R. (1985). Baby Fae: a beastly business. *Journal of Medical Ethics*, 11, 178–83.

Leaf, A. (1980). The M.G.H. trustees say no to heart transplants. *New England Journal of Medicine*, 302, 1087–8.

Manninen, D. L. and Evans, R. W. (1985). Public attitudes and behavior regarding organ donation. *Journal of the American Medical Association*, 253, 3111–15.

Medical World News (1988). Heart transplant: second decade reveals promise, future hurdles (editorial). *Medical World News*, 52–60.

Miller, M. (1987). A proposed solution to the present organ donation crisis based on a hard look at the past. *Circulation*, 75, 20–8.

Murray, T. H. (1986). Divided loyalties for physicians: social context and moral problems. *Social Science and Medicine*, 23, 827–32.

Murray, T. H. (1987). Gifts of the body and the needs of strangers. *Hastings Center Report*, 17, 30–8.

New York State Task Force on Life and the Law (1988). Transplantation in New York State: The procurement and distribution of organs and tissues (New York City, January 1988).

The National Task Force on Organ Transplantation. (1986). *Organ transplantation: issues and recommendations* (US Department of Health and Home Services, Washington DC).

President's Commission for the Study of Ethical Problems in Medicine and Biomedical and Behavioral Research: Defining Death (1981) (US Government Printing Office, Washington, DC), pp. 31–42.

Prottas, J. (1988). Shifting responsibilities in organ procurement: a plan for routine referral. *Journal of the American Medical Association*, 260, 832–3.

Rawls, J. (1971). *A theory of justice* (Harvard University Press, Cambridge MA).

Rescher, N. (1969). Allocation of exotic lifesaving medical therapy. *Ethics*, 79, 173–86.

Scharschmidt, B. F. (1984). Human liver transplantation: analysis of data on 540 patients from four centers. *Hepatology*, 4, 95S–101S.

Sells, R. A. (1989). Ethics and priorities of organ procurement and allocation. *Transplantation Proceedings*, 21, 1391–4.

Shaw, B. W. Jr, Wood, R. P., Gordon, R. D., Iwatsuki, S., Gillquist, W. P., and Starzl, T. E. (1985). Influence of selected patient variables and operative blood loss on six-month survival following liver transplantation. *Seminars in Liver Disease*, 5, 385–93.

Singer, P. A., Siegler, M., Whitington, P. F., Lantos, J. D., Emond, J. C., Thistlethwaite, J. R., *et al.* (1989). Ethics of liver transplantation with living donors. *New England Journal of Medicine*, 321, 620–2.

Stuart, F. P., Veith, F. J., and Cranford, R. E. (1981). Brain death laws and patterns of consent to remove organs for transplantation from cadavers in the United States and 28 other countries. *Transplantation*, 31, 238–44.

Tancredi, L. (1985). Some ethical dilemmas in emergency psychiatry. In *Emergency psychiatry at the crossroads* (eds F. R. Lipton and S. M. Goldfinger). (Jossey-Bass, San Francisco.)

Welch, H. G. and Larson, E. B. (1988). Dealing with limited resources: the Oregon decision to curtail funding for organ transplantation. *New England Journal of Medicine*, 319, 171–3.

Willard, L. D. (1980). Scarce medical resources and the right to refuse selection by artificial chance. *Journal of Medical Philosophy*, 5, 225–9.

Winslow, G. R. (1982). *Triage and justice: the ethics of rationing life-saving medical resources* (University of California Press, Berkeley).

9   Organ donation and procurement

S. Youngner

The psychosocial and ethical problems of live and cadaveric organ donations are separate and unique. There are also two general categories of cadaver donors; those who are dead by traditional standards and those 'beating-heart' cadavers who are dead according to a new criterion, the irreversible loss of all brain function.

Organs from cadavers

Some organs or tissues can be successfully retrieved from persons who have died traditional deaths, that is, their hearts have irreversibly stopped pumping blood and their breathing has irreversibly ceased. Deprived of oxygen and nutrients, the major organs and organ systems (e.g., brain, liver, kidney, gastrointestinal tract) quickly become irreversibly damaged and unsuitable for transplantations. Other tissues and organs, such as corneas and bone, are more resilient, and may be obtained during a period following death.

Inadequate organ donation is the rate-limiting step in the organ procurement shortage. Each year there are some 20 000 potential donors (i.e., patients maintained on ventilators) who have suffered catastrophic brain injuries resulting in irreversible loss of all brain function. Of these, only 10–20 per cent become donors. Even when patients have signed donor cards, families have final veto power and health professionals must always honour their refusals. However, some of these refusals might have been avoided. Health professionals have been too reluctant, in many cases, to present families with the option of organ donation despite public opinion polls in which the overwhelming majority of citizens endorse organ transplantation. By 1988, a large majority of American states had legal requirements that hospitals routinely give families of 'brain-dead' patients the donation option. Yet, in spite of these efforts, the number of organ donors declined for the first time in 1989. The reasons are complex, but when we look at the experience of personnel working in these areas, several pertinent observations are apparent.

The persistence of the adjective brain-dead in clinical and lay parlance suggests that there may be confusion about whether such patients really are dead. Ordinarily, we regard death as an absolute, all-or-nothing state. However, this notion of death seems less applicable to patients who are maintained on ventilators, but who have an irreversible loss of brain function. These individuals constitute a new class of dead patients in whom a considerable amount of life remains. Confusion about this concept persists and may be associated with concerns that organ retrieval kills the patient.

The confusion about brain death amongst health professionals is further illustrated by a study conducted at four Cleveland hospitals (Youngner *et al.* 1989). A sample of 195 physicians and nurses likely to be involved in organ procurement for transplantation was interviewed regarding their knowledge, personal concepts, and attitudes concerning brain death and organ donation. Although 95 per cent of those questioned personally believed that brain-dead patients were dead, only 35 per cent identified the correct legal and medical criteria for determining death. Most respondents (58 per cent) did not use a coherent concept of death consistently. Of the 95 per cent who personally thought brain-dead patients were dead, fully one-third gave explanations indicating they really believed them to be alive (e.g. 'They will die soon no matter what you do' or 'Their quality of life is unacceptable').

In addition, organ retrieval surgery is mutilating, particularly in cases of 'total body' donations. Such mutilation may seem disrespectful to the dead, even if it serves worthwhile goals. Respect for the dead in general, and for dead bodies in particular, is consistent with our cultural and moral traditions. This is true for bodies that lie in graves that are centuries old. Feelings about recently dead bodies, in which the status of the soul or person is unclear (from both psychological and religious perspectives), are even more complicated and potentially problematic.

Finally, even the most invasive and disfiguring medical and surgical interventions might be justified by the intended benefit to the patient. However, the rationale for organ retrieval involves the welfare of the recipient rather than that of the donor. Health professionals may be concerned that using brain-dead patients for this purpose may represent a deviation from their usual role and a conflict of interest regarding the needs of the donor and the recipient.

These three observations are a cause for profound ambivalence about organ donation and retrieval among health professionals and lay persons alike. On the one hand, the idea of giving organs to save the lives of potential recipients is uplifting. On the other hand, the thought of taking organs from the dead bodies of loved ones, patients, or our imagined dead selves may be disturbing. Potential organ donors and their families who are enthusiastic about donation in theory may fail to implement these lofty sentiments because of the concerns about transplantation described above. In fact, only 14 per cent of the adult population signs donor cards (Manninen and Evans 1985), and families refuse donation in some of these cases.

'Required request' laws were developed following early indications that 80–90 per cent of those who were asked agreed to donate organs. However, required request laws have not been a great success. Some families who were not approached in the past were correctly perceived by health professionals to be opposed to the donation. Asking these families simply results in more negative responses. Also, health professionals themselves may be ambivalent about organ retrieval and confused about brain death. Such individuals will not be enthusiastic about informing and asking grieving families to consent to organ donation by the patient.

Paradoxically, despite initial widespread recognition of brain-death and near-universal acceptance of organ transplantation, inadequate procurement of cadaveric organs continues to be a serious problem. Confusion about brain death, worry that organ retrieval may exploit brain-dead patients, and concern about the proper treatment of dead bodies all contribute to the organ shortage. Better education and acceptance over time may help to resolve these problems. However, more coercive policies, which ignore or trample on fears and sensibilities, however irrational, may only make matters worse.

Brain death

The major organs such as heart, liver, kidney, pancreas, and intestines must come from brain-dead patients who are being maintained on ventilators. In 1968, an *Ad Hoc* Committee (1968) at Harvard Medical School recommended that brain death be recognized as a new standard for declaring death. One of the Committee's stated motives was to facilitate organ transplantation. Since the publication of the Harvard Committee's recommendations, brain death has been legally recognized in almost every jurisdiction in the United States. Despite this seeming widespread acceptance, problems remain which have a direct bearing on organ retrieval. Before discussing these problems further, some of the clinical characteristics of brain death will be reviewed.

The medical and legal criterion for declaring a patient dead, using brain-oriented criteria, is the irreversible loss of all function in the brain, including the brain stem. Such patients are inevitably the victims of sudden and catastrophic events such as trauma (automobile accidents, gunshot wounds), intracranial events such as ruptured aneurysms, or global central nervous system ischaemia. Due to the development of critical care units with mechanical ventilators, patients who would have previously died rapid traditional deaths can now be maintained for hours or days. Maintenance of individuals in this state allows the successful retrieval of healthy organs.

The concept of brain death is supported by the following characteristics of patients who are being supported by medical technology, after they have suffered irreversible loss of all brain function:

1.   The clinical diagnosis of irreversible loss of all brain function is relatively easy to make, except in newborns and young infants. It can be made quickly at the bedside by a competent neurologist, neurosurgeon, or other critical care physician.

2.   Once the diagnosis has been made, the prognosis is entirely predictable and dismal, despite maximum efforts. The patient will never regain consciousness, will develop asystole, and will die by traditional criteria usually within hours or days. There have been no reported exceptions to this outcome in hundreds of cases reported in the literature. In no other medical condition can we so accurately predict, not only the certainty, but also the timing of death.

3.   Even if the notion of brain death is not fully accepted, the quality of life in the short time remaining before traditional death is unacceptable. The patient is unconscious and maintained only with maximum invasive intervention.

These characteristics of brain-dead persons, and the fact that they are an excellent source of major organs for transplantation, have facilitated a public policy which recognizes irreversible loss of all brain function as an acceptable criterion for declaring death and taking organs. However, the psychological, cognitive, and cultural ramifications of organ retrieval are immense.

Cognitive dissonance and brain-dead patients

Patients with irreversible loss of all brain function may be legally dead, but they still contain a great deal of life (Youngner *et al.* 1985). Their hearts beat spontaneously, pumping oxygenated blood throughout their bodies and allowing organs to metabolize nutrients, produce urine, etc. Their chests move up and down (albeit due to a ventilator) and they are warm and retain a healthy colour. These reminders of human life may affect our behaviour toward this new class of dead persons. Our technological interventions to maintain these individuals may be even more aggressive than those used to treat other patients who are more clearly alive. Brain-dead patients are closely monitored and any deviations in such physiological functions as blood pressure, blood oxygen saturation, or heart rate are quickly and efficiently corrected by attentive physicians and nurses. Some of these patients are even candidates for cardiopulmonary resuscitation when a clearly living and conscious patient in the next bed may have been designated as 'do-not-resuscitate'.

It has been estimated that 95 per cent of organ donors are declared dead in the intensive care unit. Caring for these patients and their families is a demanding and stressful task for health professionals. Despite the criteria of brain-death being met, nurses may find themselves comforting such patients or warning them before painful procedures. Although patients are legally dead when irreversible loss of all brain function has been determined, this time is rarely noted as the time of death on death certificates. Instead, death is recorded as the time when the ventilator is disconnected in the operating room. Instead of being sent to the morgue, as are other dead patients, brain-dead patients are sent to the operating room.

Brain-dead patients also present a unique set of problems and paradoxes for operating room personnel. At first, these patients appear not unlike the usual patient who is quite alive, but fully anaesthetized. They are cleaned and draped just like living patients. Sterile technique is just as rigorous. An anaesthetist is at the patient's head and monitors vital signs, adjusting ventilator settings, oxygen levels, and blood pressure. Surgeons are careful to tie off bleeders and may indeed administer blood in the course of surgery, which itself may take several hours. After long hours of arduous surgery, the anaesthetist must turn off the ventilator, thus halting all the remaining life functions. The surgeons who do not leave the operating room with the viable organs then close the body cavities, generally in one pass, using coarse retention sutures and large needles. Other surgeons may then appear on the scene to retrieve bones, eyes, and skin. These procedures are particularly disfiguring and invasive. Nurses may witness teams of orthopaedic surgeons working simultaneously on each arm and leg, removing long bones with saws and chisels and replacing them with broom handles or wooden dowels. Removal of skin and eyes may seem equally gruesome. These realities of organ retrieval can be extremely distressing to operating room personnel. Nurses may experience terror at being left alone in the operating room to clean up, put in a plastic bag, and deliver to the morgue a corpse from which all major organs as well as eyes, skin, and bones have been removed.

Organs from living donors

Living donors are an important source when the needed organs are paired (e.g. the kidneys) or when the tissues are replenishable (e.g. bone marrow). Living donors may be divided into two categories: genetically related and genetically unrelated. Unrelated donors may in turn be divided into two categories: emotionally related (e.g. a spouse) or strangers.

Living–related donors

About 20 per cent of the kidney transplants in the United States each year use kidneys from living donors; by far the greatest number of these donors are genetically related. Kidneys from living–related donors have several potential advantages for the recipient. Enhanced allograft compatibility results in greater longevity for both organ and recipient and decreased morbidity for the recipient. However, this difference in results with living–related and cadaveric kidney donations has diminished as techniques for matching immunological compatibility and preventing graft rejection have improved. None the less, a small advantage for live donation persists.

The waiting period for cadaveric kidneys may be as long as two years for certain blood types. Decreased quality of life on dialysis during this period of time may be psychologically damaging and associated with financial instability, and social dysfunction. Potential recipients often must carry beepers, knowing that they may be called at any minute or not for months. This uncertainty precludes effective planning in other aspects of life and may reinforce the loss of control experienced by the patient.

The advantages of living–related kidney donation for the recipient are real, but not overwhelming. These advantages must be weighed against the advantages and disadvantages to the donor. Removal of a kidney is major surgery entailing general anaesthesia and considerable pain and discomfort. The risk of perioperative mortality for the donor is estimated to be 0.06 per cent (Singer 1990). A larger number of donors may experience complications from the surgery. In a multi-centre study of 536 kidney donors (using a mailed questionnaire), Smith *et al.* (1986) identified 97 (18.1 per cent) donors who reported 142 medical problems which they considered to be significant and a result of the retrieval surgery. Evaluation revealed that only 24 of these were complications directly caused by kidney donation, including 22 cases of postoperative infection and two cases in which donors developed pneumothorax during surgery. No clear-cut long-term sequelae have been identified. Emphasizing such morbidity and pointing out that 20 persons have died donating kidneys, Starzl (1985) has argued that this risk is not worth taking, considering the improved efficacy of transplants from cadaveric donors. However, most centres consider the chance of serious complications to be small enough to justify the donation.

Potential donors may feel coerced into donating, and true informed consent cannot be realized. Psychological morbidity from the donation may include resentment about the pressure to donate, anxiety about the surgery and hospitalization, and depression following the loss of an organ and disturbed family relationships. Gifts often imply obligations for the recipient. Misunderstandings about the nature and extent of such obligations may cause tension or conflict. However, most studies suggest that organ donors have found the experience to be a positive one. Enhanced psychological well-being may result from making a gift of life to a loved one.

Smith *et al.* (1986) reported that of 536 kidney donors, 84 per cent believed that they had been adequately informed about all aspects of the donation. Some 23 per cent of donors reported that donation had caused financial hardship. A substantial majority said that neither their families (86 per cent) or health professionals (94 per cent) had attempted to influence their decision. Fourteen per cent reported direct pressure, particularly not to donate. The authors noted that individuals were more likely to receive pressure from their family to donate if the recipient was a parent, while family pressure not to donate was substantially more prevalent if the recipient was a sibling. One-third of the 27 study subjects who were divorced or separated at the time of the study indicated that donation was one of many reasons for the failed marriage. Less than 2.0 per cent of donors reported a decrease in the quality of their relationship with the recipient. It is significant that 97 per cent of all study subjects reaffirmed their decision regardless of the graft's success or the financial distress they experienced. Smith *et al.* (1986) conclude that 'transplantation from a living–related donor continues to be an attractive therapeutic alternative for patients with end-stage renal disease, associated with few negative social and medical consequences'.

A five to ten year follow-up study comparing the psychological sequelae in fourteen kidney donors with those in nine persons who were refused on medical grounds showed no difference in psychiatric morbidity (Sharma and Enoch 1987). Eight of nine donors expressed positive feelings about the donation. One patient reported feeling neglected after the operation. The authors concluded that, irrespective of outcome, the majority of donors feel positively toward kidney donation.

Fellner and Marshall (1968) studied twelve kidney donors and reported a follow-up of ten of these donors one decade later (Marshall and Fellner 1977). One of the interesting observations in the first study was that eight of the twelve initial subjects made their donation decision immediately. The other four subjects were aware of considerable ambivalence, but consented passively to the evaluation during the selection process, finally committing themselves only after they were identified as the most suitable donor. In regard to informed consent, all donors reported that they had 'not really been very curious or interested in what the doctors were telling them' (Fellner and Marshall 1968). The authors concluded that 'the donors avoided the predecision conflict, either by making a split-second decision, or alternatively, by letting the selection process decide for them. In all cases, the decision was upheld and the subjects remained committed to their course of action. Once the decision had been made, the donor carefully refrained from considering further data and engaged in maneuvers which permitted him to never vary in his decision or even to question it'. Other authors have commented on these seemingly spontaneous decisions by donors. For example, Bernstein and Simmons (1974) reported that of 26 potential adolescent donors (ages 16–20) 50 per cent made a '. . . rapid, instantaneous decision, that is they volunteered to donate immediately upon hearing of the need and did not reconsider this decision later'.

Fellner and Marshall (1968) also commented on 'the impressive increase in self-esteem and perceived life style changes as a long-term result'. They attribute these phenomenon to: the donor's belief in the good of what they were doing for the recipient; their positive (actual or symbolic) relationship with their physician; the positive emotional reinforcement from recipient and family; and the considerable attention paid to them by friends, acquaintances, and the news media.

A decade later, when Marshall and Fellner (1977) reassessed ten of the twelve original donors, only one reported a sense of increased vulnerability and limitations on his life. This was a man whose brother had died $4\frac{1}{2}$ years after donation. The donor complained of constant pain in his wound site and a diminished sex life which he partially attributed to the surgery. The authors also noted that, 'the donors whose recipients had died expressed more negative feeling and ambivalence about donation'. However, asked if they would do it over again, all stated that they would. Despite the decrease in attention over the years, study subjects felt they were still benefiting in terms of psychological or personal growth. Many used phrases to describe their enhanced well-being quite similar to the ones they had used ten years earlier. While acknowledging the conscious presence of ambivalence, especially if the recipient had died, the authors conclude that 'it is clear that, at least among our group of subjects, the donation has had a considerable positive, long-lasting impact upon the donors' lives. The idea that donors lose a kidney but get nothing in return is untenable.'

These positive reports do not confirm the caveats and cautions published early in the history of living–related kidney donations. Kemph (1966), for example, reported on donor status in twelve renal transplants. He concluded that 'although all donors were consciously altruistic, there was considerable unconscious resentment toward the recipients in some cases and toward those hospital personnel who requested or encouraged the transplant. They had given something and got nothing in return.' Unfortunately, Kemph does not reveal how this 'unconscious resentment' was expressed or detected. Nor does he give clinical examples. By contrast, Simmons *et al.* (1977) report improved self-esteem and positive long-term outcome in donors.

However, questionnaires or structured interviews with large numbers of patients may not detect subtle discontent or ambivalence. For example, Bernstein and Simmons (1974) reported that only 5 of 26 potential adolescent donors, '. . . were concerned about the surgical procedure'. This figure seems to minimize a concern about surgery that would be quite normal and expected, leading Mattson (1974) to question the depth of information gathered.

Thus, while the overall evidence convincingly presents a positive psychological outcome for living–related donors, there may still be potential conflicts, stresses, and regrets for the individual donors. Recognition that such problems exist does not argue against living donors, but emphasizes the need for individualized approaches.

Living–unrelated donors

Living–unrelated donors pose many of the same problems as do living–related donors. Unrelated donors are either emotionally related (like spouse or friend) or strangers. The motivations for a spouse to donate a kidney to a husband or wife are self-evident. But why would a stranger want to donate? Our society is generally suspicious of strangers who offer to put themselves at risk. Some have criticized this attitude, arguing that genuine altruism is often the motivating factor and should be honoured (Fellner and Schwartz 1971). As the organ shortage becomes more acute, attitudes toward more unconventional donors may change.

Conclusions

Organ transplantation involves not only putting organs in human beings to help them live; it also necessitates taking organs out from the bodies of others, living or dead. For each category there is a unique set of psychological and social problems, problems which reach to the core of human relationships and notions about respect for the body. Psychiatrists can contribute to the organ transplantation enterprise by helping patients and health professionals to understand and cope constructively with some of its more troubling aspects.

References

Ad Hoc Committee of the Harvard Medical School to Examine the Definition of Brain Death (1968). A definition of irreversible coma. *Journal of the American Medical Association*, 205, 337–40.

Bernstein, D. M. and Simmons, R. G. (1974). The adolescent kidney donor: the right to give. *American Journal of Psychiatry*, 31, 1338–42.

Fellner, C. H. and Marshall, J. R. (1968). Twelve kidney donors. *Journal of the American Medical Association*, 206, 2703–7.

Fellner, C. H. and Schwartz, S. H. (1971). Altruism in disrepute: medical versus public attitudes toward the living organ donor. *New England Journal of Medicine*, 284, 582–5.

Kemph, J. P. (1966). Renal failure, artificial kidney and kidney transplant. *American Journal of Psychiatry*, 122, 1270–4.

Manninen, D. L. and Evans, R. W. (1985). Public attitudes and behavior regarding organ donation. *Journal of the American Medical Association*, 253, 3111–15.

Marshall, J. R. and Fellner, C. H. (1977). Kidney donors revisited. *American Journal of Psychiatry*, 134, 575–6.

Mattson, A. (1974). Discussion of Bernstein and Simmons article, "The adolescent kidney donor". *American Journal of Psychiatry*, 131, 1342–3.

Sharma, V. K. and Enoch, M. D. (1987). Psychological sequelae of kidney donation. A 5–10 year follow up study. *Acta Psychiatrica Scandinavica*, 75, 264–7.

Simmons, R. G., Klein, S. D., and Simmons, R. C. (1977). *The gift of life: the social and psychological impact of organ transplantation.* (Wiley, New York).

Singer, P. A. (1990). A review of public policies to procure and distribute kidneys for transplantation. *Archives of Internal Medicine*, 150, 523–7.

Smith, M. D., Kappell, D. F., Province, M. A., Hong, B. A., Robson, A. M., Dutton, S., *et al.* (1986). Living–related kidney donors: a multicenter study of donor education, socioeconomic adjustment, and rehabilitation. *American Journal of Kidney Diseases*, 8, 223–33.

Starzl, T. E. (1985). Will live organ donations no longer be justified? *Hastings Center Report*, 15, 5.

Youngner, S. J., Allen, M., Bartlett, E. T., Cascorbi, H. F., Hau, T., Jackson, D. L., *et al.*

(1985). Psychosocial and ethical implications of organ retrieval. *New England Journal of Medicine*, 313, 321–4.

Youngner, S. J., Landefeld, C. S., Coulton, C. J., Juknialis, B. W., and Leary, M. (1989). 'Brain death' and organ retrieval: A cross-sectional survey of knowledge and concepts among health professionals. *Journal of the American Medical Association*, 261, 2205–10.

10   Religious and spiritual perspectives on organ transplantation

D. Dixon

Organ transplantation brings to the fore several fundamental issues of religious concern. These issues are of primary importance for the devout, as both donor and recipient, but have also had a broad influence upon the attitudes of many persons and social groupings towards the transplant process. Prominent among these are the basic beliefs regarding the afterlife, the sanctity of the body, and the relationship between the body and the soul. Indeed, given that such issues are of central importance to most major theological systems, it could be said that few interventions in all of medicine rival organ transplantation in their implications for religious dogma and piety.

Any discussion of the religious perspective necessarily requires first an understanding of the pertinent beliefs of the major faiths. Of course, no brief survey can do justice to the variegated nature of each tradition, and general statements regarding theological doctrine must of necessity simplify and compromise. Indeed, there is as likely to be as much disagreement regarding fundamental issues within each religion as between different religions. With due acknowledgement of this limitation, a select sample of the major world faiths will be examined in regard to their approach towards organ transplantation. The sample will include representatives from the three main 'families' of religion—the Abrahamic religions, the religions arising from the Indian subcontinent, and the religions of the Far East.

The religions of Abraham

Judaism, Christianity, and Islam each trace their roots back to the patriarchal figure Abraham, who is mentioned in the sacred writings of all three, and who lived presumably in Syria and Palestine around 2000 BC. Beyond shared historical relations and cultural continuities, the Abrahamic religions also find common ground in their insistence on monotheism, their view of humanity as God's highest creation, and their understanding of the world as being divinely created, but not as being divine in itself (Ludwig 1989, pp. 75–8). Beyond such common visions, of course, each religion has acquired its own distinctive world view, with varying assertions, rituals, and theological constructs.

Judaism

The construct of most relevance for developing a Jewish understanding of the implications of organ transplant is the Jewish law. The term 'Halakhah', meaning 'way', refers to the code of law which addresses how a Jew should live his/her daily life. This law arises from the Hebrew scriptures which contain the written Torah, and is detailed in the Talmud, which contains the oral Torah.

It is a common misunderstanding to regard Jewish law as a static prescriptive or a corpus of external legalism, the observance of which demands little or no spiritual depth. On the contrary, Halakhah is a code of life whose observance effects spiritual transformation and whose very essence is one of dynamism, tension, and flexibility. This tension derives, in part, from the immutability of the scriptural and Talmudic tenets on the one hand, and the ongoing need to understand and apply these same tenets to new and specific circumstances on the other. The continuing process of interpretation and application is the challenge that has faced rabbinic scholars throughout the generations to the present time. It is within the context of Jewish law as an animate and dynamic agency that organ transplantation should be understood.

The relevant issues in transplantation are particularly suited for the dialectic of rabbinic interpretation (Weiss 1988). There are inherent tensions between the Halakhic obligations to respect the corpse on the one hand and to preserve life on the other, to protect the healthy and to heal the sick. Transplantation places these obligations in direct conflict and Halakhic prioritization is demanded. Cadaveric donation requires dissection of the dead body, whereas the living donor may place his or her own health in jeopardy. In this regard, Jewish law is quite clear. Life is of supreme value such that its preservation and safe-keeping overrides virtually all other considerations. The law commands an attitude of kindness towards others which manifests itself in actions which enhance life. That does not mean that the risk for the living donor is overlooked or that the respectful regard for the dead is suspended. Instead, the Halakhic opinion holds that these considerations be viewed in relation to the life of a prospective recipient. By this reckoning, organ donation is permissible if the procedure may prolong or save the life of the recipient, and if the donation is voluntary and will not result in the death of the donor. Likewise, cadaveric donation may proceed for the same reasons, given that the 'brain death' of the donor has been established. In essence, Jewish law is of and for the living, and Halakhic opinion emerges from the ongoing dialectic to reflect this emphasis. As Weiss (1988) has stated, the process itself, with its difficulties, uncertainties and demands, displays the inherent spiritual tension and yearning for the divine that is Halakhah.

The Jewish perspective is to be understood primarily in this realm of Halakhic argumentation, rather than as part of theological constructs regarding the afterlife. Indeed, while orthodox Judaism asserts a belief in bodily resurrection, most non-orthodox Jews are more agnostic regarding the afterlife (Ludwig 1989, p. 122).

Islam

In contrast to Judaism, Islamic faith holds belief in resurrection as being of great theological import. However, except for this strong emphasis on bodily resurrection, the conflict facing Islamic jurists is quite similar to the Halakhic debate of Judaism. Islamic doctrine espouses a deep respect for the value of life and the nobility of life-saving acts, but also emphasizes directives in the sacred writings against corporal mutilation and a need for hasty burial. Islamic law is clear that cremation or mutilation of the body is prohibited, citing traditions of the Prophet Muhammad that underscore the sanctity of the body. In the situation of organ transplant, these laws collide with honourable and altruistic desires to preserve and enhance life. The matter in Islam is further complicated by the doctrine of bodily resurrection which states that a person's various body parts will be held accountable for the actions of that person on the day of judgement (Sachedina 1988). This issue is one of central importance in the Islamic theological debate.

Owing to the views on resurrection and the sanctity of the body, the conclusion to be drawn on the basis of the Qur'ān, the sacred book of Islam, and the Hadith, the collected traditions about the Prophet, would likely be a disinclination towards organ transplantation. In fact, some Muslim jurists have espoused such a view as being most consistent with Islamic law (Sachedina 1988). However, this opinion does not reflect the majority view of Muslim theologians, who consider organ transplantation permissible if the risk incurred by the donor may result in the saving of another's life, and does not constitute an intentional forfeiture of life on the part of the donor. That such differing views can be derived is owing to the varying emphases of the different schools of law within Sunni Islam. Each bases its jurisprudence on the Qur'ān and the Hadith, but differs from one another in its use of the juridical processes of analogical reasoning and communal consensus. Given the understandable silence about transplantation in early Islamic revelation, a Muslim acceptance of the procedure would necessarily involve the use of such juridical processes (Nigosian 1987; pp. 24–5, 130–5). For instance, passages in the Qur'ān stress that God can bring back decomposed or destroyed bodies, the emphasis being that no one is absolved from divine reckoning regardless of the remoteness or mode of death. By analogy, the argument can be set forth that God therefore can accomplish his purposes regardless of each individual organ's ultimate earthly destination, and regardless of the status of the donor or recipient as devout or not. More conservative scholars are less inclined to accept this reasoning, again citing earliest Islamic revelation. Still others take a middle road in their acceptance of organ transplantation, with the proviso that the organ be buried separately if the recipient is ultimately cremated (Sachedina 1988).

Christianity

Belief in bodily resurrection is also held within Christianity. Given the relative ease with which many Christians donate and receive organs, it might be assumed that Christianity does not assert a belief in bodily resurrection of the sort proclaimed by Islam. But this is not the case. The apostle Paul, in one of the earliest Christian writings on the subject, clearly emphasized a belief in bodily resurrection. This view was in contradistinction to the Hellenistic view that only the soul was immortal (1 Corinthians 15: 1–58).

How then is the permissive attitude of Christians towards transplantation explained? To begin with, Christianity has never had a true orthodoxy. The New Testament, the sacred scripture which contains the earliest extant theological formulations, bears witness to a host of influences extending well beyond the parent Judaism and which includes Platonism, Stoicism, Cynicism, and Gnosticism. These influences have, at times, contributed to contradictory teachings. While the centre of the New Testament unquestionably is Jesus of Nazareth of first century Palestine, the New Testament itself is very much a product of the Hellenistic world and preserves the eclecticism of Greek thought. Therefore, despite Paul's protestations in his letter to the Corinthians, the soul–body dualism of Greek philosophy none the less formed an integral part of Christian thinking. This concept had much to do with the ready acceptance and rapid spread of the Christian belief in the Holy Spirit (Perrin and Duling 1982, pp. 7–15).

Christianity, from the very outset, presented a diverse array of opinions, emphases, and constructs. This diversity has undeniably contributed to an extraordinary theological richness and vigour, but has also divided Christianity with respect to many issues. The specific issue of bodily resurrection reflects this diversity. While Christians profess a belief in resurrection of the body, other forces (e.g. dualistic concepts) have been brought to bear, so that most Christians do not regard resurrection as being dependent, literally, upon corporal integrity at the point of death.

Other aspects of the Christian faith are also relevant to transplantation. In the actions of Jesus, Christians see concrete examples of self-donating love for friend, family, and enemy. As well, the principle Christian sacrament, known as the Eucharist, invites the devout to share in the body and blood of Jesus, using bread and wine as a re-enactment of the Last Supper. For many Christians, the Eucharist can be understood as a paradigm for organ transplantation, the donating and sharing of body and blood in the context of self-sacrifice and compassion (May 1988).

It must be stressed that this self-sacrifice does not entail the intentional oblation of one's life. This stipulation is common to all the Abrahamic religions: that donation be carried out only in those conditions where the expected results are benefit for the recipient, and recovery for the live donor. The emphasis is on the value of life and the goodness of humanity as God's highest creation. It is this emphasis that constitutes a common thread by which each of Judaism, Islam, and Christianity meet this extraordinary theological challenge.

Religions arising from India

Like the Middle East, India has been the birthplace of many religious tradi-tions. Two of the most important and influential of these are Hinduism and Buddhism. In addition to geographical kinship, Hinduism and Buddhism share a historical development dating back to the first millennium BC. They differ from the Abrahamic religions in their view of the divine not as a personal creator God, although gods do play an important role, but as an ultimate sacred reality that transcends temporal, transient existence. Human existence is seen as an endless cycle of lifetimes, the samsara, which has as its ultimate goal the achievement of liberation from the cycle. During existence, the individual can be placed in touch with the sacred by various rituals such as meditation, which help the devout to obtain detachment from the passing world and liberation from samsara (Ludwig 1989, pp. 245–8).

Hinduism

Unlike the Abrahamic religions, Hinduism does not trace its roots back to a specific founder or specific historical events. Rather, events considered sacred in the foundation of Hinduism take place in a metaphysical time frame. They describe the actions of gods and goddesses, heroes and heroines, that occur beyond the realm of conventional history. Despite their trans-cendental essence, however, the gods share with humans the need to be liberated from the continuous cycle of birth and death. For Hindus, the ultimate divine reality that transcends this samsara is Brahman, and within each person exists the true self, the atman, which is also eternal and is identical with Brahman. Knowing the atman effects release from the samsara, a liberation known as moksha. The body, with its senses and physical desires, is considered an illusory self.

This goal of moksha must be considered side by side with another ultimate reality of Hindu theology, the Dharma. The Eternal Dharma refers to the cosmic order of the universe, and translates into a social order with prescrip-tions regarding proper behaviour and duty. The concern of Dharma, which is maintenance of the proper social order, and the concern of moksha, which is achievement of liberation from samsara, are, in certain instances, at odds with one another. However, this tension upon which Hinduism is built may be illustrated in the approach to organ transplantation (Ludwig 1989, pp. 249–300).

On the surface, organ transplantation is not problematic in Hinduism. Hindu beliefs regarding the imperishability of the atman, and the need to transcend the empirical self, together create little obstacle to organ donation. But the donor does not necessarily give up an organ with single-minded detachment, nor does the recipient accept the organ because of a misplaced appreciation of bodily well-being. On the contrary, the perspective of Dharma emphasizes that the present world and life are valuable, that the maintenance of social order enhances the well-being of all humanity, and that the attitude of compassion is a great virtue. Thus the acts of both donating and receiving an organ can be seen as promoting the Dharma of this world. Thus, while moksha priorities facilitate organ donation, Dharma priorities contextualize the acts of donating and receiving as both ennobling and socially valuable. At their logical extremes, however, the priorities ultimately conflict: the Hindu receives the life-saving organ and so can continue to live according to his or her Dharma, yet the organ is very much a part of the empirical self that must finally end in the oneness of Brahman.

Organ transplantation therefore presents the classic struggle between Dharma as ultimate and Brahman as ultimate that is at the essence of Hinduism. This perspective suggests a comparison with Judaism where the inherent conflict and debate of Halakhah was seen as an animating, spiritual force. While the specific issues in conflict are quite different, both Hinduism and Judaism demonstrate that a tension between theological constructs can be an acknowledged and even fundamental aspect of piety, as well as a medium of creative formulation in meeting new challenges.

Buddhism

Some of these same theological constructs are also found in Buddhism, a religion which traces its roots back to Siddhartha Gautama (the Buddha) who lived 2500 years ago in north-east India. At that time, the early formation of Hinduism was well under-way, and the spiritual perspective expounded by the Buddha clearly shows its ancient kinship with the teachings of the Hindu sages.

The Buddha, or 'Enlightened One', retained the Hindu concept of the samsara. Similarly, he emphasized liberation from the cycle of rebirth, known as the achievement of 'nirvana', as an ultimate spiritual goal. But in contrast to Hinduism, the Buddha maintained that there was nothing permanent or absolute, not even atman or Brahman. In fact, full enlightenment, the achievement of perfect wisdom and compassion, was based on the realization that no permanent self existed. This Dharma was the new truth preached by the Buddha.

What, then, is the Buddhist understanding of this impermanent self? Buddhism perceives the self as a dynamic process composed of five aggregates:

the body, sensations, perceptions, will, and consciousness. Each aggregate is dependent on the others in continual, ever-changing relationships. Given that there is nothing permanent to the self beyond these aggregates, the cycle of rebirths in the samsara is seen not as an ongoing passage of the atman, but rather as a continual chain of causation based on previous existences (Ludwig 1989, pp. 302–49). If the Hindu emphasis on transcendence to Brahman was seen as a facilitating factor in regard to organ donation, the Buddhist precept of utter impermanence, spiritual or physical, can be viewed as being even more conducive to the process.

As in Hinduism, the Buddhist attitude toward the body and samsara only forms part of an understanding of its overall perspective on transplantation. Consideration must also be given to the positive reasons (i.e. the motivation) for the receiving and donating of body organs in a universe without permanent underpinnings. It would be a misunderstanding of Buddhism to regard this emphasis on impermanence as meaning an absence for its followers of ultimate reality. On the contrary, the Dharma of the Buddha, the unconditioned truth about the nature of the universe, takes on the quality of the sacred and forms the central aspect of Buddhist worship. An essential principle of this Dharma is the doctrine of 'dependent arising'. The doctrine, simply stated, is that everything is conditioned by everything else. Just as the aggregates of the self are in a state of mutually dependent flux, so too all the components and events of the cosmos are interdependent. The actions, struggles, and quests of the person are inextricably 'universal' in their nature, influencing, and being influenced by, all that exists. The devout Buddhist, therefore, has an extraordinary sense of oneness with, and compassion for, all living things. The personal quest for enlightenment is therefore also humanity's quest, and vice versa. The corporal self, the individual's agency by which supreme enlightenment is attained, becomes at once the world's vehicle toward this same noble goal. Thus, the Dharma, the Buddhist concept of the divine, urges the devout towards acts of compassion, and interprets such acts within the context of the honourable, interdependent, and universal journey toward enlightenment (Tsuji 1988; Lesco 1991).

In sum, the Dharma of Buddhism and the Dharma of Hinduism, while quite different in emphasis, both serve similar functions as theological heuristics with regard to transplantation. While both religions emphasize the transience of the physical self, the Dharma of each affirms the spiritual importance of this present life, and lends meaning and purpose to the compassionate act of the donor and the hopeful attitude of the recipient.

Religions of the Far East

The religions of Japan and China form a loose family of traditions including Shinto, Taosim, Confucianism, and the Mahayana form of Buddhism. These faiths describe many sacred forces—gods, kami, spirits, ancestors, T'ien—and share an emphasis on there being one unified cosmos rather than a transcendent deity or a separate eternal realm. Reverence for nature and familial ancestors form a common link amongst these religions. While Taoism, Confucianism, and Shinto are examined separately, two considerations should be emphasized. First, Chinese and Japanese religions are in practice a synthesis of several different traditions. This makes the study of one or the other in isolation a somewhat artificial enterprise. Second, Mahayana Buddhism is tremendously important in the Far East, and is fundamental to the Japanese and Chinese religious outlooks (Ludwig 1989, pp. 377–80). For example, in Shinto, this overlap of belief systems is evident at the time of death. Shinto's orientation towards the present life is such that it does not emphasize specific beliefs and rituals for dealing with the dead body. Thus, most of the devout of Shinto turn to Buddhist teachings and observe Buddhist rituals upon the death of a follower (Ludwig 1989, p. 500).

Shinto

Shinto refers to the indigenous religion of Japan as distinct from the imported beliefs of Buddhism and Confucianism. The term Shinto means 'the way of the kami', the kami referring to the various spirits or divinities which populate the universe and which are worshipped at Japanese shrines. In Shinto thought, the kami also refer more generally to things or persons which call forth a sense of awe, wonder, or fear (Bloom 1971, p. 347).

It is believed that, through the kami, the life of the cosmos arose and is maintained. The world as originally created was good and human nature pure. But humanity becomes 'polluted' by wrong-doing and therefore becomes cut off from the vivifying purity of the kami. Hence, there is the enormous Shinto emphasis on the need for 'purification' to restore harmony with the kami (Ludwig 1989, pp. 487–9). Purification rituals and practices involve both the physical and spiritual aspects of existence. The physical purification performed in ritual worship entails usually only the washing of the hands and rinsing of the mouth. These rituals attest to a largely symbolic cleaning of the physical self, rather than a preoccupation with literal, corporal integrity (Ludwig 1989, p. 494). Most importantly, Shinto piety stresses that outward physical purification must be accompanied by an inner spiritual transformation; it is the pureness of heart that restores the person to his original uprightness (Ludwig 1989, pp. 487–9).

It might be supposed that such a strong concern for purification would lead to a certain reluctance regarding the mutilations involved in transplantation. In fact, contact with the dead does constitute a type of pollution according to Shinto piety. But it would be a far too literal interpretation of Shinto teaching to suppose that this should lead to a formal prohibition against organ transplantation. Indeed, the essential nature of the universe espoused by

Shinto, permeated as it is with divinity from the highest to lowest forms of life, makes the distinction between the sacred and the profane at times difficult to discern (Bloom 1971, p. 348). Thus the Shinto concern for purification does not of necessity appear to effect a resistance to transplantation. Furthermore, the broadest perspective of the Shinto outlook is so very much oriented to life, fertility, and growth, that any process that potentially promotes good health is almost *a priori* held in high regard.

Taoism and Confucianism

Turning now to the Chinese religious perspective, it is noteworthy that the survival of the two religions most crucial to its development, Taoism and Confucianism, is in question today in modern China. Nonetheless, the ancient wisdom of these two faiths formed the basis of an ethical, moral, religious, and pedagogical system that transformed Chinese society and guided that nation's world view for over 2000 years. As such, an understanding of Taoism and Confucianism still remains a prerequisite for an appreciation of the Chinese outlook on modern medicine and transplantation.

The teachings of Confucious asserted the basic goodness of all people, but cautioned against the corrupting forces of social anarchy and immorality. The emphasis was on the importance of family and society, and the centrality of jen, a term perhaps best defined by the word humaneness. Jen was considered the supreme virtue; it enabled men and women to subordinate their own desires for the good of humanity, to harmonize their inner selves with the outer world, to recognize their proper roles in family and society. Although Confucious himself spoke of heaven or T'ien as the sacred supreme moral authority, he was unconcerned with gods or spirits, and did not speculate on the nature of reality. Despite the intervening centuries, the Confucian outlook today still resists an emphasis on the afterlife or a concept of salvation by the gods. Rather, it continues to espouse the importance of jen and proper social relationships as the path to spiritual transformation (Bloom 1971, pp. 275–83). Taken on its own terms, there is nothing in Confucianism that would suggest a resistance toward transplantation. Indeed, its primary focus on concerns that are worldly would indicate an approval of the process. But, as stated at the outset of this section, the teachings of a single Chinese religion cannot accurately reflect the reality of the Chinese belief system. The precepts of Taoism need also be considered, as they are interwoven with other teachings in forming the underpinnings of overall Chinese beliefs and attitudes.

Religious Taoism maintains that spiritual happiness derives from a harmonization between the self and the divine forces of the cosmos. The human body is seen as a microcosm of the universe, with its parts corresponding both to various regions of the universe, and to various divine forces governing these regions. Such forces can be called upon to inhabit the body, to bring about renewal and vitality. A traditional Taoist emphasis has been on physical health, even on immortality, and Taoist priests have developed elaborate rituals and techniques for the purpose of channelling the life-enhancing gods into the body. In contrast to Confucianism, Taoism is concerned with gods and goddesses, and the role these divinities play in people's lives. As well, Taoism stresses the continued existence of the soul after death, and the ongoing interdependence between the living and the dead (Ludwig 1989, pp. 433–5).

It is largely from these Taoist emphases that the Chinese funeral rituals are derived. These are the most serious of all Chinese rituals. They involve, among other things, the careful preparation of the body and the mourning period— processes which are usually carried out in the home of the deceased, and which may go on for weeks or even months before the actual burial (Ludwig 1989, pp. 449–50).

These funeral rites bring out many of the difficulties that are encountered when an attempt is made to establish a unified Chinese religious perspective on organ transplantation. For instance, while Confucianism itself places little emphasis on an afterlife, most of its followers would nonetheless bury their dead in accordance with the usual Chinese tradition with its Taoist under-pinnings. Does this then mean that the Chinese religious attitude toward the body is that of Taoism, with its beliefs in divine spirits inhabiting organs and its great concern for the correct preparation of the corpse prior to burial? If so, do such beliefs translate into an approval or disapproval of organ transplantation?

These questions are extraordinarily difficult to answer at present. While the Taoist views on the body, afterlife, and physical well-being might in theory form the basis for a fascinating theological interpretation of organ transplanta-tion, the reality is that both Taoism and Confucianism are waning as formal religious forces in China. Both religions have been seriously weakened in their abilities to undertake new theological challenges, engage in new doctrinal debate, and assimilate the implications of modern technology into ancient dogma. Such demands tax even the most robust of theological systems (Ludwig 1989, p. 461).

The question thus remains as to how the pious of China will ultimately come to regard their rich religious heritage, and how they will ultimately choose to apply it to organ transplantation. Should Confucian precepts be regarded as philosophical considerations, or should they form the basis of a comprehensive religious outlook? Should Taoist funeral rituals be regarded as cultural tradi-tion, or as representations of sacred attitudes towards the body? Should Taoism and Confucianism be regarded as vestiges of the past, or dynamic belief systems of the present? These questions, all relevant to the religious perspective on organ transplantation, remain open.

In fact, the whole issue of organ transplantation remains quite open not just for Confucianism and Taoism, but for Shintoism as well. The task these religions have been presented is a daunting one: the placement of organ transplantation within the respective theological frameworks of complex belief systems. However, there is reason to believe that the life-affirming aspects of the Far Eastern faiths will prove a guiding and clarifying force in this process. Despite all of the theological complexity and present uncertainty, the religions of the Far East all espouse a path of spiritual transformation which stresses health and vitality, and places enormous value on the present earthly life.

Conclusions

Each of the major faiths that have been discussed espouses an implicit or explicit explanation of the nature of the universe. Further, in each has developed a repertoire of theological constructs by which the role and activity of humanity in this universe can be understood. Such explanations and constructs are highly varied, and have yielded different approaches to the dilemmas of organ transplantation. However, the religious perspectives do find common ground beyond the reach of formal theological dogma and nuance, in their respective glorifications of life and benevolence. These assertions have generally taken precedence above all other prescriptions in regard to transplantation, even in those faiths where orthodox theological precepts have appeared quite tentative about the issue. It is by these fundamental priorities, which are shared by each of the religious traditions discussed, that an overall permissive approach to organ transplantation is best appreciated. It seems as if each religion, in its own way, articulates a sacred reality understood implicitly by all humanity: that life is holy, and that acts of self-giving touch on the divine.

References

Bloom, A. (1971). Far eastern religious traditions. In *Religion and Man*, Ed. W. R. Comstock, 251–394.

Lesco, P. A. (1991). The bodhisattna ideal and organ transplantation. *Journal of Religion and Health*, 30, 35–41.

Ludwig, T. M. (1989). *The sacred paths*. (Macmillan, New York).

May, W. F. (1988). Religious obstacles and warrants for the donation of body parts. *Transplantation Proceedings*, 20, 1079–83.

Nigosian, S. (1987). *Islam: the Way of Submission*. Thorsins Publishing, New York.

Perrin, N. and Duling, D. C. (1982). *The New Testament: an introduction*. (Harcourt Brace Jovanovich, New York).

Sachedina, A. A. (1988). Islamic views on organ transplantation. *Transplantation Proceedings*, 20, 1084–8.

Tsuji, K. T. (1988). The Buddhist view of the body and organ transplantation. *Transplantation Proceedings*, 20, 1076–8.

Weiss, D. W. (1988). Organ transplantation, medical ethics, and Jewish law. *Transplantation Proceedings*, 20, 1071–5.

PART II

11   Kidney transplantation

G. Rodin and S. Abbey

Each new type of transplantation raises unique psychiatric and psychosocial issues. These are determined, in part, by the pathophysiologic processes associated with the underlying medical disease, the organ transplanted, and the relative risks to the health and life of the patient. However, there is also significant commonality amongst the psychiatric problems associated with different transplant procedures. This chapter presupposes that, as the most common and widely researched type of transplant, the kidney transplant offers valuable experience which assists with the understanding of the overall process and may guide the study of more recently available procedures. During the last 30 years, the status of kidney transplantation has evolved from an experimental procedure used in a small number of highly selected patients to its current status as a safe and effective treatment which is considered optimal for many patients with endstage renal disease (ESRD). Kidney transplants were initially associated with a significant risk of graft failure, as still occurs with newer forms of transplantation. It may be assumed that similar developments are likely to occur with newer forms of transplantation. The changing role of the psychiatric consultant in the management of the renal transplant patient will be reviewed.

Historical aspects

The need for psychiatric assistance in the management of renal transplant patients has changed as the frequency and safety of this procedure have increased. In large part, these changes have been due to improvements in medical treatment during the past several decades, particularly in the field of transplant immunology. As a result of these developments, approximately 7000 renal transplants per year were being performed in the United States by 1984 (Levey *et al.* 1986). The following year, almost one-third of all enrollees in the United States ESRD Medicare program who were under the age of 55 had functioning grafts (Eggers 1988). Patient survival one year after cadaveric transplantation is now approximately 90 per cent and is equal to or greater than survival on dialysis (Levey *et al.* 1986). Graft survival from living–unrelated donors was recently reported to be more than 90 per cent after four years (Sollinger *et al.* 1986). As the success rate with the procedure has improved, it has been demonstrated repeatedly that the quality of life with functioning grafts is clearly superior to that which is usually achieved with dialysis (Johnson *et al.* 1982; Evans *et al.* 1985; Rodin *et al.* 1985). As a result, what began as a revolutionary but experimental treatment for a life-threatening medical condition has now become the routine approach for most young and middle-aged patients with renal failure (Levey *et al.* 1986).

During the early stages of renal transplantation, psychiatric consultation was often regarded as an integral part of the preoperative evaluation of transplant candidates. This practice is no longer routinely indicated, but it may be informative to review some of the reasons that previously led to regular psychiatric assessment. These factors included: uncertainty on the part of staff regarding the selection of candidates for a new procedure; concern about informed consent of potential transplant recipients; assessment of informed consent of live donors; and the 'strangeness' of transplanting the organ of one individual into the body of another.

Concern about case selection is heightened during the introduction of a new treatment because of the potential medical and surgical risks. This emphasis on patient selection is usual in this circumstance and is commonly motivated by the desire both to achieve a successful outcome for individual patients, and to obtain a broader acceptance of a new treatment by the medical community and by the public. The viability of a new programme may itself be a factor if continued funding depends upon good outcome statistics. In this context, psychiatric assessment may be regarded as an important aspect of evaluation for a procedure which involves some risk, utilizes a relatively scarce resource, and requires that patients comply with treatment in the postoperative period. Psychiatric consultants were frequently asked to predict which kidney transplant candidates were most likely to suffer from significant postoperative psychiatric morbidity. This opinion helped to determine which patients were regarded either as unsuitable for the procedure or who would require specific psychiatric or medical attention in the postoperative period. Unfortunately, such predictions were often based upon little or no scientific evidence.

Intense interest by the physician in a procedure may sometimes interfere with a balanced approach toward obtaining voluntary and informed consent. In this regard, there may be significant differences in the way physicians and surgeons evaluate treatments compared to their patients. For example, it has been suggested that patients may be more risk-aversive than physicians with regard to selecting medical treatments (Wennberg 1990). Also, physicians may be more focused on medical morbidity, whereas patients may be more concerned about potential quality of life. In the case of ESRD, there may have been significant incentives to providers or institutions that result from assigning patients either to dialysis or transplantation. These factors may create potential conflicts of interest between patients and their health care providers. In this context, nephrologists or transplant surgeons may feel less assured of their own neutrality and therefore may have been more likely to request consultation for assessment of informed consent and mental competence. Informed consent by patients with ESRD may also have been of concern because of the relatively frequent occurrence of cognitive impairment and organic mental syndromes (Nissenson *et al.* 1977; Stewart and Stewart 1979; Dubovsky and Penn 1980; Fricchione 1989) which may affect mental competence.

Other developments have also altered the need for psychiatric consultation for renal transplant applicants. Decisions by family members to donate a kidney involve potential conflicts of interest as well as risks to individuals who will not directly benefit medically. Concern about the risk to kidney donors has perhaps become even greater today since the success rate with cadaveric transplants now approximates that with transplants from living related donors. This issue has recently aroused interest due to attempts at live donor liver transplants (Strong *et al.* 1990). Finally, when kidney transplantation was first initiated, fantasies and anxieties about the transplanted organ were reported commonly. As transplantation has become more routine, less symbolic significance has been attached by both patients and health care providers to the procedure. This has resulted in less apprehension about kidney transplants overall and much less hesitation in recommending the procedure for virtually all patients who are medically suitable. These factors have led to a marked decline in the frequency of psychiatric consultation for these transplant candidates.

Many of the dilemmas which the conscientious liaison psychiatrist faced during this initial period now occur with the newer forms of transplantation. Psychiatrists and other mental health professionals are again called upon to offer opinions without the benefit of adequate systematic research. Whereas the assessment and treatment of psychiatric disorders is based upon scientific principles, there is much less information available to predict behaviours such as adjustment to transplant or compliance with treatment recommendations. There is always the danger in this context that opinions provided will be based on personal bias and value judgements rather than on scientific information. Such opinions may unfairly affect a patient's opportunity to receive a life-saving treatment. Beliefs that psychiatric disorders will adversely affect adjustment to a medical or surgical procedure are not necessarily justified. Indeed, it has been suggested that there are no absolute psychiatric contraindications whatsoever to renal transplant surgery (Surman 1981, 1987).

Preoperative aspects

The essential questions faced by the psychiatric consultant undertaking the preoperative assessment of a transplant candidate are whether there are psychiatric factors which will compromise the patient's ability to cope with and comply with the treatment plan, and whether there is an increased risk of psychiatric complications. There have been few data upon which predictions of psychiatric morbidity could be made and even less information about the effects of interventions to reduce this morbidity.

Psychiatric disorders

When predictive data have not been available, clinicians have been forced to rely on cross-sectional data and clinical observations. Many studies of this nature exist and have shown that dialysis patients, including those on waiting lists for transplantation, are at risk for depressive symptoms (Rodin and Voshart 1987), depressive disorders (Craven *et al.* 1987), and from organic mental syndromes (Nissenson *et al.* 1977; Stewart and Stewart 1979; Dubovsky and Penn 1980). However, a dramatic fall in the frequency of depressive symptoms was noted in these same patients by six months after a successful renal transplant (Rodin *et al.* 1985). The occurrence in the early literature of severe mood and other psychotic disorders in the immediate post-transplant period was often due to the use of high-dose steroids for immunosuppression. The occurrence of postoperative organic mental disorders appears to have lessened in kidney transplant recipients due to the introduction of newer immunosuppressant regimens and lower dosage administrations. Individual vulnerabilities probably also contribute, since those with a previous or current history of affective or psychotic disorders appear to be at increased risk for such complications (Wilson *et al.* 1968; Penn *et al.* 1971; Dubovsky and Penn 1980). It has also been reported that the rate of suicide in dialysis patients is increased compared to the general population (Abram *et al.* 1971). Indeed, Fricchione (1989) has emphasized the importance of assessing active and passive suicidal ideation as well as the likelihood that self-harm behaviour will occur in the event of graft failure.

There has been little systematic attention to the frequency or impact of substance abuse in renal transplant patients. However, it has been suggested that a past history of heroin addiction is not necessarily an impediment to successful renal transplantation or even to ongoing compliance with immuno-suppressant medication (Gordon *et al.* 1986). Personality disorders have also been of concern because of their association with treatment noncompliance (Penn *et al.* 1971; Dubovsky and Penn 1980; Fricchione 1989) or, in the case of paranoid personality, with an increased risk of psychotic symptoms in the postoperative period (Short and Harris 1969; Penn *et al.* 1971; Dubovsky and Penn 1980). However, there are scant systematic data about the relationship between personality characteristics and adjustment to renal transplantation.

ESRD is associated with a number of disturbances which cause organic brain dysfunction, including metabolic disturbances related to the uraemic state and the underlying diseases (Nissenson *et al.* 1977; Stewart and Stewart 1979; Dubovsky and Penn 1980). Dialysis encephalopathy has been docu-mented to improve with transplantation (Morales-Otero *et al.* 1988). Dubovsky and Penn (1980) have noted that organic brain syndrome secondary to uraemia may easily be misdiagnosed as a functional disorder triggered by the psychological stress of kidney failure. They suggested that this condition may have interfered with some patients receiving a transplant. Indeed, 12 per cent of patients transplanted at their centre had previously been refused a transplant on psychiatric grounds at other centres. However, no psychiatric difficulties were observed in these patients after transplantation did take place. They concluded that the patients' difficulties were the result of undetected organic brain disease which improved with transplant.

Special groups have been identified who present for transplant with a particular vulnerability to psychosocial complications. These include children and adolescents who more often demonstrate problems with noncompliance, self-esteem, body-image, delayed psychosocial and psychosexual development, and family relationships (Bernstein 1971; Lilly *et al.* 1971; Zarinsk 1975; Bouras *et al.* 1976; Korsch *et al.* 1978; Stewart 1983; Rovelli *et al.* 1989). Also, psychiatric problems in diabetics may be common because of their increased medical complications and disability. It has been suggested that the psychiatric morbidity in these patients parallels their medical course (Simmons *et al.* 1977; Gulledge *et al.* 1983). Simmons *et al.* (1981) found that diabetic transplant recipients were more depressed, felt less in control and were more dependent when compared with other transplant recipients in long-term follow-up. As transplants of all kinds become more common and staff resources remain relatively scarce, it is necessary to identify high-risk patients who are most likely to benefit from or to require psychiatric intervention.

During the initial phase of development of renal transplantation, there were believed to be absolute psychiatric contraindications to transplantation. However, with the increased success of the procedure, more psychiatric experience with these patients, and greater availability of donor organs, it has become less clear whether psychiatric illness should preclude transplantation. Cramond (1971) proposed that the only absolute psychiatric contraindications to kidney transplant are a severe pre-existing schizophrenic psychosis which had proved to be intractable to psychiatric therapy, and severe degrees of intellectual retardation. But it may be argued that even these patients may be better able to cope as transplant recipients than if maintained chronically on dialysis. This is certainly a possibility if adequate social and professional supportive services are available. Improved psychiatric management has allowed for successful transplantation of patients with both severe psychoses and intellectual retardation (Surman 1987). Levy (1986) suggested that patients with a history of depression or psychosis would be better served by dialysis in light of the risk of severe steroid-associated psychiatric symptoms. However, this hypothesis demands validation prior to implementation into practice, as current evidence clearly shows that most patients function better medically and emotionally with a transplant as opposed to dialysis. It is likely that these patients would suffer as much or more with dialysis, owing to the psychological and potential cognitive complications associated with this procedure.

Prediction of compliance

Maintenance of transplant recipients on immunosuppressive medication is an essential component of a successful outcome with the transplanted organ. It has been noted in several centres that noncompliance is a significant cause of graft loss (Didlake *et al.* 1988; Rovelli *et al.* 1989). Noncompliance with immunosuppressive medications, as a cause of transplant rejection, was first reported by Owens *et al.* (1975) who were primarily interested in understanding the immunology of transplantation. Najarian (1975), in commenting on this report, noted that at least 6 of 700 renal transplant patients in his setting had discontinued their medication for 'a variety of emotional and sociopathic reasons' and all but one of the six subsequently experienced a severe rejection episode. Shortly thereafter, Uehling *et al.* (1976) provided detailed case descriptions of five living–related donor recipients who had demonstrated significant noncompliance. Two of these recipients died. The cause of noncompliance was attributed in that report to 'serious emotional problems' (e.g. depression, alcohol abuse) or to 'powerful religious convictions'.

Partial noncompliance with immunosuppressant medication may be common and is not necessarily associated with graft rejection. Uehling *et al.* (1976) found that more than 10 per cent of transplant recipients of grafts from living–related donors reported a major lapse in medication use and 17 per cent reported a less severe lapse. More recently, Didlake *et al.* (1988) reviewed compliance with cyclosporin regimens in 531 kidney transplant recipients. They found major noncompliance (resulting in graft loss) in 2.8 per cent of the sample and minor noncompliance (resulting in rejection episodes only) in 1.9 per cent. Those who demonstrated major noncompliance tended to be Caucasian females. Subclinical degrees of noncompliance were found to be even more common. Of 295 transplant patients who responded to a questionnaire, 13 per cent reported missing more than three doses per month.

A number of explanations have been advanced for noncompliance by renal transplant recipients. These include the cost of medication, concerns about the effects of immunosuppressants on physical appearance, and inability to accept the lifestyle limitations involved with the strict monitoring of serum levels. Also, major psychiatric disorders, including substance abuse or nonspecific psychosocial factors, such as low socio-economic status and dysfunctional families, may be associated with noncompliance in some patients (Korsch *et al.* 1978; Beck *et al.* 1980; Gulledge *et al.* 1983; Didlake *et al.* 1988; DeLone *et al.* 1989; Rovelli *et al.* 1989). There is some evidence that compliance may vary across different transplant groups (Rovelli *et al.* 1989). For example, Korsch *et al.* (1978) reported a 9 per cent noncompliance rate in a paediatric population, with all but one of the noncompliant patients being an adolescent. Noncompliance in these patients was often associated with family conflict. Beck *et al.* (1980) found noncompliance in 43 per cent of paediatric transplant recipients. Problems with compliance continued in 19 per cent of this sample, despite extensive education and counselling. Noncompliance in that study was most common in adolescent females. These recipients may have been affected particularly by the body image changes associated with corticosteroids (e.g. moon faces, fatty tissue redistribution) and cyclosporin (e.g. hirsutism). The degree of parental involvement, but not knowledge about the medications, was positively associated with compliance.

In a retrospective study of 196 recipients, Rovelli *et al.* (1989) could find no obvious explanation for noncompliance in most patients. In only a minority of noncompliant patients could this behaviour be explained by mental illness, alcohol abuse, or medication side-effects. A conscious or unconscious desire to encourage graft failure following postoperative complications, or difficulty coping with the uncertainty of rejection, are less obvious motivators of noncompliance. In other cases, firm convictions that the graft will fail, or a breakdown in the doctor–patient relationship, may contribute to noncompliance.

Valid and reliable predictors of noncompliance are not yet available (Didlake *et al.* 1988), and future research must include prospective studies to define such predictors. In the interim, observing patients prior to transplant to assess their compliance to dialysis treatment or other medical regimens may be the best available indicator of post-transplant compliance. DeLone *et al.* (1989) have described the usefulness of such compliance trials pre-transplant. They have required the successful completion of such trials, which include compliance contracts and psycho-educational groups for poorly compliant patients, prior to activating a patient's name on the transplant waiting list. However, noncompliance may develop postoperatively in patients who had been compliant with dialysis and pre-transplant medical care (Armstrong and Weiner 1981–2; Didlake *et al.* 1988; Rovelli *et al.* 1989). Armstrong *et al.* (1981) found noncompliance in over 2 per cent of their transplantation group. They described in detail two cases of noncompliance in adolescents who had been 'generally compliant' prior to transplant but became noncompliant postoperatively, when the successfully functioning transplant posed a threat to their 'regressed life-styles' (Armstrong and Weiner 1981–2). It remains unclear whether psychological factors or observed behaviour will be the best predictors of post-transplant compliance. Possibly, behavioural variables (e.g. observed noncompliance) will prove more specific predictors of future noncompliance. However, it should not be assumed that compliance with treatment pre-transplant necessarily implies compliance following surgery.

A substantial risk of noncompliance with the post-transplant medical protocol may be reason to defer transplantation until a later date. However, this decision requires careful consideration of the individual clinical situation. Some patients may have greater difficulty adhering to the more intensive regimen associated with dialysis than to the simpler requirements with a transplant. Other patients may find the structure and supportive environment of the dialysis unit more conducive to compliance than the less structured life of a transplant recipient. It is also unclear whether noncompliance in the transplant recipient is greater than in those ESRD patients managed with maintenance dialysis treatment. Dialysis may not necessarily be an alternative which is preferable to transplantation in patients who are noncompliant.

Case history   Ms P. was a 43 year old woman who had received a kidney transplant one year prior to referral for psychiatric assessment. Psychiatric assessment was requested due to a history of erratic and demanding behaviour since transplant, multiple somatic complaints, and poor compliance with physician appointments and laboratory investigations.

The patient reported that 17 years previously she had been diagnosed with a bipolar mood disorder. Lithium had been prescribed initially, but Ms P. had discontinued this drug, stating that it had 'erased' her personality. Although she had a subsequent history of at least two major depressive episodes and was chronically hypomanic when not depressed, no other treatment for mood disorder had ever been initiated.

Three years prior to consultation, dialysis was begun for chronic renal failure secondary to focal glomerulonephritis. While on dialysis, Ms P. had become known to the nephrology staff as a 'character' who was often gregarious, at times irritable and demanding, and always very talkative. However, she was adherent to the dietary and medical protocols associated with dialysis, made friendly acquaintance with several of the nursing staff and other dialysis patients, and held a full-time job as a nursing aid at a residence for the elderly.

Following transplant, Ms P. began to refuse to take her immunosuppressant medication and stated that she 'knew' that she did not need it. The staff became frustrated by trying to manage a patient whom they had come to believe wanted to lose her new kidney. Interpersonal difficulties also occurred in her workplace causing her to be dismissed. Finally, staff had requested a psychiatric opinion.

At the time of psychiatric assessment, classic signs and symptoms of mania were evident. Ms P. agreed to in-patient psychiatric care and carbamazepine was prescribed as a mood stabilizer. Over the next several weeks, she improved greatly, becoming less talkative and less demanding, and was able to co-operate better with medical and nursing staff. The patient admitted that while she was pleased overall to have been transplanted, she had felt lost since the procedure and missed the social and professional supportive network of the hospital dialysis treatment centre.

Had this patient been assessed preoperatively, she could have been diagnosed with a mood disorder and identified as at some risk of poor compliance. This assessment might have allowed prophylactic interventions. In retrospect, the supportive structure of the dialysis unit had helped her to avoid clinically significant behavioural disturbances. The loss of this environment and the administration of corticosteroids postoperatively likely also contributed to a worsening of mood disorder and consequent noncompliance.

Postoperative aspects

The most common psychiatric disorders in the immediate postoperative period are delirium and organic mood syndromes. The renal transplant patient is susceptible to delirium based on a number of factors, most particularly immunosuppressive medications (Fricchione 1989). Prednisone-associated delirium has been described (Wilson *et al.* 1968; Penn *et al.* 1971; McCabe and Corry 1978; Dubovsky and Penn 1980) as has a cyclosporin-induced cognitive change (Bertoli *et al.* 1988). Organic mood syndromes secondary to steroids were more problematic prior to the introduction of cyclosporin, which has allowed a reduction in steroid doses. There are reports of both mood elevation (euphoria ranging to mania) (Short and Harris 1969; Penn *et al.* 1971; MacDonald 1972; Dubovsky and Penn 1980; Surman 1987) and depression, nonpsychotic and psychotic (Wilson *et al.* 1968; Short and Harris 1969; Penn *et al.* 1971; Blazer *et al.* 1976; McCabe and Corry 1978; Dubovsky and Penn 1980; Stewart 1983; Surman 1987; Morales-Otero *et al.* 1988). Anti-hypertensive drugs have also been implicated in the development of organic mood syndromes (Blazer *et al.* 1976; McCabe and Corry 1978; Dubovsky and Penn 1980).

There have been a number of reports of mood disorders that developed beyond the immediate postoperative period (Wilson *et al.* 1968; Ferris 1969; Short and Harris 1969; Penn *et al.* 1971; Blazer *et al.* 1976; McCabe and Corry 1978). These syndromes have been attributed to a variety of factors, including steroid and antihypertensive medication. McCabe and Corry (1978) reported that seven of eight patients who developed a secondary depression due to steroids or to antihypertensives improved when treated with a tricyclic anti-depressant. Blazer *et al.* (1976) described six patients who developed depressive symptomatology of psychotic proportion between five weeks and seven months following renal transplantation. Half of these cases were associated with threatened rejection and all required somatic treatment, which included electroconvulsive treatment in half of them.

Many transplant patients who are distressed do not suffer either from an organic brain syndrome or a major mood disorder. The most appropriate psychiatric diagnosis for many of these patients is that of an adjustment disorder. The degree of distress is often correlated with the severity of physical symptoms and the occurrence of postoperative complications (Fricchione 1989). However, adjustment problems may also occur with patients who have improved and are now required to shift out of the sick role. In some cases, particularly amongst adolescent patients (Bernstein 1971; Lilly *et al.* 1971; Korsch *et al.* 1973; Nylander *et al.* 1985) or patients with narcissistic vulnerability (Levy 1986), the effects of steroids on physical appearance may be profoundly distressing. Postoperative depressive symptoms may also be common, as Dubovsky and Penn (1980) suggest, in patients who have unrealistically high expectations preoperatively. Such patients may have difficulty accepting that transplantation is an alternative treatment rather than a cure for endstage renal disease. Finally, it should be noted that during the early postoperative phase, organic mental symptoms and syndromes may easily be mistaken for an adjustment disorder. A high index of suspicion for organic symptoms is required during this period, because the management differs when the presenting symptoms are mediated primarily by biological mechanisms.

Pharmacotherapy has not posed a particular problem in the treatment of psychiatric disorders in transplant patients (Fricchione 1989). Lithium is associated with nephrotoxicity, and carbamazepine may be a preferable substitute as a mood stabilizer for the patient with bipolar mood disorder. However, this anticonvulsant may stimulate hepatic metabolism of cyclosporin and result in lower serum levels of this drug. Careful monitoring of both carbamazepine and cyclosporin levels are required while the drugs are being titrated.

Adjustment and rehabilitation

The literature suggests that most recipients adjust successfully to renal transplantation, but that there is a subgroup with psychiatric difficulties. However, there have been no large-scale systematic longitudinal studies of psychiatric outcome in renal transplant recipients. Also, much of the literature has focused on the description of symptoms rather than the prevalence of psychiatric disorders. Many studies have also been limited by including only patients referred for psychiatric consultation, although conclusions have sometimes been generalized inappropriately to the entire transplant population.

Early studies of renal transplant recipients suggested that most recipients managed well, after passing through the initial postoperative period. Colomb and Hamburger (1967) reported on 9 of 44 recipients referred for psychiatric assessment by their physicians because their behaviour was considered abnormal following transplant. One patient was significantly depressed in association with physical complications, and the other eight patients were anxious about their future and their health. Cramond (1967) reported on five kidney transplant recipients. None of these patients was clinically depressed, but four of the five recipients had received living–related donor organs and felt obligated and resentful toward the donor. Ferris (1969) also noted that psychological complications were more common in patients with living–related donor transplants than in patients with cadaveric transplants. This group reported that emotional difficulties were much less common in recipients with single transplants compared to those who have had multiple transplants. Short and Harris (1969) found that initial psychological symptoms due to high steroid doses were common, but that ultimate psychological adaptation was good in 19 transplant recipients of kidneys from living–related donors.

Kemph (1970) reported on a series of 37 recipients who had experienced some 'interesting psychodynamic effects' from the transplant (e.g. feelings of guilt, results on projective testing related to themes of robbing or being robbed) but 'no permanent, severe psychological impairment'. Cramond (1967) described a poor psychological outcome in 20 per cent of 34 recipients, characterized by being housebound, with low-grade depression and the sense of waiting for the next disaster to strike. Penn *et al.* (1971) reported that significant psychopathology was present preoperatively in 50 of 292 renal transplant recipients, of whom 36 developed postoperative psychiatric difficulties. A further 58 recipients developed postoperative psychiatric problems *de novo* in patients without identified preoperative psychopathology.

More recent studies have employed psychometric instruments to study adjustment in transplant recipients. Kalman *et al.* (1983) administered the General Health Questionnaire (GHQ) to 57 of 98 transplant recipients five or more years after transplantation: 33 per cent of respondents scored as psychiatric cases on this measure and psychological help was sought by almost as many. Petrie (1989) found that 27 per cent of respondents (response rate 96 per cent) in a New Zealand transplant programme scored as psychiatric cases on the GHQ. This proportion was not significantly different from general practice attendees, but was lower than the rate of 43 per cent for dialysis patients. Psychiatric status has also been addressed in some studies of quality of life post-transplantation. Kaplan De-Nour and Shanan (1980) found that 36 per cent of transplant recipients experience psychiatric complications at one year following transplant, although they did not specify the problems in this group. Simmons *et al.* (1981) assessed psychosocial adjustment five to nine years following transplant, using psychometric instruments, and found that mild scores for depression were reported by 71 per cent of recipients, and mild anxiety by 45 per cent.

Suicide attempts have also been reported in transplant recipients. Penn *et al.* (1971) reported four suicides in transplant recipients, two of whom had been assessed preoperatively because of depressive symptoms. Simmons *et al.* (1977) reported that there was one successful suicide and 10 attempted or threatened suicides in a sample of 208 transplant recipients. Amongst patients who attempted suicide, there was an over-representation of adolescents and individuals with diabetes. Others have also noted the problem of self-harm in adolescent transplant recipients (Lilly *et al.* 1971). However, graft failure is not a consistent precipitant, since half of those who attempted suicide had a successfully functioning graft. Overall, suicide must be regarded as a potential complication in these and other patients who are exposed to the long-term stress associated with a chronic and unpredictable medical condition. Some transplant recipients are aware of a distressing sense of physical vulnerability or fragility, that they may suddenly become ill at any time. For some, passive or active self-harm may be a reaction to this distress, or, alternatively, an unconscious attempt to exercise control over a negative event which is expected to occur anyway.

Graft failure

Early investigators hypothesized that psychological factors might contribute to organ rejection and death following transplant. Eisendrath (1969) reported that of eleven patients who died following renal transplantation, eight had experienced significant feelings of abandonment by their families or a marked degree of panic and pessimism about their surgical outcome. Three of these patients died following rejection episodes, and the remainder from other complications. Viederman (1975) described a patient who developed an episode of acute rejection five weeks after transplantation in the context of learning of the death of a man who had been a father figure for him. However, these case reports have not subsequently been substantiated by systematic research. Steinberg *et al.* (1981) found that attempts to predict rejection based on psychological factors were largely unsuccessful.

Carosella (1984) has noted that there is 'no standard emotional reaction' to an unsuccessful transplant. Some recipients may be depressed, while others may feel relief with the end of the uncertainty regarding rejection, and may welcome the return to the familiarity of dialysis. Streltzer *et al.* (1983–4) studied 25 patients who suffered transplant failure and found that all but one made a good readjustment to chronic dialysis. Fourteen of them openly grieved the loss of their kidneys, and 10 denied any psychological difficulties. Rodin *et al.* (1985) undertook the first systematic study of graft failure comparing 13 patients whose grafts had failed with 42 who had successful transplants and 38 still on the waiting list. They found that while an unsuccessful transplant was associated with some deterioration in subsequent physical activity, there was no deterioration in psychosocial functioning in patients with graft failure, as measured by the Sickness Impact Profile, and there was a reduction in depressive symptoms as measured by the Beck Depression Inventory.

Living–related donor transplants

Prior to the development of sophisticated immunological techniques to match cadaveric kidneys to recipients and to minimize rejection, the results with living–related donor transplantation were far superior to cadaveric transplants in terms of both graft and recipient survival. Since most of the early transplants were from living–related donors, the family and social dynamics of donation have been a major topic of inquiry (Kemph 1966; Colomb and Hamburger 1967; Cramond 1967; Fellner and Marshall 1968; Wilson *et al.* 1968; Kemph *et al.* 1969; Cramond 1971; Simmons *et al.* 1971).

Preliminary reports suggested that the decision to donate a kidney was a spontaneous one made with little hesitation (Fellner and Marshall 1968,

1970). Subsequent studies challenged this view and explored the complexities underlying the process of decision-making, including conflict, ambivalence, and indecision; the development of family conflict; the role of the spouse as advocate; and the decision not to donate (Kemph *et al.* 1969; Cramond 1971; Simmons *et al.* 1971). Simmons *et al.* (1971, 1977) noted the paucity of social norms that apply to family organ donation and the resulting problems which develop. A number of authors noted that occasionally the 'black sheep' of the family would offer to donate a kidney in an attempt to become reinstated within the family (Kemph *et al.* 1969; Fellner and Marshall 1970) or that a vulnerable family member (e.g. retarded, mentally ill) was put forward as the possible donor (Simmons *et al.* 1971). Families were observed to exclude potential donors from consideration based on individual or family dynamics (Fellner and Marshall 1970). It has been noted that direct refusal to donate is infrequent, but that indirect refusal by not attending scheduled laboratory testing sessions, doctors appointments, or avoiding contact with the patient or other family members is much more common (Short and Harris 1969; Fellner and Marshall 1970; Simmons *et al.* 1971). While there is considerable variation in the donor's attitude toward the recipient, depending upon the history of their relationship, it has been noted that the donor typically undergoes an increase in his or her emotional investment in the recipient (Kemph *et al.* 1969; Fellner and Marshall 1970). Previous unresolved conflicts were often re-awakened in the context of the transplantation (Kemph *et al.* 1969; Simmons *et al.* 1971).

Initially, the routine psychiatric assessment of potential donors was suggested to identify donors who might require special attention in the peri-operative period, have contraindications to the procedure (Colomb and Hamburger 1967; Cramond 1967), or for whom informed consent was in question. Current practices regarding psychiatric assessment of donors vary. Some programmes continue to use routine psychiatric assessment while others obtain psychiatric consultation only when there is a specific indication.

Fellner and Marshall (1970) observed that a frequent theme in discussions of the ethics of organ transplantation from living donors is that the organ donor is subjected to risk and receives 'nothing in return'. Research has suggested that in fact donors do report benefits including heightened self-esteem and self-concept (Kemph 1966; Fellner and Marshall 1968; Eisendrath *et al.* 1969; Fellner and Marshall 1970; Fellner 1971; Kamstra-Hennen *et al.* 1981; Sharma and Enoch 1987). Some donors experience the act as one of the most meaningful experiences of their lives, and one that brought about beneficial changes within themselves (Fellner and Marshall 1970).

Case studies have suggested that there is a low rate of psychiatric sequelae in living donors. Kemph (1970), reporting on a series of 37 living–related donors, observed that all donors went through a process of mourning with some depressive symptoms after surgery. It was suggested that this depression was related to grieving for the lost body part and for the loss of the attention of the transplant team as the focus changed from the donor to the recipient (Cramond 1967; Kemph 1970; Levy 1986). Eisendrath *et al.* (1969) found, based on an 88 per cent response rate to a mailed questionnaire to living–related donors, that 13 of the 57 donors reported some depression or anxiety. Bennett and Harrison (1974) reporting on a series of 300 donors from 1954 through 1973, found that only one donor had experienced a major postoperative psychosis. Twelve donors had been under psychiatric care at the time of the surgery but eleven of them showed no subsequent worsening in their psychiatric status. The majority of respondents indicated that there was either no change or else an improvement in their psychological status after donating a kidney. Only 6 per cent reported some deterioration afterward in the form of being more anxious or irritable. Blohme *et al.* (1981) similarly found that of 214 living–related donors from 1965 to 1980, approximately 2 per cent suffered post-operative psychiatric complications and an additional 2 per cent experienced prolonged psychosocial problems afterward. The latter were reported to be associated with preoperative difficulties in adjustment or with failure of the graft. Simmons *et al.* (1977) reported that positive feelings about the donation were reported by donors up to nine years after the transplant. By two years after the donation, only 5 per cent of 230 living–related donors reported negative feelings about the transplant. These donors tended to have been ambivalent about the transplant, or to have had low self-esteem or feelings of unhappiness beforehand.

Hirvas *et al.* (1976) found emotional disturbances in almost 20 per cent of living–related donors, which tended to be associated with donations to siblings, graft failures, and other psychosocial stressors. However, Stiller *et al.* (1985) reported that the risk of significant psychological or emotional sequelae in living–related donors was much lower, in the range of 2 per cent. Sharma and Enoch (1987), in a five to ten year follow-up study, compared 14 donors with 9 potential donors who had been rejected on medical grounds. They found one case of psychiatric disorder in each group. They concluded that the psychiatric disorder was unlikely to be related to the kidney transplant and that the procedure does not cause long-term adverse psychological sequelae for living–related donors. The outcome in transplants using recipients of living–unrelated or emotionally-related donors has also been studied. Of 22 unrelated donors, Sadler *et al.* (1971) found that there were no psychological complications at five year follow-up. All donors reported increased self-esteem and none voiced any regrets about the donation.

Conclusions

Kidney transplantation has become a standard and optimal treatment for many patients with endstage renal disease. In the early phase of its development, the frequency of both medical and psychiatric complications, graft failure, and the scarcity of the resource, led to the practice of routine psychiatric evaluation preoperatively. This helped to identify patients at high risk, and to treat many psychiatric complications of this procedure. These complications include neuropsychiatric and organic mood disorders related to the surgical procedure, the underlying and associated medical diseases, and the immunosuppressant medication. In addition, adjustment following transplant was affected by the possibility of graft failure, the changes in physical appearance, and other complications related to steroids, and the psychological response to the introduction of a foreign organ. The latter is reported to be less often the cause of disturbing fantasies since transplant has become more commonplace. There was much initial concern about the psychological impact of the procedure on living donors. However, the rate of both psychiatric and physical complications in donors appears to be low and, in fact, many donors report feelings of enhancement.

In the early phase of renal transplantation, psychiatric consultants were involved because of their professional expertise in the diagnosis and treatment of psychiatric complications. However, they were often asked to predict compliance or adjustment to the procedure. Unfortunately, there was little scientific evidence upon which to base such predictions so that judgements were liable to be unreliable or influenced by personal value judgements. The most important lesson from that experience is that all health professionals need to delineate clearly which of their opinions are speculative and which are based upon a body of scientific information. Further, such consultants need to specify, with both patients and with the treatment team, whose interests they serve. With the introduction of a new treatment, these may be at cross purposes. At present, clinicians may be confident about their ability to diagnose and treat psychiatric illness, and to assist in the process of adjustment to a stressful procedure, but should be cautious about their ability to predict the future behaviour of individual patients.

References

Abram, H. S., Moore, G. L., and Westervelt, F. B. (1971). Suicidal behavior in chronic dialysis patients. *American Journal of Psychiatry*, 127, 119–24.

Armstrong, S. H. and Weiner, M. F. (1981–2). Noncompliance with post-transplant immunosuppression. *International Journal of Psychiatry in Medicine*, 11, 89–95.

Armstrong, S., Johnson, K., and Hopkins, J. (1981). Stopping immunosuppressant therapy following successful kidney transplantation: Two-year followup. In *Psychonephrology I: Psychological factors in hemodialysis and transplantation* (ed. N. B. Levy), pp. 247–54. (Plenum, New York).

Beck, D. E., Fennell, R. S., Yost, R. L., Robinson, J. D., Geary, D., and Richards, G. A. (1980). Evaluation of an educational program on compliance with medication regimens in pediatric patients with renal transplants. *Journal of Pediatrics*, 96, 1094–7.

Bennett, A. H. and Harrison, J. H. (1974). Experience with living familial renal donors. *Surgery, Gynecology & Obstetrics*, 139, 894–8.

Bernstein, D. M. (1971). After transplantation: The child's emotional reactions. *American Journal of Psychiatry*, 127, 1189–93.

Bertoli, M., Romagnoli, G. F., and Margreiter, R. (1988). Irreversible dementia following ciclosporin therapy in a renal transplant patient. *Nephron*, 49, 333–4.

Blazer II, D. G., Petrie, W. M., and Wilson, W. P. (1976). Affective psychoses following renal transplant. *Diseases of the Nervous System*, 37, 663–7.

Blohme, I., Gabel, H., and Brynger, H. (1981). The living donor in renal transplantation. *Scandinavian Journal of Urology and Nephrology*, 64S, 143–51.

Bouras, M., Silvestre, D., Broyer, M., and Raimbault, G. (1976). Renal transplantation in children: A psychological survey. *Clinical Nephrology*, 6, 478–82.

Carosella, J. (1984). Picking up the pieces: The unsuccessful kidney transplant. *Health and Social Work*, 9, 142–52.

Colomb, G. and Hamburger, J. (1967). Psychological and moral problems of renal transplantation. In *Psychological aspects of surgery* (ed. H. S. Abram), pp. 157–77. (Little, Brown, Boston).

Cramond, W. A. (1967). Renal homotransplantation: Some observations on recipients and donors. *British Journal of Psychiatry*, 113, 1223–30.

Cramond, W. A. (1971). Renal transplantations: Experiences with recipients and donors. *Seminars in Psychiatry*, 3, 116–32.

Craven, J. L., Rodin, G. M., Johnson, L., and Kennedy, S. H. (1987). The diagnosis of major depression in renal dialysis patients. *Psychosomatic Medicine*, 49, 482–92.

DeLone, P., Trollinger, J. H., Fox, N., and Light, J. (1989). Noncompliance in renal transplant recipients: Methods for recognition and intervention. *Transplantation Proceedings*, 21, 3982–4.

Didlake, R. H., Dreyfus, K., Kerman, R. H., Van Buren, C. T., and Kahan, B. D. (1988). Patient noncompliance: A major cause of late graft failure in cyclosporine-treated renal transplants. *Transplantation Proceedings*, 20, 63–9.

Dubovsky, S. L. and Penn, I. (1980). Psychiatric considerations in renal transplant surgery. *Psychosomatics*, 21, 481–91.

Eggers, P. W. (1988). Effect of transplantation on the Medicare end-stage renal disease program. *New England Journal of Medicine*, 318, 223–9.

Eisendrath, R. M. (1969). The role of grief and fear in the death of kidney transplant patients. *American Journal of Psychiatry*, 126, 381–7.

Eisendrath, R. M., Guttmann, R. D., and Murray, J. E. (1969). Psychologic considerations in the selection of kidney transplant donors. *Surgery, Gynecology & Obstetrics*, 129, 243–8.

Evans, R. W., Manninen, D. L., Garrison, L. P., Jr, Hart, L. G., Blagg, C. R., Gutman, R. A. *et al.* (1985). The quality of life of patients with end-stage renal disease. *New England Journal of Medicine*, 312, 553–9.

Fellner, C. H. (1971). Selection of living kidney donors and the problem of informed consent. *Seminars in Psychiatry*, 3, 79–85.

Fellner, C. H. and Marshall, J. R. (1968). Twelve kidney donors. *Journal of the American Medical Association*, 206, 2703–7.

Fellner, C. H. and Marshall, J. R. (1970). Kidney donors: The myth of informed consent. *American Journal of Psychiatry*, 126, 1245–51.

Ferris, G. N. (1969). Psychiatric considerations in patients receiving cadaveric renal transplants. *Southern Medical Journal*, 62, 1482–4.

Fricchione, G. L. (1989). Psychiatric aspects of renal transplantation. *Australian and New Zealand Journal of Psychiatry*, 23, 407–17.

Gordon, M. J. V., White, R., Matas, A. J., Tellis, V. A., Glicklich, D., Quinn, T., *et al.* (1986). Renal transplantation in patients with a history of heroin abuse. *Transplantation*, 42, 556–7.

Gulledge, A. D., Buszta, C., and Montague, D. K. (1983). Psychosocial aspects of renal transplantation. *Urologic Clinics of North America*, 10, 327–35.

Hirvas, J., Enckell, M., Kuhlback, B., and Pasternack, A. (1976). Psychological and social problems encountered in active treatment of chronic uraemia: II. The living donor. *Acta Medica Scandinavica*, 200, 17–20.

Johnson, J. P., McCauley, C. R., and Copley, J. B. (1982). The quality of life of hemodialysis and transplant patients. *Kidney International*, 22, 286–91.

Kalman, T. P., Wilson, P. G., and Kalman, C. M. (1983). Psychiatric morbidity in long-term renal transplant recipients and patients undergoing hemodialysis: A comparative study. *Journal of the American Medical Association*, 250, 55–8.

Kamstra-Hennen, L., Beebe, J., Stumm, S., and Simmons, R. G. (1981). Ethical evaluation of related donation: The donor after five years. *Transplantation Proceedings*, 13, 60–1.

Kaplan De-Nour, A. and Shanan, J. (1980). Quality of life of dialysis and transplanted patients. *Nephron*, 25, 117–20.

Kemph, J. P. (1966). Renal failure, artificial kidney and kidney transplant. *American Journal of Psychiatry*, 122, 1270–4.

Kemph, J. P. (1970). Observations of the effects of kidney transplant on donors and recipients. *Diseases of the Nervous System*, 31, 323–5.

Kemph, J. P., Bermann, E. A., and Coppolillo, H. P. (1969). Kidney transplant and shifts in family dynamics. *American Journal of Psychiatry*, 125, 1485–90.

Korsch, B. M., Negrete, V. F., Gardner, J. E., Weinstock, C. L., Mercer, A. S., Grushkin, C. M., *et al.* (1973). Kidney transplantation in children: Psychosocial follow-up study on child and family. *Journal of Pediatrics*, 83, 399–408.

Korsch, B. M., Fine, R. N., and Negrete, V. F. (1978). Noncompliance in children with renal transplants. *Pediatrics*, 61, 872–6.

Levey, A. S., Hou, S., and Bush, H. L., Jr. (1986). Kidney transplantation from unrelated living donors: time to reclaim a discarded opportunity. *New England Journal of Medicine*, 314, 914–16.

Levy, N. B. (1986). Renal transplantation and the new medical era. *Advances in Psychosomatic Medicine*, 15, 167–79.

Lilly, J. R., Giles, G., Hurwitz, R., Schroter, G., Takagi, H., Gray, S., *et al.* (1971). Renal homotransplantation in pediatric patients. *Pediatrics*, 47, 548–57.

McCabe, M. S. and Corry, R. J. (1978). Psychiatric illness and human renal transplantation. *Journal of Clinical Psychiatry*, 39, 393–400.

MacDonald, D. J. (1972). Psychotic reactions during organ transplantation. *Canadian Psychiatric Association Journal*, 17, SS15–SS17.

Morales-Otero, L. A., Gonzalez, Z. A., and Santiago-Delpin, E. A. (1988). Neurological complications after kidney transplantation. *Transplantation Proceedings*, 20, 443–5.

Najarian, J. S. (1975). Editorial comment on Owens *et al. Archives of Surgery*, 110, 1451.

Nissenson, A. R., Levin, M. L., Klawans, H. L., and Nausieda, P. L. (1977). Neurological sequelae of end stage renal disease (ESRD). *Journal of Chronic Diseases*, 30, 705–33.

Nylander, W. A., Jr, Sutherland, D. E. R., Bentley, F. R., Simmons, R. L., and Najarian, J. S. (1985). Fifteen to twenty-year follow-up of renal transplants performed in the 1960's. *Transplantation Proceedings*, 17, 104–5.

Owens, M. L., Maxwell, J. G., Goodnight, J., and Wolcott, M. W. (1975). Discontinuance of immunosuppression in renal transplant patients. *Archives of Surgery*, 110, 1450–1.

Penn, I., Bunch, D., Olenik, D., and Abouna, G. (1971). Psychiatric experience with patients receiving renal and hepatic transplants. *Seminars in Psychiatry*, 3, 133–44.

Petrie, K. (1989). Psychological well-being and psychiatric disturbance in dialysis and renal transplant patients. *British Journal of Medical Psychology*, 62, 91–6.

Rodin, G. and Voshart, K. (1987). Depressive symptoms and functional impairment in the medically ill. *General Hospital Psychiatry*, 9, 251–8.

Rodin, G., Voshart, K., Cattran, D., Halloran, P., Cardella, C., and Fenton, S. (1985). Cadaveric renal transplant failure: The short-term sequelae. *International Journal of Psychiatry in Medicine*, 15, 357–64.

Rovelli, M., Palmeri, D., Vossler, E., Bartus, S., Hull, D., and Schweizer, R. (1989). Noncompliance in renal transplant recipients: evaluation by socioeconomic groups. *Transplantation Proceedings*, 21, 3979–81.

Sadler, H. H., Davison, L., Carroll, C., and Kountz, S. L. (1971). The living, genetically unrelated, kidney donor. *Seminars in Psychiatry*, 3, 86–101.

Sharma, V. K. and Enoch, M. D. (1987). Psychological sequelae of kidney donation: A 5–10 year follow up study. *Acta Psychiatrica Scandinavica*, 75, 264–7.

Short, M. J. and Harris, N. L. (1969). Psychiatric observations of renal homotransplantation. *Southern Medical Journal*, 62, 1479–82.

Simmons, R. G., Hickey, K., Kjellstrand, C. M., and Simmons, R. L. (1971). Donors and non-donors: The role of the family and the physician in kidney transplantation. *Seminars in Psychiatry*, 3, 102–15.

Simmons, R. G., Klein, S. D., and Simmons, R. L. (1977). *The gift of life: the social and psychological impact of organ transplantation*. (Wiley, New York).

Simmons, R. G., Kamstra-Hennen, L., and Thompson, C. R. (1981). Psychosocial adjustment five to nine years posttransplant. *Transplantation Proceedings*, 13, 40–3.

Sollinger, H. W., Kalayoglu, M., and Belzer, F. O. (1986). Use of the donor specific transfusion protocol in living unrelated donor–recipient combinations. *Annals of Surgery*, 204, 315–21.

Steinberg, J., Levy, N. B., and Radvila, A. (1981). Psychological factors affecting acceptance or rejection of kidney transplants. In *Psychonephrology I: psychological factors in hemodialysis and transplantation* (ed. N. B. Levy), pp. 185–93. (Plenum, New York).

Stewart, R. S. (1983). Psychiatric issues in renal dialysis and transplantation. *Hospital and Community Psychiatry*, 34, 623–8.

Stewart, R. S. and Stewart, R. M. (1979). Neuropsychiatric aspects of chronic renal disease. *Psychosomatics*, 20, 524–31.

Stiller, C. R., Lindberg, M. C., Rimstead, D., Robinette, M. A., Shimizu, A. G., and Abbott, C. R. (1985). Living related donation. *Transplantation Proceedings*, 17S, 85–100.

Streltzer, J., Moe, M., Yanagida, E., and Siemsen, A. (1983–4). Coping with transplant failure: Grief vs. denial. *International Journal of Psychiatry in Medicine*, 13, 97–106.

Strong, R. W., Lynch, S. V., Ong, T. H., Matsunami, H., Koido, Y., and Balderson, G. A. (1990). Successful liver transplantation from a living donor to her son. *New England Journal of Medicine*, 322, 1505–7.

Surman, O. S. (1981). Renal transplantation and the current treatment of end stage renal disease: A psychiatric medicine perspective. In *Psychiatric medicine update: Massachusetts General Hospital reviews for physicians* (ed. T. C. Manschreck), pp. 155–78. (Elsevier, New York).

Surman, O. S. (1987). Hemodialysis and renal transplantation. In *Massachusetts General Hospital handbook of general hospital psychiatry* (eds T. P. Hackett and N. H. Cassem), pp. 380–402. (PSG Publishing Co., Littleton, MA).

Uehling, D. T., Hussey, J. L., Weinstein, A. B., Wank, R., and Bach, F. H. (1976). Cessation of immunosuppression after renal transplantation. *Surgery*, 79, 278–82.

Viederman, M. (1975). Psychogenic factors in kidney transplant rejection: a case study. *American Journal of Psychiatry*, 132, 957–9.

Wennberg, J. E. (1990). Outcomes research, cost containment, and the fear of health care rationing. *New England Journal of Medicine*, 323, 1202–4.

Wilson, W. P., Stickel, D. L., Hayes, C. P., Jr, and Harris, N. L. (1968). Psychiatric considerations of renal transplantation. *Archives of Internal Medicine*, 122, 502–6.

Zarinsky, I. (1975). Psychological problems of kidney transplanted adolescents. *Adolescence*, 10, 101–9.

12 Heart transplantation

R. Frierson, J. Tabler, and R. Spears

Heart transplants involve many physiological and psychological challenges (McAleer *et al.* 1985; Frierson and Lippmann 1987; House and Thompson 1988). The candidate must accept the presence of a terminal illness, that a heart transplant is necessary to preserve life, and that there is uncertainty regarding acceptance or rejection for transplantation. Such individuals must assimilate an enormous amount of information in a matter of days, and emotionally re-invest in the possibility of life extension (Frierson *et al.* 1990). Given the potential for adverse psychological reactions, recent attention has been focused on the development of appropriate psychosocial screening instruments to identify those candidates at risk for impairment either during or following the procedure.

Many heart transplant programs now include a psychiatric or psychological assessment as part of the multi-disciplinary evaluative process. After completing this evaluation, the consulting psychiatrist may offer an opinion as to whether the candidate is psychologically suitable for the procedure (Thompson 1983; Mai *et al.* 1986; Kuhn *et al.* 1988). Further, as the psychological implications of heart transplantation have begun to receive more attention in the scientific literature, the consultation psychiatrist has become an integral part of the treatment team. In this role, the transplant psychiatrist is involved in assessing the patient's past and present psychological functioning, identifying persons with clinically significant psychopathology for whom compliance may be a problem, educating of patients and their families regarding emotional aspects of transplantation, assessing the candidate's support systems to enable future mobilization of these resources, and instituting proper treatment of psychiatric complications related to transplantation (Frierson and Lippmann 1987).

Most studies of the psychological aspects of heart transplantation suggest that adjustment to the procedure occurs in a series of stages (see Table 12.1) (Allender *et al.* 1983; Watts *et al.* 1984; Kuhn *et al.* 1988). Each stage poses '... unique adaptive tasks', and the candidates' ability to meet these challenges is the key to a successful psychological outcome (Kuhn *et al.* 1988). This chapter will examine the psychological challenges of heart transplantation, discuss the various stages of the procedure and their associated tasks, and offer treatment recommendations for managing the emotional reactions exhibited by these individuals.

Stages of psychological adjustment

The transplant proposal and evaluation

When first told that a heart transplant is a treatment option, patients' reactions vary according to a number of factors, including the candidate's personality style; previous experiences with surgery; the time interval between proposal and planned surgery; duration of illness; the degree of denial; and the availability of family support. Many react with marked apprehension and disbelief (Watts *et al.* 1984). While patients may have recognized deterioration of their health, for some patients the word transplant embodies their worst fears and undermines denial of the life-threatening nature of their disease. At this point, patients must decide about a procedure that many of them still consider experimental and itself life-threatening. Further contributing to uncertainty is that, in most instances, the initial proposal is made by a physician with little practical knowledge of the procedure. Applicants may have to wait for weeks before having the opportunity to ask questions directly of a heart transplant team.

The personality style of the candidate is perhaps the most important predictor of response to the proposal for transplant (Geringer and Stern 1986; Kuhn *et al.* 1988). Antisocial individuals may react to the fear of transplant by angry outbursts and challenges to physician authority (Kuhn *et al.* 1988). Dependent individuals may become regressed and tax the patience of the medical and nursing staff. Obsessive/compulsive persons may become immersed in minute details as a means of defending against anxiety. Histrionic patients may be preoccupied with the dramatic nature of a heart transplant and not give their decision adequate consideration. Finally, paranoid candidates may perceive transplantation as an assault on their person, and react with hostility or noncompliance (Kuhn *et al.* 1988). These reactions each have the potential to create strife between the candidate, his family, and medical staff. The psychiatrist's role during the transplant proposal stage is to encourage the patient to express fears openly, and to advise the care-givers and family not to react personally to maladaptive behaviour. In most cases, this stage terminates with increasing wishes for the transplant and a growing fear of not being accepted for surgery.

The evaluative stage begins when the applicant agrees to the assessment and continues through to his acceptance as a candidate (Kuhn *et al.* 1988). Anxiety and fear about dying are often superseded by concerns of possible rejection as a candidate. As a result, patients often try to present themselves as psychologically healthy, yet physically infirm, to increase their potential for acceptance (Kuhn *et al.* 1988). As candidates are seen by a variety of evaluators, the initial euphoria begins to give way to more practical considerations, such as the stringent transplant protocol, financial considerations, and even the

TABLE 12.1 Stages of heart transplantation

Stage	Major tasks	Emotional responses	Outcome
Proposal of a transplant	accept the severity of their condition reinvest in the possibility of an exten-sion of their lives make a decision about undergoing the evaluation	disbelief apprehension marked anxiety grief	strong wish for transplant fear of not being accepted as a candidate
Evaluation	assimilate an enormous amount of information in a matter of days consider practical implications of transplant as euphoria fades present themselves as psychologically healthy	initial euphoria overwhelmed anxiety fear of rejection	approval granted time frame for transplant discussed thoughts turn to donor
Waiting for a donor	adapt to feelings of loss of control stay alive until a donor is found deal with intensified fears of death maintain a sense of hope and optimism	frustration impatience anger fear of death re-emerges sense of guilt relief	appropriate donor found euphoria re-emerges anticipation and fear of surgery appear

Perioperative stage	manage anxieties about surgery begin recuperation from the procedure adjust to changes in cognition that might occur	intense euphoria (often medication augmented)	positive physiological changes noted tribulations of waiting are forgotten discharge eagerly awaited
In-house convalescence	incorporation of the heart into the sense of self engage in exercise and other rehabilitative tasks manage anxiety about first endocardial biopsy deal with biopsy rejection	concern about the donor helplessness post-euphoria let-down intense anxiety possible discouragement and depression	becomes part of a network of heart recipients and waiting candidates serves as a role model for others
Post-discharge adjustment	leave the security of hospital deal with celebrity status and notoriety compliance re-integrate into the family structure adapt to changes in appearance manage sexual concerns	separation anxiety sense of abandonment feeling of uniqueness depression possible suicidality sense of rebirth	Gradual loss of 'patienthood' and re-emergence as an integrated person

amount of pain and physical deformity. Many patients had not initially considered the possibility that after deciding on a heart transplant, they could be considered unsuitable for the procedure.

During the evaluative period, the psychiatrist must be alert for signs of ambiguity about surgery and must not be distracted from his professional assessment by the candidate's attempt to idealize himself psychologically. In those instances where the patient qualifies medically for a transplant, but not psychologically, the psychiatrist must deal with their personal reaction to denying a patient a procedure that could ultimately save his life (Frierson and Lippmann 1987).

Waiting for a donor

One author has referred to this stage of heart transplantation as '. . . dancing with death' (Kuhn *et al.* 1988). This is a period of intense dependency and loss of control for the patient. As health continues to deteriorate, fate is in the hands of a person he or she has never met (the potential donor) and the members of the transplant team, on whom he may be totally dependent. In addition, patients may feel resentful when other candidates who have not waited as long, or highly publicized transplant hopefuls, receive a heart before they do (Frierson and Lippmann 1987). These situations may lead to frustration and behavioural disturbances. Pharmacological management of anxiety may be required.

Most patients describe the waiting period as interminable, and their behaviour during this stressful time may provide an indicator of future coping ability (Frierson and Lippmann 1987). The fear of death again predominates, and patients find themselves in the unsettling position of hoping someone else dies before they do. Other features during this stage may include a desire to remain in the security of the intensive care unit, insomnia related to the fear of nocturnal demise, and ruminations about circumstances, such as a fatal accident, that might lead to a heart becoming available (so-called 'donor weather' or 'rainy day syndrome') (Frierson and Lippmann 1987; Kuhn *et al.* 1988). These phenomena have been similarly described in candidates for lung transplants (Craven *et al.* 1990) and probably represent manifestations of death anxiety occurring in a situation with an uncontrollable and ambiguous outcome.

The psychiatrist's role during this stage is to treat whatever adverse behavioural consequences of waiting become evident. Often such conservative interventions such as home passes, relaxation training, peer group support from others who are waiting, and exposure to heart recipients who are doing well, are helpful. More serious psychiatric manifestations, such as psychosis and clinical depression should be treated pharmacologically. The management of these occurrences will be discussed later in this chapter.

Surgery and the perioperative period

This is a fairly brief phase that begins when a donor heart is found and ends with transfer out of the intensive care unit (Kuhn *et al.* 1988). It is characterized by euphoria at the realization that transplant is about to become a reality. Months of seeming inactivity are replaced by hectic preparations for surgery. The positive outlook generally continues immediately after surgery as patients begin to notice improvement in their physical condition. Medications such as corticosteroids and opioid analgesics may add to the elevated mood. During this stage, patients often seem oblivious to the tasks that lie ahead.

Adaptation and rehabilitation

By the time of discharge from hospital, the patient has often become part of a network of heart transplant recipients and candidates (Kuhn *et al.* 1988). Serving as a role model for individuals still awaiting a donor may enhance self-esteem and herald entry into the final stage. The support network may then shift from the transplant team to the patient's family. For many patients, leaving the security of the hospital is an anxiety-laden event, and frequent visits back to the hospital occasionally result. At home, the new recipient is often subjected to celebrity status. Some patients, especially those with histrionic, narcissistic, and antisocial features, enjoy this. Others find it an unwelcome intrusion upon their privacy.

A first major task during this stage is incorporation of the new heart into one's sense of self. Patients often refer to the organ as 'the' heart rather than as 'my' heart (Frierson and Lippmann 1987). Some persons regard it as if it had a mind of its own (Frierson and Lippmann 1987). Such comments as '. . . the heart is rejecting me', or 'I don't think the heart can tolerate that', are not unusual. For the first time since the waiting period, the patients' thoughts turn to the donor. They fantasize about the life and death of this person and harbour fears, often left unspoken, that they will assume some of the characteristics of the deceased (Frierson and Lippmann 1987; Tabler and Frierson 1990). Our experience has been that these concerns are especially intense if the information such as the donor's sex, race, sexual preference, or cause of death is made known.

The degree of incorporation is also related to patient expectations from the procedure. Some view the transplanted organ as 'bionic' and feel a sense of re-birth (Frierson and Lippmann 1987; Tabler and Frierson 1990). One such individual fantasized that his donor had been 'sexually prolific', and that he had no choice but to '. . . live up to his reputation'. Other patients become obsessed with protecting the heart and are reluctant to engage in the rehabilitative process. Muslin (1971) has described three stages of internalization composed of a foreign body stage, when the transplanted organ is 'new, separate, or sticking out', a partial incorporation stage, when the patient begins to talk less about the organ's newness, and the final stage, characterized by a lack of awareness of the new organ, unless the patient is asked specifically about it.

Problems with incorporation vary widely with the organ being transplanted. The heart is believed to embody symbolically many more of the donor characteristics than the bone marrow, for example (Lesko and Hawkins 1983). In addition, the fact that the donor has died, accentuates problems with integration. Some psychiatric patient populations have particular difficulties with incorporation. These include schizophrenics, and those with borderline intellect, for whom such abstract concepts are difficult, and persons with serious personality disorders, especially borderline types, whose personal sense of identity is already diminished (Frierson and Lippmann 1987).

Compliance is also a major task for patients. Separated from the accustomed routine of the hospital, the patient must rely on his own initiative to take medication and attend clinic appointments. In addition, the individual must resist the temptation posed by the availability of alcohol, illicit drugs, nicotine, and prohibited foods. Some patients feel the urge to test the heart to see if indulgences they had avoided for months can now be tolerated. Patients whose previous cardiac decompensation was secondary to coronary artery disease are particularly susceptible to this behaviour. This may be related to the fact that their original disease was behaviourally based (poor eating habits, smoking, lack of exercise, poor stress management, etc.). Our experience has been that coronary artery disease patients are more prone to noncompliance than those with heart disease of other aetiologies.

Other patients, especially those whose cardiac decompensation was precipitous, are simply unaccustomed to taking multiple medications at scheduled times. Returning to the hospital for rehabilitation and clinic appointments is also perceived as intrusive and cumbersome. Some individuals feel such activities remind them of a time when they were ill and most vulnerable. Occasionally, transplanted patients have even expressed regrets about having had the procedure, but these feelings are generally transitory. We have found peer support groups and scheduled recreational activities, such as alumni picnics, to be non-threatening ways to monitor psychologic adaptation of discharged patients. Support groups for spouses are also important in this regard.

Regression is also a characteristic of the post-discharge stage. For those patients who seem to have many return visits to the transplant centre for questionable indications, separation anxiety is often a contributing factor. We have seen some discharged transplanted patients who became envious of the attention that candidates and new recipients still receive. One man angrily complained that the transplant team lost interest in him once the surgery was completed and he had become '. . . just another statistic'. The only means by which this patient could assure that he would not be forgotten would be to return to the hospital as often as possible. He eventually responded well to supportive psychotherapy and antidepressant medication. Allowing some recipients to remain associated with the team as a role model for others can maintain their sense of belonging while also enhancing their identity as healthy and more autonomous persons.

Adjustment to a heart transplant is further characterized by several other stressors. Convinced that they will now live longer, patients turn their attention to the quality of that life (Hunt 1985; Lough *et al.* 1985; Brennan *et al.* 1987). It is during this time that body image concerns may increase (Castelnuovo-Tedesco 1973, 1978; Henker 1979; Tabler and Frierson 1990). Rapid weight gain, facial puffiness, hirsutism, chest wall deformities, and surgical scars all contribute to these concerns. Additionally, the recipient's spouse had often already begun the process of emotional detachment before transplantation was proposed, and may have begun to adjust to life without the patient. Status within the family was invariably altered by being absolved of normal duties, whether as breadwinner or sexual partner (Tabler and Frierson 1990). A major task for the spouse following transplant is to reinvest emotionally in the patient whose life has unexpectedly been extended. Discharged patients frequently comment that '. . . something's missing', or '. . . she's just going through the motions'. Conversely, some spouses remember the pain of the grieving process, and hold back emotionally because '. . . I don't ever want to go through that again'. Thus, the heart recipient often returns home eager to become involved in activities there, only to realize that such involvement may not be needed.

More recent investigations have examined sexual concerns following heart transplant (Tabler and Frierson 1990). Patients are generally reluctant to discuss sexual problems with members of the transplant team, but such concerns are often present (Wise 1978; Gravesen 1986; Merrill *et al.* 1990; Tabler and Frierson 1990). Concerns may be manifested by lewd jokes about sexual activities or flirting with hospital personnel (Tabler and Frierson 1990). Some individuals feels that to expect satisfactory sexual functioning after having had their life extended may be asking too much. Others perceive discomfort on the part of their physicians when sexual matters are discussed (Merrill *et al.* 1990). One study (Tabler and Frierson 1990) revealed that post-transplant sexual confidence and performance are commonly impaired by altered roles and responsibilities between spouses, concerns about sexual attractiveness, loss of autonomy, physiological effects of medication, depressed mood, performance anxiety, and fear of coital death. Sexual difficulties in this study included both avoidance of sexual opportunities or intensified sexual desire, and fears that one might assume the sexual behaviour of the anonymous donor. The medical staff must be sensitive to the sexual concerns of transplant patients, whether verbally expressed or not. Full reintegration into the family structure is thus the most difficult challenge for the transplanted patient during this final stage.

Psychiatric disorders

Depressive disorders

There is a high incidence of depressive symptoms among transplant patients in general (Kraft 1971; Christopherson 1979; Basch 1973). Penn *et al.* (1971) reported that one-third of almost 300 kidney recipients had postoperative emotional difficulties (mainly depression) and that seven of these patients eventually committed suicide. Lunde (1969) noted that after a heart transplant, one out of nine individuals developed a clinical depression, including two with minor mood and cognitive alterations and three with psychotic depression. Most studies suggest that completed suicide is much more common in kidney than heart recipients (Penn *et al.* 1971). As with other transplanted persons, those cardiac patients with a previous history of depression are more prone to a recurrence of same.

Most depression that occurs in the context of cardiac transplantation is transitory in nature. In these instances, reassurance and support should suffice. On some occasions, however, depression can be so severe as to compromise the patient's recovery. In particular, lack of motivation, apathy, sleep disorders, poor appetite, and recurrent thoughts of death require prompt and aggressive pharmacological intervention. Because the traditional antidepressants have a lag time of 2–3 weeks, their use is often impractical (Glassman and Bigger 1981; Himmelhoch 1981; Davidson and Wenger 1982; Cavanaugh *et al.* 1983). Treatment modalities with a quicker onset of antidepressant action include electroconvulsive therapy, and psychostimulants (Katon and Raskind 1980; Moore 1981; Tesar 1982; Fernandez *et al.* 1987; Craven 1989). We have found psychostimulants to be beneficial in treating depression both before and after surgery. Methylphenidate in divided doses and dextroamphetamine, usually as a single dose because of its longer half-life, can produce positive changes in mood, appetite, sleep, and energy level in 24–48 hours. Such side effects as myocardial depression, constipation, and urinary retention are avoided (Katon and Raskind 1980; Moore 1981; Tesar 1982; Fernandez *et al.* 1987). We have maintained patients on psychostimulants for many months without evidence of habituation. These agents should be best avoided in patients who are highly anxious or prone to psychosis.

An organic mood disorder must be ruled out before transplant patients are treated with an antidepressant. Cerebrovascular accidents, anaemia, hypothyroidism, and some medications (e.g. cyclosporin) can induce depression. Corticosteroids and certain anti-hypertensives are especially prone to produce changes in mood (Erman and Guggenheim 1981; Ling *et al.* 1981).

Anxiety disorders

Anxiety is a universal finding across heart transplant centres. Given the relative novelty of the procedure and the constant proximity of death, such a finding is not unexpected. Many of the physiological manifestations of anxiety, such as tachycardia, tachypnea, shortness of breath, chest tightness, dysphagia, and diaphoresis occur commonly. Thus, deterioration of the individual's medical condition must be entertained before these symptoms are attributed to anxiety. Anxiety is especially high following transplant proposal, during the evaluative and waiting periods, and at the time of the first biopsy. Symptoms can range from transitory nervousness to panic episodes.

In most instances of anxiety related to transplants, reassurance or brief counselling are sufficient. Most patients do not have at their disposal the coping skills they have used previously. This is especially true for those patients who are action-oriented. Earlier, we mentioned the advisability of utilizing behavioural techniques such as progressive muscle relaxation, medi-tation, bio-feedback, and imagery for treating simple anxiety in these patients. However, some patients may be apprehensive to work with these techniques or may have problems with relaxation induced worries and anxiety. In the event that such an approach is either unproductive or unavailable, pharmacological intervention may be necessary. We advocate the use of short-acting benzo-diazepines such as lorazepam and oxazepam. Alternatives include hydroxyzine and buspirone, although the latter agent has about a two-week delay in the onset of anxiolytic action. Given the tremendous stress of cardiac transplanta-tion, it is difficult to label any degree of anxiety, regardless of its intensity, as pathological. However, these symptoms may certainly be both uncomfortable and problematic, and require treatment.

Organic brain disorders

The occurrence of a transient confusional state after heart transplantation is common (Abram 1971; Murray 1978; Watts *et al.* 1984; House and Thompson 1988). Delirium following this type of transplant demonstrates either typically an early or delayed pattern. Early onset delirium after a heart transplant is similar in aetiology to altered mental states seen after other types of major surgery. Causes include: pulmonary hypofunction with possible cerebral hypoxia, acid base imbalance, and atelectasis; altered cerebral blood flow during surgery, including such occurrences as microinfarction; pulmonary and wound infections; medications used during the immediate postoperative period, especially analgesics, hypnotics, anti-hypertensives, histamine recep-tor antagonists, and corticosteroids; altered cardiac rates and rhythms that decrease effective stroke volume; fluid overload; and altered metabolic para-meters (e.g. electrolyte abnormalities). The 'delayed' delirium typically occurs in the third to fifth week and often follows increased immunosuppression for rejection.

The treatment of post-transplant delirium involves discovery and correction of the underlying cause, and medical management of the behaviour in the interim. In some instances, such as those caused by medications that cannot be discontinued or reduced in dosage, the psychiatric intervention should be directed toward management until alterations in medication can be made. We have found intravenous haloperidol, often in high doses, to be most effective in managing the behaviour of acutely delirious patients after cardiac transplantation. The occurrence of extrapyramidal symptoms, commonly seen with this agent, seem to be less likely by the intravenous route. As in all instances of delirium, the use of psychotropic medication should be an adjunct to, and not replacement for, correction of the underlying cause.

Summary and conclusions

While many similarities exist, heart transplantation differs in some respects from other organ replacement procedures. These include the almost mystical significance of the heart as the centre of life. In most transplant centres, candidates for a donor heart are subjected to a more detailed psychosocial evaluation than are those who receive other organs, and problems with incorporation of the alien organ into the sense of self are more complicated than with non-cardiac transplantations.

Adjustment to heart transplantation proceeds according to the demands of the medical circumstances. Adaptation following surgery may be complicated for some patients, particularly those with a prolonged period of disability prior to surgery. Reintegration into family, vocational, and social roles may be challenging for heart transplant recipients. Sexual difficulties appear common in this group and may not be readily discussed with transplant team personnel.

References

Abram, H. S. (1971). Psychotic reactions after cardiac surgery: a critical review. *Seminars in Psychiatry*, 3, 70–8.

Allender, J., Shisslak, C., Kaszniak, A., and Copeland, J. (1983). Stages of psychological adjustment associated with heart transplantation. *Journal of Heart Transplantation*, 2, 228–31.

Basch, S. H. (1973). Damaged self-esteem and depression in organ transplantation. *Transplantation Proceedings*, 5, 1125–7.

Brennan, A. F., David, M. H., Buchholz, D., Kuhn, W. F., and Gray, L. A. Jr. (1987). Predictors of quality of life following cardiac transplantation. *Psychosomatics*, 28, 566–71.

Castelnuovo-Tedesco, P. (1973). Organ transplant, body image, psychosis. *Psycho-analytic Quarterly*, 42, 349–63.

Castelnuovo-Tedesco, P. (1978). Ego vicissitudes in response to replacement or loss of body parts: certain analogies to events during psychoanalytic treatment. *Psycho-analytic Quarterly*, 47, 381–97.

Cavanaugh, S., Clark, D. C., and Gibbons, R. D. (1983). Diagnosing depression in the hospitalized medically ill. *Psychosomatics*, 24, 809–15.

Christopherson, L. (1979). Cardiac transplantation: need for counselling. *Nursing Mirror*, 149, 34–6.

Craven, J. L. (1989). Methylphenidate for cyclosporine-associated organic mood disorder (letter). *American Journal of Psychiatry*, 146, 553.

Craven, J. L., Bright, J., and Dear, C. L. (1990). Psychiatric, psychosocial, and rehabili-tative aspects of lung transplantation. *Clinics in Chest Medicine*, 11, 247–57.

Davidson, J. and Wenger, T. (1982). Using antidepressants in patients with cardio-vascular disease. *Drug Therapy*, 12, 196–7.

Erman, M. K. and Guggenheim, F. G. (1981). Psychiatric side effects of commonly used drugs. *Drug Therapy*, 11, 55–64.

Fernandez, F., Adams, F., Holmes, V. F., Levy, J. K., and Neidhart, M. (1987). Methyl-phenidate for depressive disorders in cancer patients: an alternative to standard antidepressants. *Psychosomatics*, 28, 455–61.

Frierson, R. L. and Lippmann, S. B. (1987). Heart transplant candidates rejected on psychiatric indications: experience in developing criteria for proper patient selec-tion. *Psychosomatics*, 28, 347–55.

Frierson, R. L., Tabler, J. B., Lippmann, S. B., and Brennan, A. F. (1990). Patients who refuse heart transplantation. *Journal of Heart Transplantation*, 9, 385–91.

Geringer, E. S. and Stern, T. A. (1986). Coping with medical illness: the impact of personality types. *Psychosomatics*, 27, 251–61.

Glassman, A. H. and Bigger, J. T. Jr. (1981). Cardiovascular effects of therapeutic doses of tricyclic antidepressants: a review. *Archives of General Psychiatry*, 38, 815–20.

Gravesen, R. (1986). How do you get patients to talk about sexual problems? *Medical Aspects of Human Sexuality*, 14, 50–60.

Henker, F. O. III (1979). Body image conflict following trauma and surgery. *Psycho-somatics*, 20, 812–20.

Himmelhoch, J. M. (1981). Cardiovascular effects of trazodone in humans. *Journal of Clinical Psychopharmacology*, 1, 70–5.

House, R. M. and Thompson, T. L. II (1988). Psychiatric aspects of organ transplanta-tion. *Journal of the American Medical Association*, 260, 535–9.

Hunt, S. M. (1985). Quality of life considerations in cardiac transplantation. *Quality of Life and Cardiovascular Care*, 2, 308–16.

Katon, W. and Raskind, M. (1980). Treatment of depression in the medically ill elderly with methylphenidate. *American Journal of Psychiatry*, 137, 963–5.

Kraft, I. A. (1971). Psychiatric complications of cardiac transplantation. *Seminars in Psychiatry*, 3, 58–69.

Kuhn, W. F., Davis, M. H., and Lippmann, S. B. (1988). Emotional adjustment to cardiac transplantation. *General Hospital Psychiatry*, 10, 108–13.

Lesko, L. M. and Hawkins, D. R. (1983). Psychological aspects of transplantation medicine. In *New psychiatric syndromes: DSM-III and beyond* (ed. S. Akhtar), pp. 265–309 (Jason Aronson, Inc., New York).

Ling, M. H. M., Perry, P. J., and Tsuang, M. T. (1981). Side-effects of corticosteroid therapy. *Archives of General Psychiatry*, 38, 471–7.

Lough, M. E., Lindsey, A. M., Shinn, J. A., and Stotts, N. A. (1985). Life satisfaction following heart transplantation. *Journal of Heart Transplantation*, 4, 446–9.

Lunde, D. T., (1969). Psychiatric complications of heart transplants. *American Journal of Psychiatry*, 126, 369–73.

McAleer, M. J., Copeland, J., Fuller, J., and Copeland, J. G. (1985). Psychological aspects of heart transplantation. *Journal of Heart Transplantation*, 4, 232–3.

Mai, F. M., McKenzie, F. N., and Kostuk, W. J. (1986). Psychiatric aspects of heart transplantation: preoperative evaluation and postoperative sequelae. *British Medical Journal*, 292, 311–13.

Merrill, J. M., Laux, L. F., and Thornby, J. I. (1990). Why doctors have difficulty with sex histories. *Southern Medical Journal*, 83, 613–17.

Moore, D. P. (1981). Methylphenidate in depression and states of apathy. *Southern Medical Journal*, 74, 347–8.

Murray, G. B. (1978). Confusion, delirium, and dementia. In *Massachusetts General Hospital Handbook of General Hospital Psychiatry* (eds. T. P. Hackett and N. H. Cassem), pp. 93–116 (C. V. Mosby, St Louis).

Muslin, H. L. (1971). On acquiring a kidney. *American Journal of Psychiatry*, 127, 1185–8.

Penn, I., Bunch, D., Olenik, D., and Abouna, G. (1971). Psychiatric experience with patients receiving renal and hepatic transplants. *Seminars in Psychiatry*, 3, 133–44.

Tabler, J. B. and Frierson, R. L. (1990). Sexual concerns after heart transplantation. *Journal of Heart Transplantation*, 9, 397–403.

Tesar, G. E. (1982). The role of stimulants in general medicine. *Drug Therapy*, 12, 186–95.

Thompson, M. E. (1983). Selection of candidates for cardiac transplantation. *Journal of Heart Transplantation*, 3, 65–9.

Watts, D., Freeman, A. M. III, McGiffen, D. G., Kirklin, J. K., McVay, R., and Karp, R. B. (1984). Psychiatric aspects of cardiac transplantation. *Journal of Heart Transplantation*, 3, 243–7.

Wise, T. N. (1978). Sexual problem resulting from interactions between medical and psychological conditions. *Medical Aspects of Human Sexuality*, 12, 71–89.

13   Liver transplantation

O. Surman

Orthotopic liver transplantation has met with improved success following the introduction of cyclosporin and OKT3 monoclonal antibody in the 1980s and technical advances in surgery (Cosimi *et al.* 1987; Fung *et al.* 1987). In the Massachusetts General Hospital series, for example, there were 125 liver transplants between May 1983 and September 1991, 57 per cent of which continue to function at three weeks to 82 months post-transplantation. The operation remains a 'prodigious' effort, as described at the Liver Transplantation Consensus Conference (1983). However, full rehabilitation has been reported for two-thirds to four-fifths of those whose grafts are functioning at one year (Surman 1989). The frequent perioperative incidence of neuropsychiatric findings makes liver transplantation an area of special interest for psychiatrists active in general hospital consultation (House *et al.* 1983; Trzepacz *et al.* 1986; Surman *et al.* 1987a; Adams *et al.* 1987; Craven 1991).

Preoperative aspects

Almost all patients evaluated for liver transplantation are seriously ill with life expectancies of under one year. A history of recurrent oesophageal bleeding, infection, and hepatic encephalopathy is common in these patients as is coagulopathy, nutritional impairment, lethargy, and marked restriction of customary activities. Psychiatric assessment typically includes a semi-structured interview of up to 90 minutes in length. We have also used a screening questionnaire for alcohol and substance abuse, adapted from material developed at the Mayo Clinic (Davis *et al.* 1987). Neuropsychiatric testing is requested selectively, for example when dementia is suspect.

Patients who are most ill typically consider transplantation to be the only option for meaningful life extension. Among those who are somewhat more healthy there is likely to be greater ambivalence about the procedure. This may particularly be true for such patients whose functional ability has remained acceptable, even with marked progression of liver disease. In such instances the team's approach to the patient must be 'it's later than you think'. Since medical urgency is the primary factor to determine position on the waiting list, patients characteristically become sicker before coming to operation. One of the tragedies in the wait for a liver is that patients who were relatively stable at the time of initial assessment rapidly decompensate in response to a complicating illness.

Organic brain syndromes

Hepatic encephalopathy is a frequent occurrence in liver transplant candidates and results from intestinally absorbed toxic metabolites (House *et al.* 1983; Tarter *et al.* 1984). A decreased level of consciousness and the presence of asterixis on physical examination are classical signs of clinical hepatic encephalopathy. Confusion, memory impairment and lability of affect may be evident on testing of mental status, from family interviews, and discussion with nursing staff (Surman *et al.* 1987b). Impairment of concentration may be evident from a reduced capacity to read, watch television, and complete routine tasks. Diagnosis is facilitated by the use of electroencephalography and by neuropsychiatric testing, especially Trailmaking-Tests A and B (Rikkers *et al.* 1978, Trzepacz *et al.* 1986). Classification of hepatic encephalopathy has been traditionally accomplished with the criteria of Parsons-Smith *et al.* (1957). Using these criteria, our group has found that delirium occurred in 50 per cent of a series of liver transplant candidates and that stupor occurred in 15 per cent (Surman *et al.* 1987b). In the largest reported liver transplant series, Trzepacz *et al.* (1989) diagnosed delirium by DSM-III criteria in 18.6 per cent of 247 applicants.

Deterioration of mental state may leave patients unaware of the final steps to transplantation (Surman *et al.* 1987b). A small proportion of patients may demonstrate substantial cognitive impairment from the onset of liver disease (e.g. with fulminant hepatitis) which persists through to the time of transplant. Following surgery, family and staff members will need to provide information and answer questions about events which took place following the onset of confusion. These patients in particular may require counselling to help with adjustment following the transplant.

Adjustment disorders and depression

Diagnoses of adjustment disorder were made in 19.8 per cent of liver transplant applicants by Trzepacz *et al.* (1989), and major depressive episodes occurred in 4.5 per cent of cases. In our series, 25 per cent of patients had a history of previous psychiatric care, typically for adjustment disorders related to impaired health or social stress. In one instance, referral resulted from a diagnosis of biliary cirrhosis, which was made by a psychiatrist who performed liver function tests when a 47 year old woman presented with a history of insomnia and depression. Some degree of anxiety is usual in applicants for liver transplant (Surman *et al.* 1987b).

Depression was also common in adult patients studied by House *et al.* (1983). Major depressive disorder may be difficult to diagnose in the presence of end stage organ failure (Mai *et al.* 1986; Craven *et al.* 1987). As Watts *et al.* (1984) suggested, suicidal thinking, feelings of worthlessness, and constricted affect make a strong case for depression in the differential diagnosis. We have found that depressed affect is common in liver transplant applicants with hepatic encephalopathy. These patients must be distinguished from those with mood disorders.

Selection

Criteria for selection varies among centres and with the scarcity of organs. As experience becomes greater and a procedure in transplantation evolves from experimental to established standard of care, the net for inclusion of potential candidates becomes wider. Based on favourable outcome statistics, Starzl *et al.* (1989*a,b*) make a strong case for transplants in patients who are older, alcoholic, positive for human immunodeficiency virus, or those with primary cancers but without extra-hepatic spread.

Inclusion criteria and contraindications listed by the Boston Center for Liver Transplantation are provided in Tables 13.1 and 13.2. (Cosimi 1991) Although age over 60 is listed in Table 13.2 as a relative contraindication, we have performed liver transplantation for otherwise healthy patients in this age group and find that they often do very well. This may be the result of changes which occur in the immune system with aging, or possibly older patients may do better in terms of compliance with medications and follow-up visits.

To date we have performed liver transplants in 15 alcoholic patients enrolled in a prospective study. Selection of alcoholic candidates has been based on acknowledgement of loss of control over alcohol use, documentation of prior compliance with medical care, availability of psychosocial supports to sobriety such as a non-drinking significant other, absence of antisocial personality or dementia, willingness to participate in chemical dependency treatment, and other positive prognostic factors: altruism, spirituality, identification with a friend or family member in recovery (Gastfriend *et al.* personal communication). A similar approach has been advocated by Beresford *et al.* (1990) (see also Chapter 3), who conclude that length of sobriety criteria are not sufficiently predictive to rule out candidacy of alcoholic patients. An individualized approach to selection of patients with past alcohol dependency or abuse is consistent with the observations of Merrikin and Overcast (1985) who point out that to proceed otherwise could be discriminatory. Evans and Yagi (1987) suggest in their discussion of heart transplantation that transplant teams should act flexibly on criteria developed on a 'reasonable basis' when there is absence of confirmatory data. Inclusion of alcoholic patients affects the demand for livers since, for example, alcoholic hepatitis and cirrhosis are the most frequent cause of hepatic failure in the United States.

It is standard practice to assess availability of psychosocial supports for potential transplant recipients, but deficiencies in that area are not a customary

TABLE 13.1 Indications for liver transplantation

I. Chronic advanced cirrhosis
  A. Primarily parenchymal disease
    (e.g.) Postnecrotic Cirrhosis (Viral, Drug Related)
        Alcoholic Cirrhosis
        Cystic Fibrosis
        Autoimmune Liver Disease
  B. Primarily cholestatic disease
    (e.g.) Biliary Atresia
        Primary Biliary Cirrhosis
        Sclerosing Cholangitis
        Cryptogenic Cirrhosis
  C. Primarily vascular disease
    (e.g.) Budd–Chiari Syndrome
        Veno-Occlusive Disease

II. Acute fulminant hepatic failure
  A. Viral Hepatitis
  B. Drug Induced (e.g.) Halothane, Sulfa
  C. Metabolic Liver Disease (e.g.) Wilson's Disease, Reyes' Syndrome

III. Inborn errors of metabolism
  (e.g.) Glycogen Storage Disease
      α-1 Anti-Trypsin Deficiency
      Wilson's Disease

IV. Primary hepatic malignancies
  A. Hepatic ± Cirrhosis
  B. Cholangiocarcinoma
  C. Unusual Sarcomas Arising Within Hepatic Parenchyma

V. Retransplantation

---

reason for exclusion at our centre. Most often we find that one family member becomes a source of close perioperative support. Postoperative support from a significant other is vital to the morale of liver transplant recipients. The availability of this person must be planned well in advance of the procedure. Other social and financial resources may, at present, influence the availability or success of liver transplants for some patients. For example, the cost of a transplant is substantial and at our centre has averaged $122 246 per patient plus $1000 of monthly medication charges (Boston Center for Liver Transplantation 1985). These fees have usually been provided for by private insurance or government support.

Candidates from other countries often face even greater challenges in the transplant process. Guidelines of The National Task Force on Organ Trans-

TABLE 13.2 Contraindications to liver transplantation

Absolute contraindications

Extra-hepatic infection	Active drug or alcohol abuse
Extra-hepatic malignancy	Advanced cardiopulmonary disease
Multiple congenital anomalies (uncorrectable)	Renal failure (unrelated to liver disease)

Relative contraindications

Intrahepatic sepsis	Portal vein-thrombosis
Severe hypoxaemia (from left–right shunt)	Extensive hepatobiliary surgery
HB AG positive state	Age over 60

plantation limit availability of transplantation surgery to foreign nationals who seek extra-renal organs in scarce supply (Cowan *et al.* 1987).

Case history A non-English-speaking man aged 43 was within established quotas when he was referred to our centre from Japan with hepatocellular carcinoma. After undergoing exploratory laparotomy to rule out extra-hepatic involvement and to establish his candidacy for a new liver, the patient became acutely anxious. We treated him with serax and arranged for his mother to room in, so that he could benefit from the support of a loved one with whom he could converse. He appeared to respond favourably, but while still recovering from the first operation made a sudden attempt to leap from the eighth floor window of his hospital room. Miraculously, his mother and a transplant unit nurse were able to prevent his suicide. Subsequently, the patient was kept in restraint, with daily psychiatric visits and treated with haloperidol. The cause of the acute episode was impossible to ascertain, despite the help of a skilled interpreter and the participation of a Japanese physician from our hospital staff. The patient's primary physician was summoned from Japan to escort him back for psychiatric care in his own country. He responded favourably over the course of several weeks and we agreed to a re-evaluation. Moved by his perseverance, I learned a few words of Japanese and greeted him with the satisfaction of observing a significant improvement in mental status. Sadly, his psychiatric impairment had proven costly in time. Medical evaluation revealed metastatic pulmonary disease, and there was no choice but to send him home again.

One major purpose of the preoperative psychosocial assessment is to identify patients at high risk for compliance problems. Noncompliance among liver transplant recipients has been unusual in our experience, but was evident in two patients with marital stress who reported that they had missed doses of immunosuppressant medication, and in a third patient, a recovering alcoholic whose noncompliance was related to postoperative organic brain syndrome

(OBS) (Surman *et al.* 1987*a*). Noncompliance with anti-rejection medicines is none the less a significant phenomenon among organ recipients as a group, and, specifically in kidney recipients, has been responsible for graft loss in up to 5 per cent of cases (Didlake *et al.* 1988). In our experience, history of substance abuse, age less than 30, depression, and socioeconomic stress have been significant among those who lost grafts in this way (Gastfriend *et al.* 1989).

A major challenge for transplantation psychiatry is to develop valid and reliable predicators of serious postoperative psychological impairment. Predictors of likely poor outcome following a transplant are important from two perspectives. First, donor organs are a scarce resource and there is a societal obligation to avoid instances where benefit to the recipient is highly unlikely. Second, early identification of those at risk allows the opportunity to provide support services and works to minimize risk. Our programme had worked on the premise that no patient with a treatable psychological impairment should be denied the benefit of operative care on the basis of psychiatric evaluation.

Psychiatric treatment and support

Preoperative teaching is especially effective when the hepatologist, psychiatrist, and nursing staff can preview events in a way that promotes appropriate expectations and establishes postoperative responsibilities for each transplant candidate. Patient information manuals, visits from successful liver transplant recipients, and conferences for the patient, family, and surgical team are additional steps for enhancing the alliance between the patient and the transplant team. Brief counselling, cognitive behavioural techniques, and self-hypnosis have proven simple and effective for generalized anxiety and phobias, and may sometimes facilitate postoperative pain control (Surman 1987; Surman *et al.* 1987*a*,*b*).

Psychopharmacological intervention should be at a minimum, since dependence on hepatic metabolism is the rule for the commonly used psychotropics. Short-acting agents are the drugs of choice. Oxazepam is the minor tranquilizer which requires least metabolism by the failing liver and can be used for debilitating anxiety and insomnia. Lower than commonly prescribed doses are often indicated in these patients. Twenty or thirty mg of oxazepam by mouth has been enough to produce stupor when administered by an overly zealous house officer for an anxious patient with hepatic encephalopathy.

Diphenhydramine may also be helpful for severe insomnia. Neuroleptic agents are very rarely required and must be commenced in the lowest dose, for example, haloperidol 0.5 mg by mouth or intravenously, when hepatic failure is evident. If the patient has been taking antidepressants, blood levels should be followed closely with attention to clinical evidence of toxicity. Occasionally, one sees a patient with depression or chronic pain and insomnia in the absence of organic brain syndrome, particularly during an extended wait for a donor organ. One can begin antidepressants with the considerations mentioned above and increase in equivalents of doxepin or desipramine 25 mg by mouth until a satisfactory clinical response is evident. It may be best to avoid fluoxetine in these patients because of its long action and hepatic metabolism.

Medical management of hepatic encephalopathy includes the administration of lactulose for elimination of toxic metabolites from the gastrointestinal tract, as well as attention to infection, bleeding and electrolyte imbalance. Although rarely necessary, low-dose haloperidol may be temporarily of benefit when encephalopthy presents with psychotic symptoms or problematic agitation. Extreme caution and repeated examination are required in this circumstance to avoid over-treatment.

New horizons for liver transplant are posed by recent clinical accounts of partial hepatectomy from living donors to provide hepatic tissue to children in need of liver transplantation. This innovative therapy requires the same kind of careful scientific evaluation and standards that occurred when living organ donor surgery was introduced for renal failure therapy (Singer *et al.* 1989; Surman 1989; Strong *et al.* 1990).

Postoperative aspects

Operative time in the Massachusetts General Hospital series has been from six to twelve hours; and whole blood requirements range from two to over one hundred units. Following the operation, almost all recipients are awake and alert within 24 hours. Two to seven days in the intensive care unit is followed by transfer to a specialized transplantation unit. The customary hospital stay is of three to four weeks with a range of two to six weeks (Surman *et al.* 1987*b*). Those who come to transplant earlier in the course of illness have the most successful outcome (Neuberger *et al.* 1986; Surman *et al.* 1987*b*).

Liver transplantation is associated with less pain than one would expect, presumably because of operative denervation. Eisenach *et al.* (1989) have reported a significantly lower postoperative analgesic requirement among liver transplant patients than those undergoing cholecystectomy. We manage pain with parenteral morphine and then by oral administration of oxycodone. Low back pain is a common complaint and subsides with increasing postoperative mobilization (Surman *et al.* 1987*b*).

Anti-rejection medications commonly include adrenocorticosteroids, aza-thioprine, antithymocyte globulin, and OKT3 monoclonal antibody. The most dangerous complication is infection. Cytomegalovirus infection (CMV) may result from activation of latent infection or may occur as a primary infection (Rubin 1989). A syndrome of weakness and malaise may occur with CMV and mental status changes may be manifestations of CMV encephalitis. A new antiviral drug, gancyclovir, has led to reduced morbidity and mortality, but this drug is itself associated with leukopaenia, thrombocytopaenia, and neurotoxicity, especially in the setting of reduced renal function (Davis *et al.* 1990).

The side-effects of prednisone are well known, and in the early post-operative period may include nightmares, sweating, insomnia, delirium, affective psychosis, blurred vision, seizures, and emotional lability. The advent of cyclosporin has reduced total adrenocorticosteroid requirements following liver transplantation, and although steroid side-effects remain a problem, they are less prevalent than in the pre-cyclosporin era.

Cyclosporin (CYA) is of special importance to transplantation psychiatrists because of its association with neurotoxicity. Toxicity may be apparent with onset or increase of tremors, with sleep disturbance or with mental status changes characteristic of OBS. Additional signs include hypertension and laboratory indications of impaired renal function. Serum cyclosporin levels are not necessarily elevated in the setting of toxicity, but one should be aware of drug interactions that alter cyclosporin metabolism. This has been reviewed by Tilney *et al.* (1988). Among psychoactive compounds, anticonvulsants reduce CYA levels by P-450 enzyme induction (Tilney *et al.* 1988). Addition of erothromycin, ketoconazotes, or calcium channel blockers increase the risk of toxicity.

Neurologic complications attributed to cyclosporin toxicity have included seizures, cortical blindness, paralysis, and cerebellar syndromes, and have responded variably to reduced dosage and discontinuation of the drug (Polson *et al.* 1985; Adams *et al.* 1987; de Groen *et al.* 1987, 1988; Boon *et al.* 1988; Vogt *et al.* 1988; Surman 1989; Craven 1991). Cyclosporin-associated neurotoxicity is discussed more fully in Chapter 6.

Psychiatric syndromes

The rapid reversal of preoperative hepatic encephalopathy is a striking benefit of liver transplantation (Tarter *et al.* 1984; Surman *et al.* 1987*a*). One patient in our series, a 60 year old academic, was moribund and in stage IV hepatic coma at the time of transplantation. As in the case of other patients who were stuporous preoperatively, he was alert and articulate within a few days of his operation.

Organic brain syndromes which begin following liver transplant are most typically caused by rejection, infection, or neurological side-effects of immunosuppressant agents. Other factors include sleep deprivation and cerebral oedema from hepatic insufficiency. The clinical picture is quite variable and ranges from waking dreams to florid delirium and other neurological sequelae. Central pontine myelinolysis has been observed and associated with abnormalities in serum sodium (Estol *et al.* 1989).

Adjustment disorders following liver transplantation are commonly associated with rejection or complications leading to prolonged or recurrent hospitalization. Anticipation of allograft rejection may lead to anxiety in the early postoperative period, and anxiety may appear when patients confront the uncertainties attendant with discharge from hospital. Pulse doses of steroids, increased cyclosporin requirements, and febrile reaction to OKT3 may all provoke transient mood changes. Mental state changes produced by these and other organic mechanisms are often difficult to differentiate from psychologically mediated disorders of adjustment.

In our experience, depression following liver transplantation is almost invariably related to medical events (Surman *et al.* 1987*b*). Faced with a depressed liver transplant recipient one should immediately consider the possibility of infection. Cytomegalovirus, pneumocystis, and fungal infections are potentially lethal conditions which may initially present with mood changes for which the team requests psychiatric consultation. Only one of eight depressed patients whom we reported in our first forty cases was medically stable and fully active when seen for psychiatric consultation (Surman *et al.* 1987*b*).

Quality of life

Tarter *et al.* (1988) found that among 66 liver recipients, most reported satisfaction with the quality of their life in response to social adjustment questionnaires at one year following transplantation. In the series reported separately by our group and by Wolcott *et al.* (1989), 73–82 per cent of patients surviving at one year had achieved partial or complete rehabilitation. Wolcott *et al.* (1989) found lower Index of Well-Being Scores than among renal transplant recipients and reported a lower percentage return to full function than in our experience (Surman *et al.* 1987*b*). Starzl *et al.* (1989*b*) reported that 'more than 85% return to work and say that they are able to perform their jobs well'. Quality of life indices were reported as adequate in a sub-sample of liver transplant recipients surveyed by Scharschmidt (1984). However, further work is required in this area. Data are needed from the type of large multi-collaborative study reported by Evans *et al.* (1985) for endstage renal disease patients.

Conclusions

Liver transplantation is now a common procedure and is associated with meaningful life extension for a majority of recipients (Starzl *et al.* 1989*a*). It has proven to be a viable alternative for endstage liver disease. However, a relative scarcity of donor organs makes it necessary to distribute organs in an ethical manner and results in patient morbidity being its highest by the time of surgery. Major challenges for future work include the study of psychiatric and psychological predictors of poor outcome, the management of distressing emotional conditions in patients awaiting surgery, and the study of societal factors which limit the availability of donor organs. The neurotoxic side-effects of cyclosporin and the other immunosuppressants remain a poorly understood clinical phenomenon, the investigation of which may provide insights into the mechanisms by which brain dysfunction occurs.

Future directions in liver transplant surgery will also provide challenges for mental health practitioners. The transplantation of patients with alcoholic cirrhosis demands well-designed longitudinal studies of outcome predictors. Emerging interest in partial hepatectomy from living donors requires that this approach receive careful scrutiny for potential elements of coercion and for psychological outcome and well-being of participants.

References

Adams, D. H., Ponsford, S., Gunson, B., Boon, A., Hongisberger, L., Williams, A., *et al.* (1987). Neurological complications following liver transplantation. *Lancet*, 1, 949–51.

Beresford, T. P., Turcotte, J. G., Merion, R., Burtch, G., Blow, F. C., Campbell, D., (1990). A rational approach to liver transplantation for the alcoholic patient. *Psychosomatics*, 31, 241–54.

Boon, A. P., Adams, D. H., Carey, M. P., Williams, A., McMaster, P., and Elias, E. (1988). Cyclosporin-associated cerebral lesions in liver transplantation (letter). *Lancet*, 1, 1457.

Craven, J. L. (1991). Cyclosporine-associated organic mental syndromes in liver transplant recipients. *Psychosomatics*, 32, 94–102.

Craven, J. L., Rodin, G. M., Johnson, L., and Kennedy, S. H. (1987). The diagnosis of major depression in renal dialysis patients. *Psychosomatic Medicine*, 49, 482–92.

Cosimi, A. B. (1991). Personal Communication.

Cosimi, A. B., Cho, S. I., Delmonico, F. L., Kaplan, M. M., Rohrer, R. J., and Jenkins, R. (1987). A randomized clinical trial comparing OKT3 and steroids for treatment of hepatic allograft rejection. *Transplantation Proceedings*, 19, 2431–3.

Cowan, D. H., Kantorowitz, J. A., Moskowitz, J., and Rheinstein, P. H. (Eds.). (1987). *Human organ transplantation: societal, medical-legal, regulatory, and reimbursement issues*, pp. 391–401. (Health Administration Press, Ann Arbor).

Davis, L. J. Jr., Hurt, R. D., Morse, R. M., and O'Brien, P. C. (1987). Discriminant analysis of the Self-Administered Alcoholism Screening Test. *Alcoholism—Clinical and Experimental Research*, 11, 269–73.

Davis, C. L., Springmeyer, S., and Gmerek, B. J. (1990). Central nervous system side effects of ganciclovir (letter). *New England Journal of Medicine*, 322, 933–4.

Didlake, R. H., Dreyfus, D., Kerman, R. H., Van Buren, C. T., and Kahan, B. D. (1988). Patient noncompliance: a major cause of late graft failure in cyclosporine-treated renal transplants. *Transplantation Proceedings*, 20(suppl 3), 63–9.

Eisenach, J. C., Plevak, D. J., Van Dyke, R. A., Southorn, P. A., Danielson, D. R., Krom, R. A., *et al.* (1989). Comparison of analgesic requirements after liver transplantation and cholecystectomy. *Mayo Clinic Proceedings*, 64, 356–9.

Estol, C. J., Faris, A. A., Martinez, A. J., and Ahdab-Barmada, M. (1989). Central pontine myelinolysis after liver transplantation. *Neurology*, 39, 493–8.

Evans, R. W. and Yagi, J. (1987). Social and medical considerations affecting selection of transplant recipients: The case of heart transplantation. In *Human organ trans-*

plantation: societal, medical-legal, regulatory, and reimbursement issues (eds. D. H. Cowan *et al.*), pp. 27–41. (Health Administration Press, Ann Arbor).

Evans, R. W., Manninen, D. L., Garrison, L. P. Jr, Hart, L. G., Blagg, C. R., Gutman, R. A., *et al.* (1985). The quality of life of patients with end-stage renal disease. *New England Journal of Medicine*, 312, 553–9.

Fung, J. J., Markus, B. H., Gordon, R. D., Esquivel, C. O., Makowka, L., Tzakis, A., *et al.* (1987). Impact of orthoclone OKT3 on liver transplantation. *Transplantation Proceedings*, 19, 37–44.

Gastfriend, D. R., Surman, O. S., Gaffey, G., and Dienstag, J. (1989). *Substance abuse and compliance in organ transplantation*, 10, 149–53.

de Groen, P. C., Aksamit, A. J., Rakela, J., Forbes, G. S., and Krom, R. A. (1987). Central nervous system toxicity after liver transplantation: the role of cyclosporine and cholesterol. *New England Journal of Medicine*, 317, 861–6.

de Groen, P. C., Aksamit, A. J., Rakela, J., and Krom, R. A. F. (1988). Cyclosporine-associated central nervous system toxicity (letter). *New England Journal of Medicine*, 318, 789.

House, R., Dubovsky, S. L., and Penn, I. (1983). Psychiatric aspects of hepatic transplantation. *Transplantation*, 36, 146–50.

Liver Transplantation—Consensus Conference (1983). *Journal of the American Medical Association*, 250, 2961–4.

Mai, F. M., McKenzie, F. N., and Kostuk, W. J. (1986). Psychiatric aspects of heart transplantation: preoperative evaluation and postoperative sequelae. *British Medical Journal*, 292, 311–13.

Merrikin, K. J. and Overcast, T. D. (1985). Patient selection for heart transplantation: When is a discriminating choice discrimination? *Journal of Health Politics, Policy and Law*, 10, 7–32.

Neuberger, J., Altman, D. G., Christensen, E., Tygstrup, N., and Williams, R. (1986). Use of a prognostic index in evaluation of liver transplantation for primary biliary cirrhosis. *Transplantation*, 41, 713–16.

Parsons-Smith, B. G., Summerskill, W. H. J., Dawson, A. M., and Sherlock, S. (1957). The electroencephalograph in liver disease. *Lancet*, 2, 867–71.

Polson, R. J., Powell-Jackson, P. R., and Williams, R. (1985). Convulsions associated with cyclosporin A in transplant recipients (letter). *British Medical Journal*, 290, 1003.

Rikkers, L., Jenko, P., Rudman, D., and Freides, D. (1978). Subclinical hepatic encephalopathy: detection, prevalence, and relationship to nitrogen metabolism. *Gastroenterology*, 75, 462–9.

Rubin, R. H. (1989). The indirect effects of cytomegalovirus infection on the out-come of organ transplantation. *Journal of the American Medical Association*, 261, 3607–9.

Scharschmidt, B. F. (1984). Human liver transplantation: analysis of data on 540 patients from four centers. *Hepatology*, 4, 95S–101S.

Singer, P. A., Siegler, M., Whitington, P. F., Lantos, J. D., Edmond J. C., Thistlethwaite, J. R., *et al.* (1989). Ethics of liver transplantation with living donors. *New England Journal of Medicine*, 321, 620–2.

Starzl, T. E., Demetris, A. J., and Van Thiel, D. (1989*a*). Liver transplantation (first of two parts). *New England Journal of Medicine*, 321, 1014–22.

Starzl, T. E., Demetris, A. J., and Van Thiel, D. (1989*b*). Liver transplantation (second of two parts). *New England Journal of Medicine*, 321 *et al.*, 1092–9.

Strong, R. W., Lynch, S. V., Ong, T. H., Matsunami, H., Koido, Y., and Balderson, G. A. (1990). Successful liver transplantation from a living donor to her son. *New England Journal of Medicine*, 322, 1505–7.

Surman, O. S. (1987). The surgical patient. In *Massachusetts General Hospital Handbook of General Hospital Psychiatry* (2nd edn). (eds. T. P. Hackett and N. H. Cassem), pp. 69–83 (PSG Publishing Co., Littleton MA).

Surman, O. S. (1989). Psychiatric aspects of organ transplantation. *American Journal of Psychiatry*, 146(8), 972–82.

Surman, O. S., Dienstag, J. L., Cosimi, A. B., Chauncey, S., and Russell, P. S. (1987 a). Liver transplantation: psychiatric considerations. *Psychosomatics*, 28, 615–21.

Surman, O. S., Dienstag, J. L., Cosimi, A. B., Chauncey, S., and Russell, P. S. (1987 b). Psychosomatic aspects of liver transplantation. *Psychotherapy and Psychosomatics*, 48, 26–31.

Tarter, R. E., Van Thiel, D. H., Hegedus, A. M., Schade, R. R., and Gavaler, J. S. (1984). Neuropsychiatric status after liver transplantation. *Journal of Laboratory and Clinical Medicine*, 103, 776–82.

Tarter, R. E., Erb, S., Biller, P. A., Switala, J., and Van Thiel, D. H. (1988). The quality of life following liver transplantation: a preliminary report. *Gastroenterology Clinics of North America*, 17, 207–17.

Tilney, N. L., Strom, T. B., and Kupiec-Weglinski, J. W. (1988). Pharmacologic and immunologic agonists and antagonists of cyclosporine. *Transplantation Proceedings*, 20(3), 13–22.

Trzepacz, P. T., Maue, F. R., Coffman, G., and Van Thiel, D. H. (1986). Neuro-psychiatric assessment of liver transplantation candidates: delirium and other psychiatric disorders. *International Journal of Psychiatry in Medicine*, 16, 101–11.

Trzepacz, P. T., Brenner, R., and Van Thiel, D. H. (1989). A psychiatric study of 247 liver transplantation candidates. *Psychosomatics*, 30, 147–53.

Vogt, D. P., Lederman, R. J., Carey, W. D., and Broughan, T. A. (1988). Neurologic complications of liver transplantation. *Transplantation*, 45, 1057–61.

Watts, D., Freeman, A. M. III, McGiffin, D. G., Kirklin, J. K., McVay, R., and Karp, R. B. (1984). Psychiatric aspects of cardiac transplantation. *Journal of Heart Transplantation*, 3, 243–7.

Wolcott, D., Norquist, G., and Busuttil, R. (1989). Cognitive function and quality of life in adult liver transplant recipients. *Transplantation Proceedings*, 21, 3563.

14 Bone marrow transplantation

D. Wolcott and M. Stuber

Bone marrow transplant (BMT) is a complex medical procedure with both clinical and investigational indications. It is used in the treatment of life-threatening haematological and solid tumour malignances, other haemato-poietic disorders, and immunological disorders (Gale 1986). Allogeneic BMT entails administration of a pre-transplant conditioning regimen, usually a com-bination of chemotherapy and total body irradiation. The conditioning regimen aims to destroy all malignant or diseased bone marrow cells. This is followed by the intravenous infusion of bone marrow from a donor, most typically an HLA-identical sibling donor. The use of HLA-nonidentical related donors and of matched unrelated donors has been attempted to increase the bone marrow donor pool (Gale 1986).

Autologous BMT differs from allogeneic BMT in that the recipient's own bone marrow is harvested prior to the conditioning regimen, stored, and then re-infused after the conditioning regimen. Autologous bone marrow transplan-tation has been used in the treatment of a number of solid tumour malignancies and in the treatment of leukaemia.

The recipient's disease diagnosis and many other factors contribute to the use of varied chemotherapy and radiation therapy protocols in BMT con-ditioning regimens. These varying approaches to pre-treatment reflect attempts to resolve the often conflicting problems posed by recipient engraft-ment rates, the post-BMT rates of development of acute and chronic graft versus host disease, relapse rates in patients with leukaemia and other malig-nancies, and short- and long-term recipient survival rates (Champlin and Gale 1984).

BMT is followed by a several week recovery phase in hospital, a subacute phase of several months of more gradual medical recovery, and an extended phase of adjustment and rehabilitation. Transplantation is associated with a relatively high (15–20 per cent) mortality rate during the acute and subacute recovery phase. Medical complications which may occur and which contribute to acute morbidity and mortality in recipients include the acute toxicity of the conditioning regimen, graft failure, graft versus host disease, interstitial pneu-monitis, and the occurrence of infections due to a state of immunodeficiency (Champlin and Gale 1984).

The number of BMT programmes and annual number of BMTs performed has grown steadily from the late 1970s. In 1977, 169 BMT procedures were performed by about 60 international BMT programmes (Bortin and Gale 1986). In 1987, there were 240 known BMT programmes in 41 countries which performed 3964 BMTs, a 23-fold increase from one decade earlier (Bortin and Rimm 1989). Through 1987, the cumulative number of allogeneic BMTs performed in the world exceeded 21 000, and probably exceeded 30 000 by the end of 1990. As of mid-1990, the total number of unrelated donor BMTs performed is about 400, with a current annual rate of about 350 per year (R. P. Gale, personal communication).

In 1987, 32 per cent of BMT programmes were in North America, 41 per cent in Western Europe, and 14 per cent in Asia. From 1985 to 1987, 46 per cent of all BMTs were performed in North America, and 42 per cent in Western Europe. Many BMT programmes perform a relatively small number of BMTs per year. In 1987 127 out of 240 BMT programmes performed fewer than 12 BMTs each. From 1985 to 1987, 73 per cent of (non-autologous) BMTs were for leukaemia, 11 per cent for other malignant diseases, 9 per cent for severe aplastic anaemia, and 7 per cent for other diseases (Bortin and Rimm 1989).

Current data from the International Bone Marrow Transplant Registry indicate that the five year actuarial probability of survival in patients with severe aplastic anaemia receiving HLA-identical sibling BMTs during 1978–87 was 57 per cent. The most favourable five year disease-free survival rates for the common leukaemias were 43 per cent for patients with acute lymphoblastic leukaemia transplanted in first complete remission, 48 per cent for patients with acute myelogenous leukaemia transplanted in first complete remission, and 41 per cent for patients with chronic myelogenous leukaemia transplanted in the first chronic phase. Leukaemia patients who receive a BMT at a more advanced phase of their illness have a much poorer prognosis than those transplanted earlier (Bortin *et al.* 1989).

One recent study in the USA compared the cost-effectiveness of BMT as compared to conventional chemotherapy for the five year period from the time of diagnosis for the treatment of acute non-lymphocytic leukaemia. The total 5 year treatment costs were $193 000 per patient for BMT, and $136 000 per patient for chemotherapy. At the five year follow-up point the treatment costs per year of life saved were nearly equal, at $62 000 for BMT and $64 000 for chemotherapy, as the five year patient survival rate was higher with BMT (Welch and Larson 1989). This study underscores the great costs associated with treatment of non-lymphocytic leukaemia, and the need for further studies to compare the cost-effectiveness of BMT and conventional treatment for other conditions.

BMT has also been expanding rapidly within paediatrics over the past 15 years. The medical procedures and time course of paediatric transplant are similar to those described above. There are, however, differences in indications for the procedure and in survival statistics. BMT has been used successfully to treat congenital metabolic and immunological disorders, in addition to aplastic anaemia, the leukaemias, and solid tumours. Survival statistics for paediatric BMT are superior to those for adults overall (Parkman 1986). However, variations exist by (i) underlying diagnosis, (ii) stage of disease, and (iii) type of transplant (autologous, related allogeneic, matched unrelated). Two year disease-free survival after BMT for children ranges from 80 per cent (for non-transfused aplastic anaemia) to approximately 30 per cent (for stage 4 neuroblastoma) (Wiley and House 1988).

Bone marrow transplantation in adults

A number of reports have emphasized that specific psychosocial phases of BMT exist. These phases correlate with medical phases of the transplant (Brown and Kelly 1976; Popkin and Moldow 1977; Popkin *et al.* 1977) and include the pre-hospitalization phase; the transplant phase (which includes the bone marrow transplant conditioning regimen, the bone marrow infusion, the engraftment, and acute medical stabilization phase); the early recovery phase; and longer term rehabilitation and adjustment. Knowledge of the literature on psychiatric aspects of cancer (Holland and Rowland 1989), of the general literature on psychiatric aspects of organ transplantation (House and Thompson 1988; Surman 1989; Wolcott 1990), and of previous reviews of psychiatric aspects of bone marrow transplantation (Folsom and Popkin 1987; Wolcott *et al.* 1987*a*; Lesko 1989) is useful in providing clinical and research perspective on bone marrow transplant psychiatry.

Pre-hospitalization

Although few data exist concerning the patient's decision to undergo transplant, candidates commonly report that they made their decision almost instantaneously, well before detailed discussion of the procedure itself (Wolcott *et al.* 1987*a*). A rapid decision to confront life-threatening illness by undertaking an aggressive medical treatment probably more closely reflects an individual's basic character style and coping patterns than the effects of careful education about the procedure as one of several possible options.

Most individuals considered for this transplant have had a life-threatening illness for at least several months and up to many years. Exceptions to this generalization are patients with acute aplastic anaemia, who often have known of their illness only for several days or weeks, and usually have had only minimal medical treatment for their illness prior to the BMT. These patients and their families may remain in a phase of denial, disbelief, and emotional disavowal at the time of BMT recommendation. Particular attention must be directed to these patients who must decide upon BMT at a time of intense emotional and intrafamilial turmoil.

Information about the decision-making process experienced by living–related bone marrow donor candidates and of the communication processes between the transplant and donor candidates is unavailable. Data from kidney transplants suggest that the psychological outcome is usually positive for the living–related donor and recipient, even if the transplanted organ fails (Simmons *et al.* 1977). However, the circumstance of the negatively valued family member donor has been commonly observed to result in adverse psychological outcomes for the donor and the donor–recipient relationship. Many differences exist between kidney and bone marrow transplantation. In contrast to kidney transplant, the decision for BMT is not really elective, is associated with a much higher recipient morbidity and mortality rate, and results in a significant occurrence of life-threatening graft versus host disease, in which the donor's tissue directly contributes to this adverse event. Clinical experience has indicated a much higher frequency of dysfunctional communication and decision-making processes between living-related BMT candidates and donors than have been reported in living–related kidney transplant (Wolcott *et al.* 1987*a*). Further research concerning this issue is needed, but the suggestion that these families be assessed psychiatrically prior to a final decision regarding their donation appears to be well justified by these clinical impressions.

The question of whether there are psychiatric contraindications for BMT remains unsettled. No prospective studies addressing this question have been reported. The authors' position is that psychiatric contraindications to acceptance for BMT do exist. These are based on the ability to document accurately psychiatric diagnoses and/or enduring features which highly predict unacceptable BMT outcomes (e.g. serious treatment regimen noncompliance) and which cannot be managed in spite of the best available interventions (Wolcott 1990). Clinical experience indicates that based on these contraindications, only a very small minority of potential candidates would appropriately be excluded from this potentially life-saving treatment. Some transplant centres view adolescence as a relative contraindication to bone marrow transplant (Stuber, in press).

Hospitalization

In general, persons respond to the severe stressors associated with life-threatening illness with intensification of pre-existing patterns of psychological defences and with regression (Fawzy *et al.* 1977; Popkin and Moldow 1977; Popkin *et al.* 1977). Given the disruptions experienced by bone marrow transplant recipients during the hospitalization phase, the authors strongly support previous recommendations that all candidates should be psychiatrically evaluated at least upon admission for the transplant and followed throughout their hospitalization (Fawzy *et al.* 1977; Popkin and Moldow 1977).

The conditioning regimen is physically and psychologically traumatic for the recipient. Anticipatory nausea and vomiting may begin before either conditioning regimen is completed. Only a successful infusion of marrow can rescue him from the otherwise fatal toxicity of the conditioning regimen. The bone marrow infusion itself is largely anticlimactic, being commonly experienced as simply another transfusion. Many recipients experience a transient euphoria with the infusion. Some experience the infusion as a symbolic re-birth, and celebrate the date as a second birthday for the rest of their lives. For others, the infusion symbolizes a positive intertwining of their existence with their donor.

Within the first few days after the infusion, most recipients develop significant physical symptoms of nausea, vomiting, and pain from oral mucositis, and many develop early infections. They typically have sleep disturbance, require total parenteral nutrition, and demonstrate delirium. During the first 1–2 weeks post-transplant, the major clinical psychiatric issues centre around pain control, treatment of insomnia, and of delirium. Patients are rarely physically able or predisposed to engage in more than the briefest supportive psycho-therapeutic encounters during this time, but often benefit from anxiety management and relaxation-induction interventions.

By two to three weeks following transplant, the major acute physical symptoms have typically abated. The recipient and his or her family will begin to focus on concerns related to graft function and disease recurrence. At this time, recipients may have strong needs to reassert control over their lives. This may be attempted in ways which are distressing to staff members (e.g., insisting on early discharge), or which are truly counterproductive for their own recovery.

Families come to the transplant experience with highly variable relationship histories between members of the family of origin and the current family of procreation. While many families are able to cope well with the stresses of the BMT hospitalization, others decompensate and require intensive psychological support from staff members. Families with a history of parental divorce, with member(s) with substance abuse histories, with a history of estrangement between family members, or with marked intergenerational boundary and role conflicts appear to be at greatest risk during the BMT hospitalization.

Often the transplant is performed at a hospital which is at a distance from the recipient's home. Thus, patients and their families may be separated from one another or their own communities. They may face financial stresses related to housing/living costs and a reduced standard of living. Families often spend much of their time on the BMT unit and interact intensely with each other and with other bone marrow transplant recipient families. This can be very supportive and helpful. However, recipients may have multiple complications or may die during the hospitalization, resulting in physical and emotional exhaustion in family members and arousing death anxiety in other candidates and recipients. Patenaude and Rappeport (1982) have reported interview data indicating that death of another recipient on the BMT unit can result in significant manifestations of psychological trauma in the recipients, including identification with the deceased, survivor guilt, and fears of a similar fate. Some families may have disruptive effects on each other, and their behaviour may greatly increase the responsibilities of the staff members who care for the recipients.

Some recipients will have failure of engraftment, early indications of disease recurrence, early major infections, and/or early significant graft versus host disease. Decisions must then be made about another transplant or about treatment approaches which may have significant toxicity or limited efficacy. The critical individual and family choices which must be made about the aggressiveness of medical care in these situations are often anguished, and the psychiatric team can often facilitate the process of making personally appropriate life and death choices. While living–related bone marrow donors have no control over the outcome of the BMT, many feel a sense of failure or guilt if the bone marrow does not engraft, and intense guilt if clinically significant graft versus host disease occurs. Prolonged or pathological grief reactions appear common in living–related bone marrow donors when the recipient dies.

Even without major complications or graft failure, BMT requires a lengthy period of hospitalization. Many recipients are relatively young adults with whom the BMT staff may identify as a potential sibling or spouse. Recipients are quite ill and dependent on medical and nursing staff. Each of these factors contributes to the rapid development of strong bonds between staff members, the recipients and their family members. With the relatively high mortality rate of recipients, the staff are repeatedly exposed to death. These factors combine to place a great burden on staff members and contribute to professional stress or burn-out syndrome (Fawzy *et al.* 1977; Wellisch *et al.* 1977; Lesko 1989).

The time of hospital discharge is a time of relief and joy but also of further apprehension. Recipients will often begin to work through the trauma of the hospitalization only near the time of discharge. Ambivalence about discharge is the rule, as the desire to escape the hospital is counterbalanced by leaving the protective hospital environment and realistic concerns about exposure to infectious agents outside the hospital. Concerns about reproductive issues, family roles, financial problems, and vocational rehabilitation may surface at the time of discharge. The degree of concern and attention the recipient receives from the transplant team diminishes as discharge nears and represents a distressing loss for some patients.

Neuropsychiatric complications

Although no systematic studies have specifically reported the frequency of acute organic mental disorders in BMT recipients, clinical experience indicates that delirium is a common complication of the conditioning process. High dose cyclophosphamide treatment has been associated with transient water intoxication, euphoria, and feelings of unreality (de Fronzo *et al.* 1973; Lesko 1989). Sullivan *et al.* (1982) reported immediate and delayed neurotoxicity in bone marrow transplant recipients secondary to mechlorethamine (nitrogen mustard) administration. Delirium with diffuse EEG slowing occurred acutely; delayed neurological abnormalities, including communicating hydrocephalus, developed two to eight months post-transplant. Age greater than 21, cyclophosphamide treatment, and concomitant total body irradiation were associated with greater risk for development of neurotoxicity.

Patchell *et al.* (1982) reported on the incidence and aetiology of central nervous system complications in 77 adult and child recipients who died. Some 48 of 77 (62 per cent) developed neurological complications. A total of 56 per cent developed altered mental state which was most commonly due to metabolic or hypoxic aetiologies. Only six (8 per cent) of their sample developed CNS infections, with aspergillus CNS infections occurring in three (4 per cent).

Smith *et al.* (1983) reported post-BMT myasthenia gravis in one 12 year old bone marrow transplant recipient with antibodies of donor cell origin. Wade and Meyers (1983) reported the development of transient lethargy, disorientation, agitation, tremor, and hemiparaesthesias in 6 (4 per cent) of 143 bone marrow recipients treated with acyclovir for herpes virus infection. While other factors may have contributed to these neuropsychiatric symptoms, their data do suggest that acyclovir treatment may be associated with transient delirium in a small number of recipients treated with this drug. Wolcott *et al.* (1987*a*) have reported anecdotally on the development of prolonged dementia in a small number of recipients. Medications used in the prevention and treatment of graft versus host disease, including corticosteroids and cyclosporin A, have a range of neuropsychiatric side-effects including encephalopathy and organic mood syndromes (Ling *et al.* 1981; de Groen *et al.* 1987; Craven 1991).

Parth *et al.* (1989) reported results from a longitudinal study of neuropsychological findings in a small number of adult and paediatric recipients, with a donor or spouse control group. They interpreted their data to mean that BMT was not associated with impairment in gross motor performance, but that modest transient decreases in some aspects of cognitive performance did occur in the recipient as compared to control group. They emphasized that multiple other explanations, other than the neurotoxicity of the conditioning regimen itself, could account for their findings.

Andrykowski *et al.* (in press) have recently reported that increased dose of total body irradiation was associated with impaired cognitive function as assessed by two self-report measures (the Profile of Mood States confusion subscale and the alertness-behaviour subscale of the Sickness Impact Profile) in 30 long-term adult survivers of BMT. The primary areas of self-reported impairment included slowed reaction time, reduced attention and concentration, and difficulties with reasoning and problem-solving.

BMT has also been found to be associated with transiently impaired nonsuppression of cortisol levels with dexamethasone administration (Wolcott *et al.* 1987*b*), and with a modest incidence of hypothyroidism post-BMT (Champlin and Gale 1984). Based on previous work documenting adverse consequences of chemotherapy and radiation therapy in cancer patients, the long-term consequences of the conditioning regimens on the hypothalamic–pituitary–gonadal axis are of concern (Gillbert and Kagan 1980; Richards 1980; Schilskey *et al.* 1980; Sheline 1980; Chapman 1982).

The frequency, severity, time course, and determinants of neuropsychiatric sequelae of BMT, and the acute and chronic neuroendocrine function effects of BMT remain under-studied areas of psychiatric interest.

Rehabilitation and adjustment

The early post-hospitalization phase is typically characterized by persistent physical symptoms, gradual recovery of energy and endurance and normalization of sleep, appetite, and taste. Recurrent psychosocial themes in the long-term adaptation of cancer survivors have been recently reviewed. Issues include the fear of recurrence and death; relationship with the treatment team; adjustment to physical compromise; alterations in usual social relationships and social support; relative social isolation; often fundamental and persistent personal re-orientation to the meaning, goals, and priorities of one's life; and employment and insurance problems (Welch-McCaffrey *et al.* 1989). The developing literature on long-term adaptation of adult bone marrow transplant recipient survivors is consistent with each of these. Spouses, children, and other family members often demonstrate persistent concerns over the recipient's recovery and ongoing disruption in usual family relationship roles and dynamics.

The current literature indicates that, despite the challenges described, a majority of adult bone marrow transplant recipient long-term survivors report reasonable long-term adaptation. However, there are residual problems in a number of life activity domains. Hengeveld *et al.* (1988) found that 40–50 per cent of 17 bone marrow transplant recipients who were 1–5 years post-BMT reported ongoing problems in health status, sexual/reproductive function, and incomplete vocational rehabilitation. Poor adaptation occurs in 15–25 per cent of long-term survivors.

Wolcott *et al.* (1986*a*) studied 26 adult bone marrow transplant recipients who were an average of 42 months post-BMT. Of these, 15–25 per cent reported ongoing medical problems, significant emotional distress, low self-esteem, and less than optimal life satisfaction. They also found that the recipient's perception of the current quality of the recipient–donor relationship was highly correlated with the recipient's own current physical and psychosocial status. Their bone marrow transplant recipient subjects were quite vocationally active, with 35 per cent employed full-time, 23 per cent maintaining a household, and 27 per cent in school. They concluded that 15–20 per cent of adult bone marrow transplant recipient long-term survivors report levels of psychological distress that might benefit from specific intervention.

Andrykowski and colleagues have published a number of reports concerning long-term adaptation of adult bone marrow transplant recipient survivors. They studied 23 bone marrow transplant recipients who were an average of 26 months post-BMT, and found levels of mood disturbance higher than three historical comparison groups of cancer patients. Functional quality of life was somewhat better than found in cancer out-patients receiving chemotherapy. Transplant recipients transplanted at less than age 30 had less mood disturbance and better functional quality of life than those transplanted at an older age (Andrykowski *et al.* 1989*a*). A longitudinal follow-up of their original sample demonstrated persistent mood and other problems. Subjects reported progressive increases in problems related to cognitive function (difficulties with concentration, memory, forgetfulness, slowed reaction time and clumsiness), and at least 50 per cent were not working or were retired for health-related reasons. They concluded that only a minority of long-term bone marrow transplant survivors return to normal levels of functioning and that structured vocational and rehabilitation programmes are greatly needed (Andrykowski *et al.* 1989*b*).

In a follow-up analysis, this group has found that mood disturbance and psychological distress were greatest among bone marrow transplant recipients 30–60 months post-BMT as compared to groups who were either a shorter or longer interval since transplant. They hypothesized that emotional adjustment worsens as bone marrow transplant recipients become increasingly aware of and frustrated by chronic physical and functional deficits, and then ultimately improves again as patients revise their expectations and adapt to the reality of their life (Andrykowski and Henslee-Downey 1990).

Andrykowski *et al.* (1990) have recently compared quality of life in a sample of 29 pairs of bone marrow transplant recipients and renal transplant recipients matched for age, sex, and time since transplant. They concluded that both groups had impaired quality of life, and that there were few quality of life differences between the bone marrow transplant recipients and renal transplant recipients. Multivariate analyses of quality of life in the bone marrow transplant recipient group found that poorer status on several quality of life measures was related to less education, increased dose of total body irradiation during the BMT, and older age. Duration since BMT was not related to current quality of life. Of their sample, 55 per cent were employed outside of the home.

Table 14.1 shows results from a previously unpublished study of 26 adult bone marrow transplant recipients who were surveyed concerning their self-reported post-transplant rehabilitation service needs, and the extent to which their service needs had been met. Table 14.1 shows the percentage of the sample who reported having needed each service post-BMT, the percentage of the entire sample who reported their needs had been incompletely met, and the proportion of those needing each service whose needs had been met. This study indicates that overall, the overwhelming majority of those who reported service needs post-transplant also reported those needs had been inadequately

TABLE 14.1 UCLA adult bone marrow transplant recipient service needs study
($n = 26$)

Service	Needed (%)	Unmet (%)	Met: Needed ratio
Physical activity recommendations	73	50	0.32
Medical advice: return to work	73	50	0.32
Diet instruction	65	58	0.12
Patient support group	58	54	0.07
Counsel: disability benefits	58	54	0.07
Counsel: paying medical bills	54	50	0.07
Individual psychotherapy	50	42	0.15
Counsel: work patterns related health	46	39	0.17
Team–employer communication	42	35	0.18
Counsel: financial problems	42	42	0.00
Supervised exercise programme	42	42	0.00
Marital and sex counsel	39	39	0.00
Medications: depression and anxiety	39	31	0.20
Counsel: housing	39	31	0.20
Counsel: medication bills	35	35	0.00
Insomnia treatment	35	23	0.33

met. These data strongly support the need for integrated comprehensive rehabilitation programmes for adult bone marrow transplant recipients.

Wolcott *et al.* (1986*b*) studied adaptation in 18 bone marrow donors whose recipient had survived at least one year. These bone marrow donors had low levels of mood disturbance, high self-esteem, and a high degree of current life satisfaction. Donors reported little post-donation change in their relationship with their recipients. Donor-perceived quality of the donor–recipient relationship was highly correlated with perceived family approval of themselves, and was also highly correlated with recipient health status, psychological status, and recipient current social role function variables. In this sample, 4 (22 per cent) of 18 reported pre-donation doubts about donating; 100 per cent said they would donate again, and 16 per cent agreed with 'I have given something which is part of me for nothing in return'. Some 22 per cent reported post-donation medical problems, and 11 per cent reported feeling self-blame when their recipient had medical complications. Thus 10–20 per cent of living–related bone marrow donors reported some adverse medical and psychological outcomes even when their recipient was a long-term survivor. It is probable that the psychological morbidity rates in living–related bone marrow donor whose recipient does not survive are much higher. No other studies of psychological outcome in living–related bone marrow donors have yet been reported.

Bone marrow transplantation in children and adolescents

The literature in paediatric BMT is relatively limited, and consists primarily of descriptive reports of the clinical issues presenting during or immediately following hospitalization (Pfefferbaum *et al.* 1977; Gardner *et al.* 1977; Pfefferbaum *et al.* 1978; Patenaude *et al.* 1979; Wiley *et al.* 1984). However, two prospective studies have reported preliminary psychological findings (Pot-Mees and Zeitlin 1987; Stuber *et al.* 1989). Additional perspectives on the transplant of children and adolescents are provided in Chapter 4.

The medical 'late-effects' of paediatric bone marrow transplant are a topic of intense investigation (Parth *et al.* 1989; Trigg 1988). In a prospective study of children aged 3–7, anxiety symptoms related to the transplant persisted more than 12 months following the procedure (Stuber *et al.* 1989). Parents stated that the possibility of relapse continued to haunt them for at least a year, and some felt they would never fully relax about their child's health. The developing child is also subject to growth failure, learning disabilities, and infertility. Although some of these complications are amenable to medical intervention, there is considerable potential for psychiatric sequelae. Adaptive denial is often used, and can be quite helpful in avoiding an impaired self-concept. However, parents and children need guidance about when to discuss and investigate these potential late effects of treatment. In a current long-term follow-up study (Davidson and Stuber 1990), adolescent BMT survivors acknowledged infertility as a possible side-effect, but typically avoided the topic in discussions with their physicians, who were in a position to investigate the actual fertility status.

Learning difficulties pose a particular threat to long term functioning and self-esteem. Despite the significant plasticity of the developing nervous system, the potential negative impact of cranial irradiation and intrathecal methotrexate has been demonstrated in a number of studies (Wimmer *et al.* 1981). Since the toxicity appears to be dose-related, and BMT generally involves lower doses of radiation than have been studied with children undergoing cranial irradiation for leukaemia prophylaxis, the neuropsychiatric impact of paediatric BMT is still under investigation. However, it is likely that this will prove to be an area deserving intervention for children already delayed educationally by prolonged school absences.

Long-term adjustment of non-BMT paediatric cancer survivors has been found to be adequate in most recent studies (Fritz *et al.* 1988). However, most clinicians believe that there is a subtle impact which has not yet been adequately described. A current study of adolescent survivors six to ten years post-BMT, examining role and identity formation, may help to explain the ways in which this experience and its sequelae are incorporated into the developing personality (R. B. Davidson, personal communication). As matched familial marrow donors are most frequently siblings, research should also investigate the impact of donation on long-term adjustment and development. When problems with engraftment, relapse, or graft versus host disease occur, additional attention may be needed to help the donor child manage guilt and anger over the failure of this precious gift (Wiley *et al.* 1984).

There is growing interest in the long-term psychosocial and medical impact of treatment for paediatric cancer, including transplantation (Kazak 1989). However, until recently there were not sufficient numbers of survivors to investigate the possibility of specific developmentally-determined vulnerability. Age-dependent variation in cognitive understanding and developmental tasks at the time of transplant could be predicted to result in variability in psychological as well as medical response. Improved understanding of the impact of BMT on the developing body and personality will assist future clinicians as they assist children and families through the lengthy and difficult process.

Conclusions

While there is a gradually accumulating body of knowledge concerning long-term quality of life outcomes and neuropsychological function in bone marrow transplant recipients, even this body of research is still remarkably small. There is essentially no systematic data concerning pre-transplant mental status of bone marrow transplant recipients or living–related bone marrow donor candidates, of in-hospital psychiatric or behavioural outcomes of BMT recipients or their family members, of the prevalence of critical long-term psychiatric outcomes in BMT recipients, or of long-term effects of BMT on marital relations. The effects of BMT on development of brain function and personality in paediatric BMT recipients also needs much further study.

Given the relatively large number of individuals who now undergo BMTs, the increasing number of long-term survivors, and the important clinical, psychiatric, and neuropsychiatric questions which the procedure poses, rapid growth is required in both the amount and sophistication of research into the psychosocial aspects of this procedure.

References

Andrykowski, M. A. and Henslee-Downey, P. J. (1990). Emotional adjustment in adult survivors of allogeneic bone marrow transplant (BMT): beyond the 'honeymoon effect'. *Psychosomatic Medicine*, 52, 239.

Andrykoswki, M. A., Henslee, P. J., and Barnett, R. L. (1989*a*). Longitudinal assessment of psychosocial functioning of adult survivors of allogeneic bone marrow transplantation. *Bone Marrow Transplantation*, 4, 505–9.

Andrykowski, M. A., Henslee, P. J., and Farrall, M. G. (1989*b*). Physical and psychosocial functioning of adult survivors of allogeneic bone marrow transplantation. *Bone Marrow Transplantation*, 4, 65–71.

Andrykowski, M. A., Altmaier, E. M., Barnett, R. L., Otis, M. L., Gingrich, R., and Henslee-Downey, P. J. (1990). The quality of life in adult survivors of allogeneic bone marrow transplantation: Correlates and comparison with matched renal transplant recipients. *Transplantation*, 50, 399–406.

Andrykowski, M. A., Altmaier, E. M., Barnett, R. L., Burish, T. G., Gingrich, R., and Henslee-Downey, P. J. (in press). Cognitive dysfunction in adult survivors of allogeneic bone marrow transplantation: Relationship to dose of total body irradiation. *Bone Marrow Transplantation*, 6, 269–76.

Bortin, M. M. and Gale, R. P. (1986). Current status of allogeneic bone marrow transplantation: a report from the international bone marrow transplant registry. In *Clinical Transplants* (ed. P. Terasaki), pp. 17–25. (UCLA Tissue Typing Laboratory, Los Angeles).

Bortin, M. M. and Rimm, A. A. (1989). Increasing utilization of bone marrow transplantation. II. Results of the 1985–1987 survey. *Transplantation*, 48, 453–8.

Bortin, M. M., Horowitz, M. M., and Rimm, A. A. (1989). Report from the international bone marrow transplant registry. *Bone Marrow Transplantation*, 4, 221–8.

Brown, H. N. and Kelly, M. J. (1976). Stages of bone marrow transplantation: a psychiatric perspective. *Psychosomatic Medicine*, 38, 439–46.

Champlin, R. E. and Gale, R. P. (1984). The early complications of bone marrow transplantation. *Seminars in Hematology*, 21, 101–8.

Chapman, R. M. (1982). Effect of cytotoxic therapy on sexuality and gonadal function. *Seminars in Oncology*, 9, 84–94.

Craven, J. (1991). Cyclosporine-associated organic mental syndromes in liver transplant recipients. *Psychosomatics*, 32, 94–102.

Davidson, R. B. and Stuber, M. L. (1990). Post traumatic stress disorder and identity formation among adolescent bone marrow transplant survivors (abstract). Annual Meeting of the Academy of Psychosomatic Medicine, Phoenix, Arizona, November, 1990.

Fawzy, F. I., Wellisch, D. K., and Yager, J. (1977). Psychiatric liaison to the bone marrow transplant project. In *The family in mourning* (eds. C. Hollingsworth, R. O. Pasnau), pp. 181–9. (Grune & Stratton, New York).

Fritz, G. K., Williams, J. R., and Amylon, M. (1988). After treatment ends: Psychosocial sequelae in pediatric cancer survivors. *American Journal of Orthopsychiatry*, 58, 552–61.

de Fronzo, R. A., Braine, H., and Colvin, O. M. (1973). Water intoxication in man after cyclophosphamide therapy. *Annals of Internal Medicine*, 78, 861–9.

Folsom, T. L. and Popkin, M. K. (1987). Current and future perspectives on psychiatric involvement in bone marrow transplantations. *Psychiatric Medicine*, 4, 319–29.

Gale, R. P. (1986). Potential utilization of a national HLA-Typed donor pool for bone marrow transplantation. *Transplantation*, 42, 54–8.

Gardner, G., August, C., and Githeus, J. (1977). Psychological issues in bone marrow transplantation. *Pediatrics*, 60, 625–31.

Gillbert, H. A. and Kagan, A. R. (eds) (1980). *Radiation damage to the nervous system: a delayed therapeutic hazard*. (Raven Press, New York).

de Groen, P. C., Aksamit, A. J., Rakela, J., Forbes, G. S., and Krom, R. A. (1987).

Central nervous system toxicity after liver transplantation: The role of cyclo-sporine and cholesterol. *New England Journal of Medicine*, 317, 861–6.

Hengeveld, M. W., Houtman, R. B., and Zwaan, F. E. (1988). Psychological aspects of bone marrow transplantation: A retrospective study of 17 long-term survivors. *Bone Marrow Transplantation*, 3, 69–75.

Holland, J. C. and Rowland, J. H. (eds) (1989). *Handbook of psychooncology* (Oxford University Press, New York).

House, R. M. and Thompson, T. L., II. (1988). Psychiatric aspects of organ transplan-tation. *Journal of the American Medical Association*, 260, 535–9.

Kazak, A. E. (1989). Families of chronically ill children: A systems and social-ecological model of adaptation and challenge. *Journal of Consulting and Clinical Psychology*, 57, 25–30.

Lesko, L. M. (1989). In *Handbook of psychooncology* (eds J. C. Holland and J. H. Rowland), pp. 163–73. (Oxford University Press, New York).

Ling, M. H. M., Perry, P., and Tsuang, M. T. (1981). Side effects of corticosteroid therapy: psychiatric aspects. *Archives of General Psychiatry*, 38, 471–7.

Parkman, R. (1986). Current status of bone marrow transplantation in pediatric oncology. *Cancer*, 58, 569–72.

Parth, P., Dunlap, W. P., Kennedy, R. S., Lane, N. E., and Ordy, J. M. (1989). Motor and cognitive testing of bone marrow transplant patients after chemoradio therapy. *Perceptual and Motor Skills*, 68, 1227–41.

Patchell, R. A., White, C. L., III, Clark, A. W., and Beschorner, W. E. (1982). Central nervous system complications of bone marrow transplantation: a clinical and pathological study. *Annals of Neurology*, 12, 80.

Patenaude, A. F. and Rappeport, J. M. (1982). Surviving bone marrow transplantation: the patient in the other bed. *Annals of Internal Medicine*, 97, 915–18.

Patenaude, A. F., Symanski, L., and Rappeport, J. (1979). Psychological costs of bone marrow transplantation in children. *American Journal of Orthopsychiatry*, 49, 409–22.

Pfefferbaum, B., Lindamood, M., and Wiley, F. (1977). Pediatric bone marrow trans-plantation: psychosocial aspects. *American Journal of Psychiatry*, 134, 1299–1301.

Pfefferbaum, B., Lindamood, M., and Wiley, F. (1978). Stages in pediatric bone marrow transplantation. *Pediatrics*, 61, 625–8.

Popkin, M. K. and Moldow, C. F. (1977). Stressors and responses during bone marrow transplantation. *Archives of Internal Medicine*, 137, 725.

Popkin, M. K., Moldow, C. F., Hall, R. C. W., Branda, R. F., and Yarchoan, R. (1977). Psychiatric aspects of allogeneic bone marrow transplantation for aplastic anemia. *Diseases of the Nervous System*, 38, 925–7.

Pot-Mees, C. C. and Zeilin, H. (1987). Psychosocial consequences of bone marrow transplantation in children: a preliminary communication. *Journal of Psychosocial Oncology*, 5, 73–81.

Richards, G. E. (1980). Effects of irradiation on the hypothalamic pituitary regions. In *Radiation damage to the nervous system: a delayed therapeutic hazard* (eds. H. A. Gillbert and A. R. Kagan), pp. 175–80. (Raven Press, New York).

Schilskey, R. L., Lewis, B. J., Sherins, R. J., and Young, R. C. (1980). Gonadal dysfunc-tion in patients receiving chemotherapy for cancer. *Annals of Internal Medicine*, 93(1), 109–14.

Sheline, G. E. (1980). Irradiation injury of the human brain: a review of clinical experiences. In *Radiation damage to the nervous system: a delayed therapeutic hazard* (eds H. A. Gillbert and A. R. Kagan), pp. 39–58. (Raven Press, New York).

Simmons, R. G., Klein, S. D., and Simmons, R. L. (1977). *Gift of Life: the psychological and social impact of organ transplantation.* (Wiley, New York).

Smith, C. I. E., Aarli, J. A., Biberfeld, P., Bolme, P., Christensson, B., and Gahrton, G. (1983). Myasthenia gravis after bone-marrow transplantation: Evidence for a donor origin. *New England Journal of Medicine*, 309, 1565–8.

Stuber, M. L. (in press). Psychologic care of adolescents undergoing transplantation. In *Textbook of adolescent medicine* (eds E. R. McNarney, R. E. Kreipe, D. P. Orr, and G. D. Comerci). (W. B. Saunders, Philadelphia).

Stuber, M. L., Nader, K., Pynoos, R., Yasuda, P., Cohen, S., and Laemmel, M. (1989). PTSD after pediatric bone marrow transplantation. Presented at the American Psychiatric Association Annual Meeting.

Sullivan, K. M., Storb, R., Shulman, H. M., Shaw, C. M., Spence, A., and Beckham, C. (1982). Immediate and delayed neurotoxicity after meclorethamine preparation for bone marrow transplantation. *Annals of Internal Medicine*, 97, 182–9.

Surman, O. S. (1989). Psychiatric aspects of organ transplantation. *American Journal of Psychiatry*, 146, 972–82.

Trigg, M. E. (1988). Bone marrow transplantation for treatment of leukemia in children. *Pediatric Clinics of North America*, 35, 933–48.

Wade, J. C. and Meyers, J. D. (1983). Neurologic symptoms associated with parenteral acyclovir treatment after marrow transplantation. *Annals of Internal Medicine*, 98, 921–5.

Welch, H. G. and Larson, E. B. (1989). Cost effectiveness of bone marrow transplantation in acute nonlymphocytic leukemia. *New England Journal of Medicine*, 321, 807–12.

Welch-McCaffrey, D., Hoffman, B., Leigh, S. A., Loescher, L. J., and Meyskens, F. L. Jr. (1989). Surviving adult cancers. Part 2: psychosocial implications. *Annals of Internal Medicine*, 111, 517–24.

Wellisch, D. K., Fawzy, F. I., and Yager, J. (1977). Life in a venus flytrap: Psychiatric liaison to patients undergoing bone marrow transplantation. In *Contemporary models in consultation—Liaison psychiatry* (eds R. Faguet, F. Fawzy, D. Wellisch, and R. O. Pasnau), pp. 29–51. (Spectrum, New York).

Wiley, F. M. and House, K. U. (1988). Bone marrow transplant in children. *Seminars in Oncology Nursing*, 4, 31–40.

Wiley, F., Lindamood, M., and Pfefferbaum, B. (1984). The donor–patient relationship in pediatric bone marrow transplantation. *Association of Pediatric Oncology Nurses*, 1, 8–14.

Wimmer, R. S., Hill, W. B., and Baird, H. W. (1981). Neurometric and psychometric evaluation of long-term survivors of childhood acute lymphocytic leukemia. *Proceedings of the American Association for Cancer Research and the American Society of Clinical Oncology*, 22, 398.

Wolcott, D. L. (1990). Organ transplant psychiatry: psychiatry's role in the second gift of life. *Psychosomatics*, 31, 91–7.

Wolcott, D. L., Wellisch, D. K., Fawzy, F. I., and Landsverk, J. (1986a). Adaptation of adult bone marrow transplant recipient long-term survivors. *Transplantation*, 41, 478–84.

Wolcott, D. L., Wellisch, D. K., Fawzy, F. I., and Landsverk, J. (1986b). Psychological adjustment of adult bone marrow transplant donors whose recipient survives. *Transplantation*, 41, 484–8.

Wolcott, D. L., Fawzy, F. I., and Wellisch, D. K. (1987*a*). Psychiatric aspects of bone marrow transplantation: a review and current issues. *Psychiatric Medicine*, 4, 299–317.

Wolcott, D. L., Fawzy, F. I., Wellisch, D. K., and Weiner, H. (1987*b*). Changes in DST before and after a bone marrow transplant conditioning regimen: A pilot study. *Psychiatric Medicine*, 4, 85–92.

15 Lung transplantation

P. Kelly, C. Bart, and J. Craven

The Toronto Lung Transplant Group (1986) performed the first truly success-ful lung transplant in 1983 and, as of September 1990, had performed 44 single and 30 double lung transplants with an overall survival rate of 64 per cent post-transplant. Lung transplant has passed through the experimental stage (Cooper 1987; Grossman *et al.* 1990) and is now regarded as an important therapeutic option for people with endstage lung disease. The importance of psychosocial factors in the health and well-being of candidates and recipients has been recognized since the early days of the lung transplant programme in Toronto. Professionals from psychiatry, social work, and psychology work closely with other members of the team to assess, support, and treat patients in the pro-gramme. This chapter describes the involvement of these professionals with the transplant team and presents data on psychosocial aspects of lung trans-plantation.

Preoperative phase

Assessment of applicants

All lung transplant applicants are given a thorough medical, physiotherapeutic, and psychosocial assessment during a two-week in-patient admission. The assessment is conducted with two goals in mind: to determine the suitability of applicants for lung transplantation, and to gather information that can guide the team in the management and support of patients who are accepted as trans-plant candidates. The assessments conducted by members of the psychosocial group address both of these goals but, in practice, rejections for psychosocial reasons alone have been rare. Consequently, the assessments by psychology, social work, and psychiatry are used primarily to identify areas of concern and to develop plans for managing the anticipated emotional and psychological needs of each accepted transplant candidate.

Table 15.1 summarizes basic demographic data and medical diagnoses for a consecutive series of 106 patients who were assessed by the lung transplant programme. The patient sample was 54 per cent female. Most patients had some high school education and were in stable relationships. Approximately one-third of the patients lived within commuting distance of the hospital, 34

TABLE 15.1 Demographic and clinical characteristics of 106 consecutive lung transplant applicants

Variable	Male	Female	Combined
Sex	49 (46%)	57 (54%)	106
Age: mean	43.2	40.2	41.5
standard deviation	13.0	10.6	11.7
Level of education			
(up to completion of)			
elementary	10.0%	4.3%	6.6%
high school	46.6%	67.4%	59.2%
post-secondary	43.3%	28.3%	34.2%
Marital status			
married or c/l	73.5%	70.2%	71.7%
never married	22.4%	22.8%	22.6%
separated, divorced, widowed	4.1%	7.0%	5.7%
Location of home			
local	28.6%	40.4%	34.9%
non-local Canadian	40.8%	28.1%	34.0%
non-local/non-Canadian	30.6%	31.6%	31.1%
Medical diagnosis			
pulmonary fibrosis	28.6%	15.8%	21.7%
COPD/emphysema	14.3%	14.0%	14.2%
alpha-1 antitrypsis deficiency	14.3%	21.1%	17.9%
cystic fibrosis	24.5%	15.8%	19.8%
other	18.4%	33.3%	26.4%

per cent were Canadians from outside the Toronto area and the remaining patients were predominantly American citizens.

Each of the three mental health professions integrated into the transplant service contributes to the psychosocial assessment of patient strengths and vulnerabilities. The psychiatric assessment involves a ninety minute semi-structured interview that elicits information relevant to psychiatric diagnosis, coping strategies, adjustment to illness and potential death, capacity for informed consent and patient's understanding of the transplant process (Craven *et al.* 1990*a*). The social work assessment focuses primarily on the quality of social support available to the applicant. All applicants for transplant are required to have a support person, because emotional and instrumental support are needed during the waiting and recovery periods. The social worker interviews the applicant, support person, and other available family members in order to assess the adequacy of social support for the patient (Bright *et al.* 1990).

The psychological assessment procedure was primarily designed to provide information about the applicant's interpersonal style, personality and coping characteristics, symptoms of psychopathology, and current mood (Kelly 1988). The assessment involves a semi-structured interview and a psychological test battery. Included in the battery are tests that assess symptoms of psychopathology: the Basic Personality Inventory (BPI) (Jackson 1989); personality functioning: the California Psychological Inventory (CPI) (Gough 1987); coping style: Health and Daily Living Form (Moos *et al.* 1985); physical and psychosocial functioning: Sickness Impact Profile (Bergner *et al.* 1976); current mood: Beck Depression Inventory (Beck *et al.* 1988), Profile of Mood States (POMS) (McNair *et al.* 1971), Speilberger State-Trait Anxiety Inventory (STAI) (Speilberger *et al.* 1970); and defensive style and subconscious perception of issues relevant to transplant: the Thematic Apperception Test (TAT) (Murray 1971) (Card order: 1, 2, 3BM, 4, 8GF, 8BM, 6BM, 12M, 10, 15, 11, 17BM).

The psychosocial assessment must take into consideration that this is a time of uncertainty and stress for most applicants and their families. Most patients realize that their life is in grave danger from lung disease. They are either fearful of being found too ill to undergo the procedure or that a previously undetected organ dysfunction will eliminate them from candidacy. Worry, insomnia, and performance anxiety during the period of assessment are common enough to be considered normal in these circumstances. Also of importance to note is that a sizeable proportion of patients have applied to the programme from places far distant from the treatment site. Many candidates have had to move their homes to Toronto while awaiting and recovering from the procedure. Patients are aware that they may have to live in the treatment area for between 9 and 24 months and this move is a significant additional burden for many patients and their families.

After the social worker, psychologist, and psychiatrist on the team each conduct an independent assessment of the patient, they meet to discuss the case and form a consensus psychosocial recommendation about the suitability of the applicant. Each professional writes an independent assessment report for the patient's hospital chart and the consensus recommendation of the psychosocial group is presented verbally to the transplant team at a case conference. During the conference, the applicant's psychosocial strengths and vulnerabilities are reviewed. Discussions related to psychosocial issues may be quite brief if the applicant is seen as acceptable without any reservations.

Psychosocial recommendations

As shown in Table 15.2, 55.5 per cent of a consecutive series of 110 applicants were assessed by the psychosocial team as having adequate coping abilities and social support and as being unreservedly acceptable. An additional 20 per cent of the applicants were viewed as likely to place manageable but greater than average demands on the programme's psychosocial resources. These patients

Table 15.2 The relationship between psychosocial recommendation and transplant team assessment decision

Psychosocial recommendations	Team decision					Total	
	Accept	Reassess later	Reject: medical	Reject: psychosocial	Reject: combined med./psych.		
Accept without reservation	44	10	7	0	0	61	(55.5%)
Accept with precautions	14	4	2	0	2	22	(20.0%)
Accept with specific criteria	7	4	2	0	3	16	(14.5%)
Reject	0	0	0	5	6	11	(10.0%)
Column totals	65	18	11	5	11	110	
	(59.1%)	(16.4%)	(10.0%)	(4.5%)	(10.0%)		

$x^2 = 89.88$; D.F. $= 15$; Prob. $= <0.0001$

included those with impoverished support networks, difficulty in understanding the demands of the programme, markedly poor interpersonal skills, or psychiatric disorder.

A further 14.5 per cent of applicants were given specific criteria to meet before their formal enrolment in the transplant programme. Examples of these criteria include abstinence from alcohol for several months, arrangement of a suitable support person, agreement to attend regularly a patient support group, or to receive individual psychotherapy. A trial of adherence to programme requirements for one or two months was also required of some patients as a behavioural test of compliance. Generally speaking, patients were very motivated to enter the programme and many met their specified criteria.

For 10 per cent of the 110 applicants, it was the recommendation of the psychosocial assessment group that the patient not to be accepted. This recommendation was based on a judgement that the applicant would be likely to require much more support or assistance than the programme could provide in order to participate adequately in the programme or else there were very serious reservations about the patient's ability to cope with the long-term requirements to monitor symptoms of rejection and reliably take immuno-suppressive medication.

Denial of enrolment to the programme was only recommended if the applicant had multiple and severe psychosocial problems and was unwilling or unable to use the supportive psychosocial services that were available adequately. For example, the psychosocial assessment group recommended rejection of one applicant who had a prolonged history of alcohol dependence, a coping style characterized by denial and marked dependency, passivity and cognitive disability. In addition, the applicant was discovered to be non-compliant and unreliable during the in-patient assessment stay.

In summary, the psychosocial group make four general types of recommendations to the transplant team: (1) accept without reservations; (2) accept with precautions; (3) accept with specific criteria; and (4) reject as unsuitable for psychosocial reasons. Table 15.2 also shows the relationship between the consensus psychosocial recommendation and the final assessment decision of the transplant team. There was a statistically significant relationship between the psychosocial recommendation and the team decision and, as the table indicates, the team always respected the opinion of the psychosocial group when relevant issues were under consideration. More specifically, none of the 61 applicants who were psychosocially rated as acceptable without reservation were rejected for psychosocial reasons and all 11 of the applicants who were rated as unsuitable on psychosocial grounds were denied enrolment in the programme. A subset of five of these patients were rejected solely because of psychosocial factors and the remaining six were rejected for a combination of psychosocial and medical reasons.

Each applicant was assessed for current and past DSM-III Axis I disorders by the consulting psychiatrist (Craven *et al.* 1990*b*). Organic brain syndromes, depressive disorders, alcohol abuse, and anxiety disorders were the most common diagnoses made. For most of these applicants, the onset of the psychiatric disorder occurred following the onset of pulmonary disease and was, in many cases, a recognizable complication of physical illness and/or its treatment. Panic and anxiety disorder not otherwise specified appear to be common in patients with respiratory disease (Karajgi *et al.* 1990). Anxiety disorders have been a frequent problem for lung transplant candidates who have presented both with symptoms characteristic of anxiety disorders (e.g. panic episodes, anticipatory anxiety, and avoidance motivation) and symptoms more specific to the medical context (e.g. suffocation phobia, heightened sensitivity to the discomfort of medical procedures, performance anxiety during medical or rehabilitative exercises, and fastidiousness with health care). Panic anxiety in patients with endstage lung disease may result from biological factors (e.g. increased PCO_2 levels (Karajgi *et al.* 1990; Gorman *et al.* 1988)) or psychosocial factors (e.g. feelings of helplessness, loss of control, or physical confinement with progressive disability). Counselling, stress management techniques or, when required, pharmacological interventions have decreased anxiety to tolerable levels. In a small number of these patients, buspirone, an anxiolytic without marked sedative or respiratory side-effects (Newton *et al.* 1986; Garner *et al.* 1989), has been of benefit and has resulted in no respiratory complications.

In order to explicate further the operational criteria for the four types of psychosocial recommendations that have been made by the Toronto Lung Transplant psychosocial group, a series of statistical analyses were conducted to identify empirically the psychiatric and psychological factors associated with the psychosocial recommendations. Table 15.3 shows that there was a statistically significant relationship between presence of a current Axis I disorder and

TABLE 15.3 The relationship between psychosocial recommendation and current DSM-III Axis 1 disorder

Psychosocial recommendation	Presence of DSM-III Axis 1 disorder at time of assessment		
	Present	Not present	Row total
Accept without reservation	2 (3.3%)	58 (96.7%)	60
Accept with precautions	5 (23.8%)	16 (76.2%)	21
Accept with specific criteria	3 (21.4%)	11 (78.6%)	14
Reject	5 (50.0%)	5 (50.0%)	10
Column totals	15 (14.3%)	90 (85.7%)	105

$x^2 = 18.4$; D.F. $= 3$ Prob. $= 0.0004$

type of psychosocial recommendation. Specifically, there was an overall prevalence rate of 14.3 per cent for the sample of 105 applicants and the rate varied from 3.3 per cent for applicants who were rated as acceptable without reservation to 50 per cent for applicants who were rated as unsuitable. This finding reflects the tendency for patients with current addictions to be declined enrolment on the waiting list. The presence of other psychiatric disorders was not, in and of itself, considered reason for disqualification. Table 15.4 shows that the relationship between lifetime history of an Axis I disorder and type of psychosocial recommendation was not significantly related. The overall prevalence rate was 41.0 per cent and the likelihood of a past Axis I disorder was equivalent across the types of psychosocial recommendation.

TABLE 15.4 The relationship between psychosocial recommendation and past DSM-III Axis 1 disorder

Psychosocial recommendation	Occurence of DSM-III Axis 1 disorder prior to time of assessment		
	Past disorder	No past disorder	Row total
Accept without reservation	19 (31.7%)	41 (68.3%)	60
Accept with precautions	11 (52.4%)	10 (47.6%)	21
Accept with specific criteria	7 (50.0%)	7 (50.0%)	14
Reject	6 (60.0%)	4 (40.0%)	10
Column totals	43 (41.0%)	62 (59.0%)	105

$x^2 = 5.2$; D.F. $= 3$ Prob. $= 0.154$

In addition to the interview-based data described above, psychometric test data were also available. For example, the applicants were administered the Basic Personality Inventory (BPI) (Jackson 1989) and California Psychological Inventory (CPI) (Gough 1987) as part of a standardized psychometric assessment battery. The BPI was designed as a replacement for the MMPI and it assesses symptoms of psychopathology on 12 sub-scales. The CPI contains sub-scales relevant to interpersonal relatedness, self-control and intellectual efficiency. On the basis of clinical impressions, it was anticipated that the applicants, on average, would score in the normal range on these tests of psychopathology and personality functioning.

As predicted, the sub-scale scores on all BPI sub-scales were within normal limits for a sample of 75 applicants. There was a subclinical elevation on a sub-scale that assessed somatic preoccupation, but the degree of elevation was appropriate for pulmonary patients with an average life expectancy of less than eighteen months. The mean CPI profiles for male and female applicants were also in the normal range on all sub-scales. For both sexes, there were minor elevations on two CPI sub-scales, Sc (Self control) and Gi (Good impression). These elevations suggest that applicants tried to present themselves in a somewhat favourable light when they were assessed, but the degree of bias was not sufficient to invalidate the test. Results of normative data from the BPI and CPI strongly supported the clinical impression that lung transplant patients, on average, are psychologically normal.

Analyses were also conducted to determine if applicants who were given different types of psychosocial recommendations could be distinguished on the basis of BPI data. During the time period when the BPI was routinely administered to lung transplant applicants, 8 of 75 applicants were rated as unsuitable for psychosocial reasons. It is noteworthy that three (37.5 per cent) of these eight unsuitable applicants refused to complete the standard psychological test battery, while none of the remaining 67 applicants refused. Of course, the three refusers were not rejected because they did not fill out the tests. Each of them also showed strong indications of significant personality disorders on the basis of psychiatric interview, history, and observational data. However, the absence of these individuals from the psychometric database means that some population differences may not be adequately represented in the sample of test completers.

On the basis of available BPI data, applicants who were rejected had significantly higher scores on the Thought Disorder sub-scale. Additionally, patients who were rated as accepted with specific recommendations had significantly higher scores on the Deviation sub-scale. These findings suggest that applicants who were rejected had greater psychopathology and/or neurocognitive problems, and that applicants who were accepted with specific recommendations were more likely to complain of specific, clinically noteworthy, symptoms or to use alcohol excessively. Results from the analysis of psychometric data therefore concur with the results of the analysis of Axis 1 disorders.

Over the last few years the lung transplant team has gained greater experience in working with psychosocially vulnerable patients and more resources have been allocated to supporting emotionally needy or challenging patients. With these programme changes, the team has felt better able to work with these patients and there is a strong impression that the criteria for psychosocial acceptance has shifted in the direction of greater likelihood of acceptance of patients with psychopathology. For example, during 1990 patients have been accepted who would, in all probability, have been rejected two years earlier. This change is consistent with our emerging philosophy that absolute psychosocial contraindications to transplant surgery probably do not exist, but that flexible and relative contraindications are acceptable and in part dependent upon the resources and experience of the transplant team (Craven *et al.* 1990; Craven *et al.* 1990*a*).

This clinical impression was investigated by testing the hypothesis that the relationship between the degree of psychopathology and the type of psycho-social recommendation has changed in the period from 1986 to 1990. In a multiple regression analysis, the dependent variable was a four point scale indicating degree of acceptance, based on the psychosocial recommendation. The first predictor variable was presence of current DSM-III Axis I disorder (0 = no, 1 = yes) and the second predictor variable was an interaction term computed by multiplying the first predictor variable by an applicant sequence number. The adjusted R^2 for the first predictor was 0.225 ($p < .0001$) and, with the entry of the second predictor the adjusted R^2 increased to 0.288. The increase in R^2 was significant at the 0.009 level. The results of this analysis support the hypothesis that the presence of a current DSM-III Axis I disorder is a significant determinant of the type of psychosocial recommendation and, as well, that the influence of the degree of psychopathology on the psychosocial recommendation has changed over the history of the lung transplant pro-gramme.

In summary, these statistical analyses support our clinical impressions that lung transplant applicants, on average, are psychologically normal. The results also support the validity of the recommendations made by the psychosocial group, since the type of recommendation varied systematically with degree of psychopathology as assessed by semi-structured interview and psychometric test scores. Perhaps the most important finding was the indication that the pro-gramme has moved in the direction of accepting applicants with more demanding psychosocial problems.

Awaiting transplant

As indicated in Table 15.2, 59.1 per cent of the patients from the consecutive series of 110 applicants were accepted as transplant candidates and enrolled into the lung transplant programme. Most of the patients who are enrolled in the programme feel an initial sense of relief and excitement for having 'passed' the assessment. However, candidates who have had less time to adjust psycho-logically to the need for a transplant sometimes feel more fear than relief when they are enrolled.

All of the candidates must face a number of common challenges. For the 29 per cent of candidates who were Americans and the 33 per cent who were non-local Canadians, the most immediate challenge was the need to arrange accom-modation and financing for a move to Toronto. After the candidates arrive in Toronto they are faced with an indeterminate wait until a suitable donor becomes available. The waiting time to transplant has averaged six to eight months with the shortest time being 2 days and the longest 21 months. Since patients who are enrolled in the programme typically have an anticipated life expectancy of less than 18 months, the risk of death before transplantation increases as the candidate's wait duration increases. In 1987, for example, 21 per cent of candidates died before transplantation. Hospitalizations for pulmonary insufficiency and infections are common and they heighten patients' anxieties that they may not live to get their chance at a 'new life'.

At least some symptoms of anxiety are ubiquitous in patients awaiting transplant. Anxiety disorders have been found in 21 per cent of candidates awaiting lung transplant and include adjustment disorder with anxious mood, panic disorder, and anxiety disorder not otherwise specified (Craven *et al.* 1990*a*). These disorders developed both in persons with a past history of anxiety or depression as well as in candidates with no previous psychiatric history. Factors which may contribute to these symptoms and disorders include the major changes in lifestyle and medical treatment required by programme involvement, geographical movement away from homes and families, and increased appreciation of the severity of illness (as evidenced by acceptance to the transplant programme). In addition, there may be a breakdown of denial regarding the dangers of their illness and impending surgery because of education by the transplant team and familiarity with candidates who die while awaiting surgery. Each of these stressors is exacerbated by the protracted and indeterminate wait for lung transplant surgery.

The prolonged waiting period stimulates a variety of fantasized and real concerns among transplant candidates (Levenson and Olbrisch 1987). Patients may become preoccupied with the wish for a donor to become available, or may fantasize about the occurrence of an accidental death which would provide an organ for their transplant. Morbid humour about benefiting from the misfortune of others provides relief for some, while others are so distressed that they attempt to suppress these thoughts and/or quietly suffer guilt and self-recrimination. Although the patients are pleased when one of them is transplanted, it is not uncommon for a candidate to be preoccupied about his or her place on 'the list' or to be concerned that other patients may be given priority over themselves.

In addition to the patient's personal concerns, the support person and other family members may also have their lives substantially disrupted, and financial or interpersonal difficulties may arise for relatives or friends during the prolonged waiting period. For example, the support person must assume responsibility for much of the candidate's personal and medical needs. At times, entire families have chosen to relocate during the waiting period to remain with the candidate. The burdens of waiting can put a prolonged strain on the relationships among the candidate, designated support person, and other family members. This strain sometimes leads to family dysfunction and psychosocial intervention is required. Some candidates have had difficulty engaging one designated friend or family member to be a support person. In such cases a rotating support system of different friends or hired staff has been used to meet the support person requirement (Bright *et al.* 1990).

While all the candidates must face a set of common practical and emotional challenges, some patients have more personal and social coping resources than others. A rough indication of this variability can be derived from Table 15.2. Of the 65 candidates who were enrolled, 67.7 per cent were judged to have good social and intrapersonal coping resources, 21.5 per cent were assessed as likely to require greater than average psychosocial support and 10.8 per cent were accepted on the condition that they meet specific criteria such as abstaining from alcohol. As the lung transplant programme has evolved, the social worker, psychiatrist, and psychologist have developed a set of interventions to support good and poor copers. The interventions are graded in therapeutic intensity and have ranged from less formal supportive interventions to twice weekly cognitive–behavioural therapy.

Some contextual support is provided by the regular involvement of patients in rehabilitative therapy and medical clinic. The candidates are encouraged to develop informal support networks with other candidates and support persons. Such a network is important to the candidates' sense of well-being because it serves as a substitute community for out-of-town patients. The candidates and their support people also derive an important sense of belonging from association with others who share their hardships and understand their concerns. Sharing instrumental activities and emotions has led to the development of close friendships among the patients. However, some candidates have found the intimacy engendered by the close contact uncomfortable and minimized their involvement with the programme. One undesirable complication of the informal network has been the ease with which rumours are communicated within the patient group.

The social worker and psychologist facilitate a weekly support group that is open to the candidates, recipients, and support persons. Attendance has generally ranged from 15–25 people. The focus of the group varies from the sharing of concrete information to emotional ventilation and support. On a regular basis, didactic sessions are offered by team members to discuss topics such as new developments in surgical techniques, donor availability, and infection control. The mutual support established and facilitated by the group has been a major aid to the candidates and their support people in their coping with the transplant process (Bright *et al.* 1990). Group concerns, wishes, and problems are also communicated to other team members through the facilitators.

The intimacy generated by the group has sometimes led to the group members feeling entitled to confidential information about other patients. Explanations regarding patient rights and confidentiality must be restated from time to time by staff to offset this behaviour. Usually the group members can get the information they want about, for example, a recently transplanted patient, because the support person of the recipient will come to the group and give a report.

Postoperative phase

Immediately following the transplant, both patients and their families are commonly euphoric. However, they often soon face the likelihood of medical or surgical complications which may be physically and emotionally exhausting. Supportive contact of the new recipient by family, friends, and medical staff is of great value during this time.

Postoperative agitation and delirium have been frequent complications following lung transplant. A study of the first 30 lung transplant recipients at this centre (Craven *et al.* 1990*b*) showed that 50 per cent of recipients demonstrated delirium and an additional 20 per cent demonstrated transient confusional states during the first two postoperative weeks. Disorientation and a fluctuating level of consciousness have repeatedly interfered with the recipients' ability to co-operate with medical procedures. Restlessness, agitation, or combativeness have contributed to problematic physiological changes in the unstable patient (e.g. decreased oxygen saturation) and have complicated the process of ventilatory weaning.

Delirium was found to be associated with the prolonged use of cardiopulmonary bypass during transplant and postoperative cyclosporin administration (Craven *et al.* 1990*b*). Bypass may produce delirium as a result of microembolism to the cerebral circulation (Lee *et al.* 1971). Because of the risk of excessive haemorrhage during lung transplant, heparin has been administered in amounts lower than is usual with bypass, and the risk of microembolism may have been increased. Anxiety, agitation, disorientation, vivid nightmares, and psychosis have been associated with cyclosporin use in liver transplant recipients (de Groen *et al.* 1987; Craven 1991) and these clinical features may be manifestations of delirium or subcortical seizure activity. These symptoms and signs have been most pronounced in lung transplant recipients whose cyclosporin levels have rapidly risen to greater than 300 micrograms per litre. Cyclosporin-associated neurotoxicity is discussed in greater detail in Chapter 7.

Due to the frequency of agitation and disorientation during the first week following transplantation, we have prepared candidates and their families for this possibility. A recent review of post-cardiotomy delirium has substantiated the benefits of this preoperative education (Smith and Dimsdale 1989). In addition, patients have been routinely administered haloperidol (1.0 milligrams IV, q4–6h) from the time of regaining consciousness. Many patients with delirium have now been well controlled with this regimen only. When more severe agitation or aggressiveness has occurred, the dose of haloperidol has been doubled in a stepwise manner to a maximum of 10 milligrams per dose and/or the dosage interval halved as required to a minimum of 30 minutes. Once resolution of acute agitation is obtained, the dose of haloperidol may be rapidly titrated downwards to the lowest amount required to maintain control over the agitation. Our experience concurs with results from similar protocols using intravenous haloperidol (Adams *et al.* 1986; Tesar *et al.* 1985). For most patients, this drug may be safely used in the intensive care unit setting and over-sedation may be largely avoided if the mental state is frequently re-assessed. Since this earlier review of our programme (Craven *et al.* 1990*b*), the implementations of the interventions described and the decreased use of cardiopulmonary bypass appear to have lessened the occurrence of delirium and agitation. Kast (1989) has recently suggested a biochemical potential for neuroleptics to inhibit the immunosuppressant activity of cyclosporin and has recommended caution when administering these drugs in combination. Although further systematic investigation is required to determine whether the proposed interaction is clinically significant, we have not found an increased frequency of rejection episodes since instituting the haloperidol protocol described above.

Organic mental symptoms associated with corticosteroids (euphoria, irritability, and anxiety) or cyclosporin (transient confusional states, visual hallucinosis, anxiety and restlessness) have also occurred during the first four postoperative weeks. Insomnia has been common for the first two post-operative weeks and has proven largely unresponsive to standard pharmaco-therapy. Explaining the aetiology and reversibility of these symptoms is reassuring and most helpful to patients. Although not often required, small bedtime doses of neuroleptics (i.e. haloperidol 0.5–2.5 milligrams qhs or perphenazine 2–4 milligrams qhs) have been effective in managing mild organic symptoms.

Patients who have experienced severe postoperative delirium may require postponement of self-medication teaching until cognitive function improves. For example, a female lung recipient experienced short-term memory deficits postoperatively that warranted instituting a behavioural programme utilizing memory aids, a daily medication diary and, eventually, involvement by a community occupational therapist to assist the recipient's home adaptation. A visuo-perceptual deficit was identified in a second lung recipient after in-accuracies in self-administered liquid cyclosporin were discovered. Tablet administered cyclosporin ensured that this recipient received a more accurate medication dosage. In both of these cases, neuropsychological test findings played an important role in clarifying that the apparent compliance problem was caused by a cognitive deficit and not by poor motivation.

A small number of lung transplant recipients have developed episodes of severe major depression. In each of these patients, depression occurred in the context of a prolonged postoperative course with multiple complications. They have been treated for depression with standard antidepressant therapy. One patient developed a depressive syndrome characterized by anergy, anorexia, inactivity, and apathy which began during the second postoperative week and, despite a good physical recovery, persisted throughout the hospital stay. This syndrome was considered to be in part a neuropsychiatric complication of cyclosporin administration and responded well to a six-week course of methyl-phenidate (Craven 1989).

Rehabilitation and adjustment

As recipients experience the reality of post-transplant life, they are challenged to find ways to cope with feelings of vulnerability and to relinquish magical expectations regarding the outcome of transplant surgery. The hope for complete independence from the health care system can be strong. However, they must adjust to accepting the continuing role of patient and minor compliance problems can arise at this time. Such problems are particularly common in young adult patients with cystic fibrosis who exhibit adolescent dynamics. A supportive but directive approach addresses the problem.

Recipients are usually able to return home after three months if their clinical course has been relatively uneventful. For many of the recipients, leaving the protective environment offered by the immediate proximity of the transplant team and the close relationships established with other transplant patients results in considerable apprehension. Unacknowledged anxiety regarding separation from the perceived security of the transplant environment has led to somatic complaints, problems in assuming independence, and over-involvement in transplant-associated activities.

After the recipients leave the hospital they may feel anxious because physicians in their home area lack the experience of the transplant team physicians. The recipients may also feel somewhat alienated in the home community because people there are unsure about what questions to ask or how to empathize with their experience. The recipient's transplant experience has generated new self-understandings which those not familiar with the transplant process are unable to appreciate. For example, relatives and former employers may inappropriately assume that the recipient has returned to a completely 'normal' life.

During the longer term, the response of the recipient's family and support person to increasing independence may not always be appropriate. Overprotection is common in cases such as cystic fibrosis where the patient has had a long history of vulnerable health and has required intense care from a family member or spouse. Conversely, too little support may be provided when the support person hopes to be released from their duties. For example, anger and guilt toward a recipient's slow postoperative course and continued dependency has resulted in depression in some family members. In instances where family problems are identified, the psychosocial group recommends, or if possible provides, interventions that focus on enhancing communication between patients and their families. Marital or family therapy can help the recipient and his or her significant others deal more effectively with the changes in roles, abilities, and family dynamics that usually follow transplantation.

Lung recipients face a number of other challenges, in addition to rebalancing family relationships, as they try to maintain a sense of personal control. For example, they must regularly submit to medical procedures such as bronchoscopy to monitor for signs of rejection. Anticipatory anxiety may develop and lead to avoidance of the procedure. A more serious challenge to the recipient's sense of control and stability has also become salient in the past year. During this time it has become apparent that 15 per cent of transplant survivors develop bronchiolitis obliterans. The condition is eventually fatal and re-transplantation is the only effective treatment. Recipients who develop the condition must deal with feelings of disappointment, anger, and vulnerability when they are confronted with the need to consider a second transplant in order to extend their lives.

Improvement in physical functioning and quality of life are the primary goals of lung transplantation, but little research has yet been conducted to assess the degree of improvement provided by transplant surgery. One study by Craven *et al.* (1990) surveyed persons who had survived at least six months following lung transplant ($n = 22$) with respect to their functional outcome and life satisfaction. A total of 82 per cent of the recipients surveyed had returned to full- or part-time employment or had made a voluntary choice to return to household duties while 18 per cent did not resume employment. However, 64 per cent of the recipients reported that their ability to work was in some way hampered by their physical health. At the same time, 72 per cent of the recipients rated their satisfaction with their physical health as good to excellent.

Other measures of satisfaction also indicated that recipients rated their physical and emotional health and overall life satisfaction highly. For example, 86 per cent reported good to excellent satisfaction with their emotional health while only 28 per cent indicated poor to satisfactory quality of life. Those who rated these indices less favourably tended to have sub-optimal medical outcomes. It is also noteworthy that several of the respondents stated that, even though they did not obtain the desired medical outcome, they were more satisfied with their lives in contrast to preoperative life satisfaction. The contrast with their severely limited functional status prior to transplantation probably accounts for this favourable appraisal (Craven *et al.* 1990). For instance, one recipient stated that her physical limitations were a 'small price to pay for being alive'.

These survey results suggested an overall trend toward improvement in the physical and emotional well-being of the lung recipients. However, these findings should be interpreted with some caution because of potential response bias in the survey (Bart 1990). For instance, recipients may have felt obligated to report high life satisfaction to the lung transplant team because of gratitude to members of the team and because the recipients must maintain contact with the team for follow-up assessment or treatment. Recipients may also have minimized their own awareness of post-transplant problems as a way to manage anxiety about their vulnerability to infection.

In order to understand fully the relationship between organ replacement and reported quality of life it will also be necessary to identify and analyse the psychological factors which mediate the effects of post-transplant physical functioning on overall life satisfaction or influence life satisfaction independent of degree of physical health. For example, as reported in some quality of life studies (Burckhardt 1985; Scheier *et al.* 1989), positive self-esteem, an internal locus of control regarding health, perceived social support, and dispositional optimism may mediate reported life satisfaction in lung transplant recipients. In addition, changes in self-concept associated with surviving a life-threatening situation probably contribute to the lung recipients' reported life satisfaction.

As Bart (1990) has emphasized, transplant patients are more than passive recipients of a surgical procedure. The patients make a conscious decision to enter the transplant process and they use a number of active cognitive strategies in their attempt to assimilate and control the changes that confront them. In this regard, most recipients make an effort to understand what has happened to them and to appraise thoughtfully the impact the transplant has had and will have for their lives. For example, one double lung recipient anticipated a finite five year survival rate for herself and attempted to put her limited, projected, lifespan in perspective. Rather than being distressed by the prospect of having only five years to live, she stated that she learned to live more in the present and appreciate each minute because she 'now knows how much each moment is worth'. Another recipient felt reconciled with death and no longer feared it. He felt he had gained valuable knowledge about life and death which he desired to share with others.

Reports of a greater sensitivity to internal states and inner resources and a changed sense of identity often accompany the perception of 'a second chance at life' for a number of recipients (Craven *et al.* 1990). Similar reactions have been reported in survivors of other life-threatening situations (Dobson *et al.* 1971; Kennedy *et al.* 1976; Rosen 1976; Noyes 1980; Daiter *et al.* 1988). For some, perceptions of rebirth or self-renewal precede experimentation with new activities and a search for alternate life directions. Experiencing these changes can be distressing, and a period of inner re-organization is required. Recipients need the opportunity to share or make public their experience in the support group, with their support persons or team members. Providing an atmosphere that supports this process has evolved as the lung transplant team has gained greater experience with the psychological effects of transplantation.

Conclusions

Psychosocial factors play a decisive role in the selection and management of lung transplant patients. The psychosocial assessment of applicants provides the Toronto Lung Transplant team with a variety of information about the patients, including their adjustment to illness, presence of psychiatric disorder, family and social supports, interpersonal and coping characteristics, perceptions of the transplant process and life after surgery, and ability to adhere to medical recommendations. This information is an important component of the overall selection criteria. With the broadening of the selection criteria for acceptance, the psychosocial data primarily facilitate the organization of personal resources or psychotherapeutic management in order to match patients' strengths and vulnerabilities.

Lung transplantation presents a number of psychosocial challenges for patients and the transplant team. Prominent psychiatric manifestations include anxiety disorders in applicants and candidates and organic brain syndromes during the early postoperative period. The variegated interventions provided by the psychosocial team assist in promoting a more positive experience and ultimately enhance the overall quality of life for those who received 'a second chance at life'.

Acknowledgement

The authors would like to thank Ms Jane Bright (MSW) of the Toronto Lung Transplant Group for reviewing this manuscript.

References

Adams, F., Fernandez, F., and Andersson, B. S. (1986). Emergency pharmacotherapy of delirium in the critically ill cancer patient. *Psychosomatics*, 27, 33–7.

Bart, C. A. (1990). Issues in transformation: cognitive factors and adjustment in organ transplant recipients. *The First Working Conference on the Psychiatric, Psychosocial and Ethical Aspects of Organ Transplantation*, Toronto, Ontario.

Beck, A. T., Steer, R. A., and Garbin, M. (1988). Psychometric properties of the Beck Depression Inventory: twenty-five years of evaluation. *Clinical Psychological Review*, 8, 77–100.

Bergner, M., Bobbitt, R. A., Carter, W. B., and Gilson, B. (1976). Validation of interval scaling: the Sickness Impact Profile. *Health Services Research*, 11, 516–28.

Bright, J. M., Craven, J., Kelly, P., and the Toronto Lung Transplant Group (1990). Assessment and management of psychosocial stress in lung transplant candidates. *Health and Social Work*, 15, 125–32.

Burckhardt, C. S. (1985). The impact of arthritis on quality of life. *Nursing Research*, 34, 11–16.

Cooper, J. D. (1987). Lung transplantation: a new era. *Annals of Thoracic Surgery*, 44, 447–8.

Craven, J. (1989). Methylphenidate for cyclosporine-associated organic mood disorder (letter). *American Journal of Psychiatry*, 146, 553.

Craven, J. (1991). Cyclosporine-associated organic mental disorders in liver transplant recipients. *Psychosomatics*, 32, 94–102.

Craven, J. and the Toronto Lung Transplant Group (1990*a*). Psychiatric aspects of lung transplant. *Canadian Journal of Psychiatry*, 35, 759–64.

Craven, J. and the Toronto Lung Transplant Group (1990*b*). Post-operative organic mental syndromes in lung transplant recipients. *Journal of Heart Transplantation*, 9, 129–32.

Craven, J., Bright, J., and Lougheed Dear, C. L. (1990). Psychiatric, psychosocial and rehabilitative aspects of lung transplantation. *Clinics in Chest Medicine*, 11, 247–57.

Daiter, S., Larson, R., Weddington, W., and Ultmann, J. (1988). Psychosocial symptomatology, personal growth, and development among young adult patients following the diagnosis of leukaemia or lymphoma. *Journal of Clinical Oncology*, 6, 613–17.

Dobson, M., Tattersfield, A., Alder, M., and McNichol, M. (1971). Attitudes and long-term adjustment of patients surviving cardiac arrest. *British Medical Journal*, 3, 207–12.

Garner, S. J., Eldridge, F. L., Wagner, P. G., and Dowell, R. T. (1989). Buspirone, an anxiolytic drug that stimulates respiration. *American Review of Respiratory Disease*, 139, 946–50.

Gorman, J. M., Fuer, M. R., Goetz, R., Askanazi, J., Liebowitz, M. R., Fyer, A. J. *et al.* (1988). Ventilatory physiology of subjects with panic disorder. *Archives of General Psychiatry*, 45, 31–9.

Gough, H. G. (1987). *The California Psychological Inventory*. (Consulting Psychologists Press, Palo Alto).

de Groen, P. C., Aksamit, A. J., Rakela, J., Forbes, G. S., and Krom, R. A. F. (1987). Central nervous system toxicity after liver transplantation: the role of cyclosporine and cholesterol. *New England Journal of Medicine*, 317, 861–6.

Grossman, R., Frost, A., Zamel, N., Patterson, G., Cooper, J., Myron, R., *et al.* (1990). Results of single-lung transplantation for bilateral pulmonary fibrosis. *New England Journal of Medicine*, 322, 727–34.

Jackson, D. (1989). *The Basic Personality Inventory*. (Sigma Assessment Systems, London, Ontario).

Karajgi, B., Rifkin, A., Doddi, S., and Kolli, R. (1990). The prevalence of anxiety disorders in patients with chronic obstructive pulmonary disease. *American Journal of Psychiatry*, 147, 200–1.

Kast, R. (1989). Blocking of cyclosporine immunosuppression by neuroleptics (letter). *Transplantation*, 47, 1095–6.

Kelly, P. (1988). The role of psychologist on a lung transplant service. *41st Annual Convention of the Ontario Psychological Association*, Toronto, Ontario.

Kennedy, B., Tellegen, A., Kennedy, S., and Havernick, N. (1976). Psychological response of patients cured of advanced cancer. *Cancer*, 38, 2184–91.

Lee, W. H., Brady, M. P., Rowe, J. M., and Miller, W. C. (1971). Effects of extracorporeal circulation upon behavior, personality, and brain function: Part II, hemodynamic, metabolic, and psychometric correlations. *Annals of Surgery*, 173, 1013–23.

Levenson, J. L. and Olbrisch, M. E. (1987). Shortage of donor organs and long waits: New sources of stress for transplant patients. *Psychosomatics*, 28, 399–403.

Moos, R. H., Cronkite, R., Billings, A. G., and Finney, J. W. (1985). *Health and Daily Living Form manual—revised*. (Social Ecology Laboratory, Stanford University, Palo Alto).

McNair, D., Lorr, M., and Droppleman, L. (1971). *Profile of mood-states manual*. (Educational and Industrial Testing Services, San Diego).

Murray, H. A. (1971). *The thematic apperception test*. (Harvard University Press, Cambridge).

Newton, R. E., Marunycz, J. D., Alderdice, M. T., and Napoliello, M. J. (1986). Review of the side-effect profile of buspirone. *American Journal of Medicine*, 80, 17–21.

Noyes, J. (1980). Attitude change following near-death experiences. *Psychiatry*, 43, 234–41.

Rosen, D. (1976). Suicide survivors: psychotherapeutic implications of egocide. *Suicide and Life-Threatening Behaviour*, 6, 209–15.

Scheier, M. F., Matthews, K., Owens, J., Magovern, G., Lefebvre, R., Abbott, R., *et al.* (1989). Dispositional optimism and recovery from coronary artery bypass surgery: the beneficial effects on physical and psychological well-being. *Journal of Personality and Social Psychology*, 57, 1024–40.

Smith, L. W. and Dimsdale, J. E. (1989). Postcardiotomy delirium: conclusions after 25 years? *American Journal of Psychiatry*, 146, 452–8.

Spielberger, C. D., Gorsuch, R., and Lushene, R. (1970). *STAI Manual for the State-Trait Anxiety Inventory ("Self-Evaluation Questionnaire")*. (Consulting Psychologists Press, Palo Alto).

Tesar, G. E., Murray, G. B., and Cassem, N. H. (1985). Use of high-dose intravenous haloperidol in the treatment of agitated cardiac patients. *Journal of Clinical Psychopharmacology*, 5, 344–7.

The Toronto Lung Transplant Group (1986). Unilateral lung transplantation for pulmonary fibrosis. *New England Journal of Medicine*, 314, 1140–5.

16 Pancreas transplantation

R. Lentz, M. Popkin, E. Colon, and D. Sutherland

Pancreas transplantation is a rapidly evolving procedure performed electively, almost exclusively in diabetic patients, and aimed at preventing or controlling severe complications of diabetes mellitus. In order to understand the patient's experience and to provide supportive services to the transplant team, the psychiatrist must be informed about complications of diabetes, the indications for pancreas transplantation, and what may be expected after transplant.

Candidates for pancreas transplantation have coped with a chronic diabetic condition. They are highly self-selected, reaching transplantation after overcoming substantial hurdles, often including the cost of the procedure. Psychiatric predictors of psychological, social, and surgical oucome of pancreas transplantation are largely unknown. The psychiatric literature on pancreas transplantation is almost non-existent. This chapter reviews basic information essential to understand psychiatric issues in diabetic patients relevant to pancreas transplantation, and reviews the University of Minnesota experience.

Medical aspects

Pancreas transplantation has been available to diabetic patients since 1966 (Sutherland 1988, 1989; Sutherland *et al.* 1989*a,b,c*). Of 2004 transplantation procedures performed up to the end of June 1990, 1215 have been done since 1986. Since 1986, actuarial one year survival rates were 87 per cent for patients and 56 per cent for transplants (i.e. insulin independence), according to the most recent analyses of the Pancreas Transplant Registry data (Sutherland *et al.* 1989*a,c*; Sutherland and Moudry-Munns 1990). These rates are significantly improved over earlier results.

At the six large pancreas transplant centres, results are better than at smaller centres, with one year graft survival rates reaching as high as 80 per cent (Sutherland 1988, 1989; Sutherland *et al.* 1989*a*). Considering procedures at all centres since 1985, one year pancreas graft survival rates are 62 per cent for simultaneous pancreas/kidney grafts, 48 per cent for pancreas grafts in non-uraemic patients with prior kidney graft, and 40 per cent for pancreas grafts alone in non-uraemic patients (Sutherland 1988, 1989; Sutherland *et al.* 1989*a*). In the United States, results are somewhat better than elsewhere with overall one year survival rates since 1987 of 69 per cent for grafts and 91 per cent for patients (Sutherland *et al.* 1989*c*).

The University of Minnesota is the only institution with a large experience in transplanting isolated pancreas grafts into non-uraemic patients. Overall one year survival rates of 276 patients transplanted since 1978 are 42 per cent for grafts and 91 per cent for patients. For the most recent 76 patients, survival rates were 56 per cent for grafts and 92 per cent for patients (Prieto *et al.* 1987; Sutherland *et al.* 1988*a*, 1989*a,b,c*; Sutherland 1989). As of June 1990, 133 non-uraemic patients have received transplants, with a 50 per cent graft survival (Sutherland *et al.* 1989*c*). Bladder drainage of the exocrine pancreatic duct improves diagnosis of rejection, especially when cadaveric donors are used (Prieto *et al.* 1987). One year graft survival rates have reached 75 per cent when bladder duct drainage was used in simultaneous pancreas–kidney grafts (Sutherland *et al.* 1989*c*).

In addition to bladder duct drainage and early control of rejection, the use of cyclosporin and other anti-rejection agents, a decreased number of technical failures, and HLA-matching have improved results. Further progress is likely (Prieto *et al.* 1987; Sutherland, 1988, 1989; Sutherland *et al.* 1988*a*, 1989*b*; Sutherland *et al.* 1989*a*). Although living–related donors are used when cytotoxic antibodies are present, most procedures use cadaveric donors (Sutherland 1989).

Indications and outcome

For endstage renal disease in diabetes, kidney transplantation is the treatment of choice (Tattersall 1989). However, malignant retinopathy, neuropathy, hypertension, large vessel disease, and premature death often accompany diabetic nephropathy (Sutherland 1988, 1989; Tattersall 1989). Five to nine years after renal transplantation, diabetic patients do much less well than non-diabetic patients physically, emotionally, and socially (Simmons *et al.* 1981). They report more hospitalization, weakness, fatigue, and difficulties with daily activities such as housework, lifting, and shopping. Similarly, diabetics report lower self-esteem, less independence and sense of control, more preoccupation with themselves, and more depression and anxiety five to nine years after renal transplantation than do non-diabetics (Simmons *et al.* 1981).

Successful pancreas transplantation leads to insulin independence and freedom from dietary and other lifestyle restrictions. These considerations alone are insufficient indications for pancreas transplantation (Sutherland 1988, 1989; Tattersall 1989). Ideally, pancreas transplantation should be done for those patients without diabetic complications, but destined to develop complications more serious than the effects of immunosuppression and anti-rejection therapy and the limited risks of surgery (Sutherland 1988). Regrettably, there are no predictors to determine who will develop the secondary lesions of diabetes (Sutherland 1988; Tattersall 1989). There are, however, current criteria for pancreas transplantation, based on the likelihood that a pancreas graft and euglycaemia may control the secondary lesions of diabetic retinopathy (Sutherland 1988, 1989; University of Michigan 1988; Tattersall, 1989). It remains possible that hormones other than insulin and islet cells other than beta cells are involved in diabetes and its complications.

Several studies have examined the effects of pancreas transplantation on the course of diabetes (Ramsay *et al.* 1988; Sutherland 1988, 1989; University of Michigan 1988; Tattersall 1989; Bilous *et al.* 1989; Kennedy *et al.* 1990). Successful transplantation does not appear to prevent possession of retinopathy beyond the background stage for two years following the transplant. However, retinopathy remains stable thereafter (Ramsay *et al.* 1988; Sutherland 1989). After a successful transplant, peripheral nerve condition velocities and motor and sensory indices of nerve function improve, and autonomic neuropathy stabilizes (Sutherland 1989; Kennedy *et al.* 1990). Assessment of the effect of pancreas transplantation on renal function may be complicated by a significant early decline in creatinine clearance due to cyclosporin (Sutherland 1988). Assessment of glomerular mesangial volume by kidney biopsy is more specific for diabetes than creatinine clearance (Sutherland 1988; Bilous *et al.* 1989). Pancreas transplantation may stabilize renal lesions in patients with albuminuria and early diabetic nephropathy with mild renal insufficiency, but without uraemia (Sutherland 1988). It does prevent recurrence of diabetic nephropathy in transplanted kidneys (Bilous *et al.* 1989).

The University of Minnesota, which has the largest experience in pancreas transplantation (over 250 cases by January 1989), has established specific selection criteria for the three pancreas recipient categories usually described in diabetics: (1) uraemic patients in need of kidney transplantation; (2) non-uraemic patients with functioning prior kidney transplants; and (3) non-uraemic patients with early nephropathy who receive pancreas grafts alone. All patients in the first category are offered simultaneous pancreas and kidney grafts, since addition of a pancreas graft may positively affect secondary diabetic complications, remove insulin requirements and dietary restrictions, and improve quality of life (Sutherland 1988, 1989). Since immunosuppression is already required for the kidney graft, and since both pancreas and kidney grafts do well when transplanted together, there is little added risk for this recipient category (Sutherland 1988, 1989; University of Michigan 1988; Tattersall 1989). Similar considerations apply to the second recipient category (Robins *et al.* 1984; Sutherland 1988, 1989).

For the third recipient category, additional criteria at the University of Michigan include albuminuria (since it heralds progressive nephropathy); the specific diabetic lesion of mesangial expansion on kidney biopsy (to a degree compatible with early nephropathy); and creatinine clearance (>70 ml/min cyclosporin will be tolerated) (Sutherland 1988, 1989). Pancreas transplantation may prevent progression of nephropathy in patients with such early nephropathy, but not with more advanced renal disease (Sutherland 1988, 1989). Most centres would not transplant a pancreas for diabetic retinopathy or for neuropathy as the sole diabetic complication, but criteria may be redefined as results improve and immunosuppressive regimens become less risky (Sutherland 1988, 1989; University of Michigan 1988; Tattersall 1989).

Some non-uraemic patients suffer from extremely labile diabetes with frequent episodes of hypoglycaemia and/or ketoacidosis, refractory to other methods of glucose control. Such patients would be considered for pancreas transplantation by some (Sutherland 1988, 1989), but not other (Tattersall 1989) physicians.

Unlike transplants of other organs, which are essentially life-saving or replacing dialysis, pancreas transplants are elective, performed largely to control secondary diabetic complications, and occasionally for labile diabetes (Evans *et al.* 1985; Sutherland 1988, 1989; House and Thompson 1988; Surman 1989). Pancreas transplantation substitutes immunosuppressant effects for diabetic sequelae. Recipients have usually endured diabetes since childhood, as well as progressive complications.

In the USA, prior to acceptance, patients must agree to pay the costs of pancreas transplantation, since Medicare and most insurers do not. For recipients of combined cadaveric pancreas/kidney grafts, where the kidney transplant is covered, additional costs of pancreas transplantation and organ procurement are approximately $35 000. For isolated cadaveric pancreas transplants, costs are approximately $60 000. These estimates exclude physician fees, follow-up care, transportation (many come long distances), lost wages, costs of complications, and expenses related to living–related donors. The average surgical cost for a related donor is about $15 000. In many instances, the costs are provided by fund-raising. These efforts impact on the patient by providing support, but also influence their expectations and psychological response to transplantation and the post-surgical course. Patients willing to persevere throughout the application and evaluation procedures are highly selected for assertiveness, high motivation, and a high level of personal and social supportive resources.

Psychiatric considerations

Pre-transplant

Candidates have been evaluated at the University of Minnesota by the NIMH Diagnostic Interview Schedule (DIS) (Robins *et al.* 1981) and by clinical psychiatric consultation of a supervised resident. The structured interview provides a reliable diagnostic database. The resident evaluation adds clinically important data about patients' support systems and family, how they have coped with prior stressors, their expectations of the procedure (including risks and potential benefits), and helps formulate an understanding of the patient's general coping style. We use a consultation model (Popkin *et al.* 1983) in the context of liaison relationships. Residents and staff provide direct verbal feedback, as indicated, to the transplant co-ordinator or surgical staff. One of us (RDL) serves on an interdisciplinary pancreas transplant co-ordinating committee which evaluates candidates. Patients are also seen by a clinical social worker assigned to the surgical department who provides social service evaluation and support.

In contrast to programmes which routinely exclude patients with major psychiatric disease, history of alcoholism, job instability, antisocial behaviour, or without specific forms of support (Knox 1980; Tattersall 1989), we do not. Our approach is to avoid discriminatory exclusions based on opinion and to work towards evaluating the effect of psychiatric conditions on psychosocial and surgical outcome. Our role is to provide information to the transplant team, not to recommend acceptance or rejection. The team may recommend stabilization or treatment for a psychiatric condition (e.g. active alcoholism), as for a medical condition, but then proceed with the transplant if otherwise appropriate.

Living–related donors receive psychiatric evaluations which emphasize general psychiatric history, coping style, response to past stressors, expectations, family issues, donor selection, and attitudes to transplantation. The same resident psychiatrist will not see both potential donor and recipient. Communication with the surgical staff and recommendations to the team follow the guidelines outlined for recipients.

Perioperative phase

Both recipients and donors are encouraged to discuss ambivalence, questions, and psychological issues in supportive psychotherapy, as indicated clinically. Medication such as antidepressants or anxiolytics may be used. For the many patients who live elsewhere, or who have local psychiatrists, recommendations are made for follow-up and co-ordination with psychiatrists or referring physicians.

Patients are seen at the time of transplant and during both routine and unscheduled admissions. Since cadaveric transplants are done urgently, these recipients are usually seen for follow-up after the transplant procedure. Issues such as depression, anxiety, delirium, rejection, immunosuppression, infection, relationships, finances, other stressors, and hospital milieu factors are similar to those for other organ transplants (House and Thompson 1988; Surman 1989). They occur, of course, in the context of long-standing diabetes.

Post-transplant

Prior publications have described psychiatric aspects of transplantation in general (House and Thompson 1988; Surman 1989). To our knowledge, there is only one report of psychiatric factors affecting surgical outcome following pancreas transplantation (Popkin *et al.* in press). Of 140 candidates with a first transplant evaluated by us from February 1984 to December 1987, 80 patients had been transplanted by December 1988. These 80 patients were evaluated at least one year post-transplant; 31 (38.8 per cent) were insulin-independent for a mean of 94.3 weeks after transplantation; 41 (61.9 per cent) had partial or complete graft failure a mean of 14.6 weeks after transplantation. Statistical analyses showed no significant relationship of psychiatric disorders commonly present on initial evaluation, such as major depressive disorder, simple phobia, generalized anxiety disorder, antisocial personality disorder, or psychosexual dysfunction, to surgical graft outcome (Popkin *et al.* 1988, in press). In contrast, lifetime prevalence rates of tobacco use disorder or alcohol abuse/dependence were significantly associated with lower duration of graft function, even if patients became abstinent prior to transplant. The mechanisms of this association remain unclear. These two disorders coexisted so commonly that their individual effect on outcome could not be distinguished. We speculate that these disorders may be markers for noncompliance, poor impulse control, or for more advanced diabetic microangiopathy. Alternatively, continued but covert use may contribute to graft failure, possibly by altering immunosuppressive compliance or efficacy (Popkin *et al.* in press). It is the policy at our centre not to transplant patients currently abusing alcohol. Alcoholic patients probably do less well after heart transplantation, whereas reports are mixed for liver transplantation (Popkin *et al.* 1988, in press). Careful attention to alcohol and tobacco use histories and to possible covert abuse is indicated in all transplant patients.

Patients' perception of support from first degree relatives was also significantly associated with surgical transplant outcome, whereas perception of support from spouses or significant others was not. It may be that recipients expect as routine, and thus undervalue, spousal support, whereas extensive familial support confers an advantage. We cannot comment on the possible mechanism by which support is related to surgical outcome. Of many other patient factors active in this population, only HLA-DR matching was related to outcome (Popkin *et al.* in press).

We have not yet systematically addressed the psychiatric or psychosocial outcome of pancreas transplantation. In addition, studies of quality of life following pancreas transplantation, similar to those of Simmons following kidney transplantation (Simmons *et al.* 1981, 1987), are just beginning at our centre.

The practice of excluding various organ transplant candidates on psychiatric grounds (Knox 1980; Tattersall 1989) is not supported by our data, except for tobacco and alcohol abuse/dependence disorders. Although we have not looked systematically at personality disorders other than antisocial personality disorder, we have followed several such patients after transplantation, including one woman with borderline personality disorder. All of these patients have done better psychiatrically following the transplant than before, and generally well overall. Similarly, although a few patients with major depression had subsequent psychiatric admissions, they too did well with appropriate treatment. Any exclusion of patients from transplantation on psychiatric grounds should be based on objective data rather than on arbitrary discrimination which prompts the stigma of mental illness.

Psychiatric aspects of transplantation in diabetic persons

Type I insulin-dependent diabetes mellitus afflicts approximately 500 000 people in North America (Harris 1982), one in 300 people under 20 years of age (Cahill and McDevitt 1981). New cases occur at a rate of 15 per 100 000 annually (Cahill and McDevitt 1981). Complications may be extensive and severe (Krolewski *et al.* 1987). Approximately 16 per cent will become blind, 21 per cent will suffer a myocardial infarction, 10 per cent a stroke, and 12 per cent will have gangrene or an amputation (Stiller *et al.* 1984). Despite the prevalence of diabetes, limited recent attention has been directed to its psychiatric aspects (Wilkinson 1981; Schwartz 1988). Existing literature can be divided into four categories: stress and personality factors, coexistence with eating disorders, cognitive dysfunction, and mood disorder (Popkin *et al.* 1989).

Information about stress and personality factors has been recently reviewed (Schwartz 1988; Popkin *et al.* 1989). Coexistence of eating disorders and diabetes is reviewed elsewhere (Rodin *et al.* 1985, 1991; Steele *et al.* 1987). Therefore, we shall concentrate on the remaining two categories.

Diabetes does affect the central nervous system and might therefore be expected to cause cognitive dysfunction (Alex *et al.* 1962; Locke 1965; Popkin *et al.* 1989). Besides metabolic effects, infection, anoxia, and large vessel disease, diabetes causes lesions of small blood vessels in the brain similar to those in other organs (Alex *et al.* 1962; Locke 1965). Diseases of large and small vessels leads to earlier, more severe central nervous system lesions in diabetes (Alex *et al.* 1962). In children, neuropsychological testing suggests that very early onset of diabetes may predispose children to subtle cognitive impairment, presumably from metabolic damage (Ryan *et al.* 1985; Rovet *et al.* 1987). In older insulin-dependent diabetics, limited data from psychometric tests show minor impairment (Lawson *et al.* 1984), although relatives of these same patients estimated 16 per cent cognitive impairment (Surridge *et al.* 1984). Other studies have shown that cognitive changes do exist in ageing diabetics with less severe non-insulin-dependent (Type II) diabetes (Perlmuter *et al.* 1984) as well as in insulin-dependent (Type I) diabetic children (Ryan *et al.* 1985; Rovet *et al.* 1987). Induced hypoglycaemia does cause cognitive impairment in subjects with early onset diabetes (Pramming *et al.* 1986). Because pancreas transplant candidates have prominent complications or poor glycaemic control, one might expect them to have measurable cognitive impairment. This has not been studied systematically or longitudinally (Popkin *et al.* 1989).

Systematic studies of mood disorders in diabetics have been largely limited to the work of Lustman (Lustman *et al.* 1983, 1986*a,b*, 1988) and of our group (Popkin and Callies 1987; Popkin *et al.* 1988, in press; Popkin 1989). In 1983, the prevalence of depression in diabetes was unknown (Lustman *et al.* 1983). In 1986, among Type I and II diabetic out-patients, Lustman reported the life-time prevalence of major depressive disorders to be 33 per cent (6 per cent in Type I patients), and of generalized anxiety disorder to be 41 per cent, both six to seven times greater than the prevalences in the Epidemiologic Catchment Area (ECA) data (Robins *et al.* 1984; Lustman *et al.* 1986*a*). The data suggested that psychiatric illness in general (lifetime prevalence 71 per cent) and depression in particular, were associated with poorer glycaemic control (Lustman *et al.* 1983). It was unclear whether depression caused or was caused by poor control, although anecdotal reports have suggested that depression increases insulin requirements (Lustman *et al.* 1986*a*; Popkin *et al.* 1989). In a five year follow-up study, recurrent depression developed in 79 per cent of Type I and II diabetic patients who were depressed at Lustman's index examination, and in only 10 per cent of comparable diabetics not initially depressed, indicating a malignant course of depression in diabetics (Lustman *et al.* 1988). Both groups had similar rates of neuropathy, retinopathy, and nephropathy.

In a cohort of Type I diabetics hospitalized on medical–surgical units and referred for psychiatric consultation, our group reported a 25 per cent incidence of affective disorder (Popkin and Callies 1987). In a different cohort of advanced Type I diabetics with moderate to severe complications, comprising all patients electively evaluated for pancreas transplantation, we found a lifetime prevalence of major depressive disorder (DSM-III criteria, Diagnostic Interview Schedule) to be 24 per cent (22.9 per cent of 45 females; 25.9 per cent of 27 males) (Popkin *et al.* 1988). This 24 per cent lifetime prevalence rate of depression in transplant candidates was several times the prevalence rates of depression for their sibling or first degree relative donors and also for Epidemiologic Catchment Area norms (Robins *et al.* 1984; Popkin *et al.* 1988). Although our prevalence rates were similar among males and females, Lustman reported a female preponderance of depression among diabetics usually seen in other depressed populations (Lustman *et al.* 1988); in other respects, our data are comparable to those of Lustman (Lustman *et al.* 1986*a*, 1988). The prevalence of depression was independent of age, duration or diabetes, and lesions of diabetic triopathy. Depression, although clinically important, is often under-recognized and under-treated in diabetic patients (Popkin and Callies 1987; Lustman and Harper 1987; Popkin *et al.* in press). Since most patients with stroke and prominent vascular disease, a population at risk for mood and organic mental disorders, were excluded from transplant evaluation, the observed prevalence rate of depression is especially noteworthy. Nevertheless, the high prevalence rate of depression may be due in part to subtle vascular changes in the brain (Popkin *et al.* 1988).

Also noted in pancreas transplant candidates was a high six month and life-time prevalence of simple phobia in females (31.3 per cent lifetime) compared to donors (0 per cent) and Epidemiologic Catchment Area data (18.4 per cent), and of antisocial personality disorder in male candidates (14.8 per cent) and donors (26.7 per cent) compared to ECA data (4.6 per cent) (Popkin *et al.* 1988). We speculate that phobia may be related to metabolic and autonomic disturbances, and antisocial personality disorder to the selection of patients who reject social restrictions and choose to be transplant recipients or donors (Popkin *et al.* 1988). Other prominent diagnoses included tobacco abuse, psychosexual dysfunction, generalized anxiety disorder, and alcohol abuse and dependence (Popkin *et al.* 1988).

Conclusions

Any consideration of the psychiatric aspects of pancreas transplantation must take into consideration both the transplant situation and also the most common underlying condition, diabetes mellitus. Data from our centre suggest that a history of alcoholism or nicotine dependence is associated with lower duration of graft survival. Further work is required to test for this relationship in pancreas and other transplant recipients, and also to investigate mechanisms of the association. Investigation of the neurocognitive status of pancreas transplant patients and the course of depression following transplantation is also recommended.

References

Alex, M., Baron, E. K., Goldenberg, S., and Blumenthal, H. T. (1962). An autopsy study of cerebrovascular accident in diabetes mellitus. *Circulation*, 25, 663–73.

Bilous, R. W., Mauer, S. M., Sutherland, D. E., Najarian, J. S., Goetz, F. C., and Steffes, M. W. (1989). The effects of pancreas transplantation on the glomerular structure of renal allografts in patients with insulin-dependent diabetes. *New England Journal of Medicine*, 321, 80–5.

Cahill, G. F., Jr. and McDevitt, H. O. (1981). Insulin-dependent diabetes: The initial lesion. *New England Journal of Medicine*, 304, 1454–65.

Evans, R. W., Manninen, D. L., Garrison, L. P., Jr., Hart, L. G., Blagg, C. R., Gutman, R. A., *et al.* (1985). The quality of life of patients with endstage renal disease. *New England Journal of Medicine*, 312, 553–9.

Harris, M. (1982). The public health impact of diabetes. In *Advances in diabetes epidemiology* (ed. E. Eschwege), pp. 17–20. (Elsevier/North-Holland, New York).

House, R. M., and Thompson, T. L. II (1988). Psychiatric aspects of organ transplantation. *Journal of the American Medical Association*, 260, 535–9.

Kennedy, W. R., Navarro, X., Goetz, F. C., Sutherland, D. E., and Najarian, J. S. (1990). Effects of pancreatic transplantation on diabetic neuropathy. *New England Journal of Medicine*, 322, 1031–7.

Knox, R. A. (1980). Heart transplants: to pay or not to pay. *Science*, 209, 570–5.

Krolewski, A. S., Warram, J. H., Rand, L. I., and Kahn, C. R. (1987). Epidemiologic approach to the etiology of Type I diabetes mellitus and its complications. *New England Journal of Medicine*, 317, 1390–8.

Lawson, J. S., Erdahl, D. L. W., Monga, T. N., Bird, C. E., Donald, M. W., Surridge, D. H. C., *et al.* (1984). Neuropsychological function in diabetic patients with neuro-pathy. *British Journal of Psychiatry*, 145, 263–8.

Locke, S. (1965). Diabetes and the nervous system. *Medical Clinics of North America*, 49, 1081–92.

Lustman, P. J. and Harper, G. W. (1987). Nonpsychiatric physicians' identification and treatment of depression in patients with diabetes. *Comprehensive Psychiatry*, 28, 22–7.

Lustman, P. J., Amado, H., and Wetzel, R. D. (1983). Depression in diabetics: a critical appraisal. *Comprehensive Psychiatry*, 24, 65–74.

Lustman, P. J., Griffith, L. S., Clouse, R. E., and Cryer, P. E. (1986*a*). Psychiatric illness in diabetes mellitus: relationship to symptoms and glucose control. *Journal of Nervous and Mental Disease*, 174, 736–42.

Lustman, P. J., Harper, G. W., Griffith, L. S., and Clouse, R. E. (1986*b*). Use of the Diagnostic Interview Schedule in patients with diabetes mellitus. *Journal of Nervous and Mental Disease*, 174, 743–6.

Lustman, P. J., Griffith, L. S., and Clouse, R. E. (1988). Depression in adults with diabetes: results of 5-year follow-up study. *Diabetes Care*, 11, 605–12.

Perlmuter, L. C., Hakami, M. K., Hodgson-Harrington, C., Ginsberg, J., Katz, J., Singer, D. E., *et al.* (1984). Decreased cognitive function in ageing non-insulin-dependent diabetic patients. *American Journal of Medicine*, 77, 1043–8.

Popkin, M. K. (1989). Depression and patients with diabetes mellitus. In *Depression and coexisting disease* (eds R. G. Robinson and P. V. Rabins), pp. 73–82. (Igaku-Shoin, New York).

Popkin, M. K. and Callies, A. L. (1987). Psychiatric consultation to inpatients with 'early onset' Type I diabetes mellitus in a university hospital. *Archives of General Psychiatry*, 44, 169–71.

Popkin, M. K., Mackenzie, T. B., and Callies, A. L. (1983). Consultation–Liaison Outcome Evaluation System: I. Consultant–consultee interaction. *Archives of General Psychiatry*, 40, 215–19.

Popkin, M. K., Callies, A. L., Lentz, R. D., Colon, E. A., and Sutherland, D. E. (1988). Prevalence of major depression, simple phobia, and other psychiatric disorders in patients with long-standing Type I diabetes mellitus. *Archives of General Psychiatry*, 45, 64–8.

Popkin, M. K., Colon, E. A., and Callies, A. L. (1989). Psychiatric disorders in patients with diabetes mellitus. In *Recent advances in psychiatric medicine* (ed. R. C. W. Hall), pp. 106–12. (Rylandic Publishing, Longwood, FL).

Popkin, M. K., Callies, A. L., Colon, E. A., Lentz, R. D., and Sutherland, D. E. R. (in press). Psychiatric diagnosis and the outcome of pancreas transplantation in patients with Type I diabetes mellitus.

Pramming, S., Thorsteinsson, B., Theilgaard, A., Pinner, E. M., and Binder, C. (1986). Cognitive function during hypoglycaemia in Type I diabetes mellitus. *British Medical Journal*, 292, 647–50.

Prieto, M., Sutherland, D. E., Goetz, F. C., Rosenberg, M. E., and Najarian, J. S.

(1987). Pancreas transplant results according to the technique of duct management: bladder verses enteric drainage. *Surgery*, 102, 680–91.

Ramsay, R. C., Goetz, F. C., Sutherland, D. E., Mauer, S. M., Robison, L. L., Cantrill, H. L., *et al.* (1988). Progression of diabetic retinopathy after pancreas transplantation for insulin-dependent diabetes mellitus. *New England Journal of Medicine*, 318, 208–14.

Robins, L. N., Helzer, J. E., Croughan, J., and Ratcliff, K. S. (1981). National Institute of Mental Health Diagnostic Interview Schedule: its history, characteristics, and validity. *Archives of General Psychiatry*, 38, 381–9.

Robins, L. N., Helzer, J. E., Weissman, M. M., Orvaschel, H., Gruenberg, E., Burke, J. D. Jr., *et al.* (1984). Lifetime prevalence of specific psychiatric disorders in three sites. *Archives of General Psychiatry*, 41, 949–58.

Rodin, G., Craven, J., Littlefield, C., Murray, M., and Daneman, D. (1991). Eating disorders and intentional insulin undertreatment in adolescent females with diabetes. *Psychosomatics*, 32, 171–6.

Rodin, G. M., Daneman, D., Johnson, L. E., Kenshole, A., and Garfinkel, P. (1985). Anorexia nervosa and bulimia in female adolescents with insulin dependent diabetes mellitus: a systematic study. *Journal of Psychiatric Research*, 19, 381–4.

Rovet, J. F., Ehrlich, R. M., and Hoppe, M. (1987). Intellectual deficits associated with early onset of insulin-dependent diabetes mellitus in children. *Diabetes Care*, 10, 510–15.

Ryan, C., Vega, A., and Drash, A. (1985). Cognitive deficits in adolescents who developed diabetes early in life. *Pediatrics*, 75, 921–7.

Schwartz, L. S. (1988). A biopsychosocial approach to the management of the diabetic patient. *Primary Care*, 15, 409–21.

Simmons, R. G., Kamstra-Hennen, L., and Thompson, C. R. (1981). Psychosocial adjustment five to nine years post transplant. *Transplantation Proceedings*, 13, 40–3.

Simmons, R. G., Marine, S. K., and Simmons, R. L. (1987). *Gift of life: the effect of organ transplantation on individual, family and societal dynamics*. (Transaction Books, New Brunswick).

Steel, J. M., Young, R. J., Lloyd, G. G., and Clarke, B. F. (1987). Clinically apparent eating disorders in young diabetic women: associations with painful neuropathy and other complications. *British Medical Journal*, 294, 859–62.

Stiller, C. R., Dupre, J., Gent, M., Jenner, M. R., Keown, P. A., Laupacis, A., *et al.* (1984). Effects of cyclosporine immunosuppression in insulin-dependent diabetes mellitus of recent onset. *Science*, 223, 1362–7.

Surman, O. S. (1989). Psychiatric aspects of organ transplantation. *American Journal of Psychiatry*, 146, 972–82.

Surridge, D.H. C., Erdahl, D. L. W., Lawson, J. S., Donald, M. W., Monga, T. N., Bird, C. E., *et al.* (1984). Psychiatric aspects of diabetes mellitus. *British Journal of Psychiatry*, 145, 269–76.

Sutherland, D. E. R. (1988). Who should get a pancreas transplant? *Diabetes Care*, 11, 681–5.

Sutherland, D. E. R. (1989). Coming of age for pancreas transplantation. *Western Journal of Medicine*, 150, 314–18.

Sutherland, D. E. R. and Moudry-Munns, K. C. (1990). International pancreas transplantation registry analysis. *Transplantation Proceedings*, 22, 571–4.

Sutherland, D. E. R., Kendall, D. M., Moudry, K. C., Navarro, X., Kennedy, W. R.,

Ramsay, R. C., *et al.* (1988*a*). Pancreas transplantation in non-uremic, Type I diabetic recipients. *Surgery*, 104, 453–64.

Sutherland, D. E. R., Moudry, K. C., Dunn, D. L., Goetz, F. C., and Najarian, J. S. (1989*a*). Pancreas-transplant outcome in relation to presence or absence of end-stage renal disease, timing of transplant, surgical technique, and donor source. *Diabetes*, 38 **(Suppl. 1)**, 10–12.

Sutherland, D. E. R., Moudry-Munns, K. C., and Gillingham, D. (1989*b*). Pancreas transplantation: Report from the international registry and a preliminary analysis of the United States results from the United Network for Organ Sharing (UNOS) registry. In *Clinical Transplants* (ed. P. Terasaki). UCLA Tissue Typing Laboratory, Los Angeles, pp. 19–43.

Sutherland, D. E. R., Dunn, D. L., Goetz, F. C., Kennedy, W., Ramsay, R. C., Steffes, M. W., *et al.* (1989*c*). A 10-year experience with 290 pancreas transplants at a single institution. *Annals of Surgery*, 210, 274–88.

Tattersall, R. (1989). Is pancreas transplantation for insulin-dependent diabetics worthwhile? *New England Journal of Medicine*, 321, 112–14.

The University of Michigan Pancreas Transplant Evaluation Committee (1988). Pancreatic transplantation as treatment for IDDM: Proposed candidate criteria before end-stage diabetic nephropathy. *Diabetes Care*, 11, 669–75.

Wilkinson, D. G. (1981). Psychiatric aspects of diabetes mellitus. *British Journal of Psychiatry*, 138, 1–9.

Index